Toxicology

Editor

JANICE L. ZIMMERMAN

CRITICAL CARE CLINICS

www.criticalcare.theclinics.com

Consulting Editor
JOHN A. KELLUM

July 2021 • Volume 37 • Number 3

ELSEVIER

1600 John F. Kennedy Boulevard • Suite 1800 • Philadelphia, Pennsylvania, 19103-2899

http://www.theclinics.com

CRITICAL CARE CLINICS Volume 37, Number 3
July 2021 ISSN 0749-0704, ISBN-13: 978-0-323-79453-4

Editor: Joanna Collett
Developmental Editor: Axell Purificacion

Critical Care Clinics (ISSN: 0749-0704) is published quarterly by Elsevier Inc., 360 Park Avenue South, New York, NY 10010-1710. Months of issue are January, April, July, and October. Business and Editorial Offices: 1600 John F. Kennedy Blvd., Suite 1800, Philadelphia, PA 19103-2899. Customer Service Office: 6277 Sea Harbor Drive, Orlando, FL 32887-4800. Periodicals postage paid at New York, NY and additional mailing offices. Subscription prices are $258.00 per year for US individuals, $890.00 per year for US institutions, $100.00 per year for US students and residents, $287.00 per year for Canadian individuals, $952.00 per year for Canadian institutions, $328.00 per year for international individuals, $952.00 per year for international institutions, $100.00 per year for Canadian students/residents, and $150.00 per year for foreign students/residents. To receive student/resident rate, orders must be accompanied by name of affiliated institution, date of term, and the signature of program/residency coordinator on institution letterhead. Orders will be billed at individual rate until proof of status is received. Foreign air speed delivery is included in all *Clinics* subscription prices. All prices are subject to change without notice. POSTMASTER: Send address changes to *Critical Care Clinics*, Elsevier Periodicals Customer Service, 11830 Westline Industrial Drive, St. Louis, MO 63146. **Customer Service: 1-800-654-2452 (US). From outside of the US, call 1-314-447-8871. Fax: 1-314-447-8029. E-mail: journalscustomerservice-usa@elsevier.com (for print support) or journalsonlinesupport-usa@elsevier.com (for online support).**

Reprints. For copies of 100 or more of articles in this publication, please contact the Commercial Reprints Department, Elsevier Inc., 360 Park Avenue South, New York, NY 10010-1710. Tel.: 212-633-3874; Fax: 212-633-3820; E-mail: reprints@elsevier.com.

Critical Care Clinics is also published in Spanish by Editorial Inter-Medica, Junin 917, 1er A, 1113, Buenos Aires, Argentina.

Critical Care Clinics is covered in *MEDLINE/PubMed (Index Medicus)*, *EMBASE/Excerpta Medica*, *Current Concepts/Clinical Medicine*, *ISI/BIOMED*, and *Chemical Abstracts*.

Contributors

CONSULTING EDITOR

JOHN A. KELLUM, MD, MCCM
Professor, Critical Care Medicine, Medicine, Bioengineering and Clinical and Translational Science, Director, Center for Critical Care Nephrology, The Clinical Research Investigation and Systems Modeling of Acute Illness (CRISMA) Center, Vice Chair for Research, Department of Critical Care Medicine, University of Pittsburgh School of Medicine, Pittsburgh, Pennsylvania, USA

EDITOR

JANICE L. ZIMMERMAN, MD, MACP, MCCM
Adjunct Professor of Medicine, Baylor College of Medicine, Houston, Texas, USA

AUTHORS

TIMOTHY E. ALBERTSON, MD, PhD
Departments of Emergency Medicine and Internal Medicine, University of California, Davis, School of Medicine, Sacramento, California, USA; Department of Internal Medicine, Mather VA Medical Center, Mather, California, USA

SAKIB AMAN, MBBS, MCPS, FCPS
Indoor Medical Officer, Department of Medicine, Dhaka Medical College Hospital, Dhaka, Bangladesh

WEDAD AWAD, PharmD
King Hussein Cancer Center, Amman, Jordan

KEITH AZEVEDO, MD
Assistant Professor, Critical Care and Emergency Medicine, Departments of Emergency and Internal Medicine, University of New Mexico Hospital, Albuquerque, New Mexico, USA

KEVIN BAUMGARTNER, MD
Fellow, Department of Emergency Medicine, Division of Medical Toxicology, Washington University School of Medicine, St Louis, Missouri, USA

HEATHER A. BOREK, MD
Assistant Professor, Division of Medical Toxicology, Department of Emergency Medicine, University of Virginia School of Medicine, Charlottesville, Virginia, USA

ANNE RAIN T. BROWN, PharmD, BCCCP, FCCM
The University of Texas MD Anderson Cancer Center, Houston, Texas, USA

HALLIE BROWN, MD
Department of Emergency Medicine, Indiana University School of Medicine, Indianapolis, Indiana, USA

NICHOLAS A. BUCKLEY, MD, FRACP
Pharmacology and Biomedical Informatics and Digital Health, Faculty of Medicine and Health, The University of Sydney, Camperdown, New South Wales, Australia

JAMES A. CHENOWETH, MD, MAS
Department of Emergency Medicine, University of California, Davis, School of Medicine, Sacramento, California, USA; Department of Internal Medicine, Mather VA Medical Center, Mather, California, USA

ANGELA L. CHIEW, PhD, FACEM
Clinical Toxicology Unit, Prince of Wales Hospital, Randwick, New South Wales, Australia

FAZLE RABBI CHOWDHURY, FCPS, MSc, PhD
Assistant Professor, Department of Internal Medicine, Bangabandhu Sheikh Mujib Medical University, Dhaka, Bangladesh

JASON DEVGUN, MD
Assistant Professor, Department of Emergency Medicine, Division of Medical Toxicology, Washington University School of Medicine, St Louis, Missouri, USA

JESSICA EVANS-WALL, MD
Department of Emergency Medicine, University of New Mexico Health Sciences Center, Albuquerque, New Mexico, USA

MARIO GANAU, MD, PhD, MBA, FRCS(Ed), FEBNS, FACS
Consultant in Neurosurgery, Neurosciences Department, John Radcliffe Hospital, Oxford University Hospitals NHS Foundation Trust, Oxford, United Kingdom

MATTHEW R. GREER, MD
Department of Emergency Medicine, University of California, Davis, School of Medicine, Sacramento, California, USA

CRISTINA GUTIERREZ, MD
Associate Professor of Medicine, Department of Critical Care, Division of Anesthesiology and Critical Care, The University of Texas MD Anderson Cancer Center, Houston, Texas, USA

CHRISTOPHER P. HOLSTEGE, MD
Chief, Division of Medical Toxicology, Professor, Departments of Emergency Medicine and Pediatrics, University of Virginia School of Medicine, Director, Blue Ridge Poison Center, University of Virginia Health System, Charlottesville, Virginia, USA

MOLLY JOHNSON, MD
Department of Emergency Medicine, University of New Mexico Health Sciences Center, Albuquerque, New Mexico, USA

DAVID B. LISS, MD
Assistant Professor, Department of Emergency Medicine, Division of Medical Toxicology, Washington University in St. Louis, St Louis, Missouri, USA

ANNETTE D. LISTA, PharmD, BCCCP
Department of Pharmacy, Houston Methodist Hospital, Houston, Texas, USA

COLLEEN McEVOY, MD
Director, Stem Cell Transplant and Oncology Intensive Care Unit, Assistant Professor of Medicine, Division of Pulmonary and Critical Care Medicine, Washington University School of Medicine, St Louis, Missouri, USA

MICHAEL E. MULLINS, MD
Associate Professor, Department of Emergency Medicine, Division of Medical Toxicology, Washington University in St. Louis, St Louis, Missouri, USA

JOSEPH L. NATES, MD, MBA
Director, Professor and Deputy Chair, Department of Critical Care, Division of Anesthesiology and Critical Care, The University of Texas MD Anderson Cancer Center, Houston, Texas, USA

LAMA H. NAZER, PharmD, BCPS, FCCM
King Hussein Cancer Center, Amman, Jordan

SHREBASH PAUL, MBBS, MCPS
Phase-B Resident, Department of Internal Medicine, Bangabandhu Sheikh Mujib Medical University, Dhaka, Bangladesh

KATHERINE A. POLLARD, MD
Departments of Emergency Medicine and Medicine, Indiana University School of Medicine, Indianapolis, Indiana, USA

LARA PRISCO, MD, MSc, AFRCA, AFFICM
Consultant in Anesthesiology and Intensive Care Medicine, Neurosciences Intensive Care Unit, Oxford University Hospitals NHS Foundation Trust, Senior Clinical Research Fellow, Nuffield Department of Clinical Neurosciences, University of Oxford, John Radcliffe Hospital, Oxford, United Kingdom

DANIEL REYNOLDS, MD
Chief Fellow, Division of Pulmonary and Critical Care Medicine, Washington University School of Medicine, St Louis, Missouri, USA

JENNIFER A. ROSS, MD, MPH
Medical Toxicology Fellow, Division of Medical Toxicology, Department of Emergency Medicine, University of Virginia School of Medicine, Charlottesville, Virginia, USA

FRANCESCA RUBULOTTA, MD, PhD, MBA, FRCA, FFICM
Associate Professor, Chief of the Critical Care Program, Department of Anesthesia, Faculty of Medicine, McGill University, Montreal, Québec, Canada; Senior Lecturer and Consultant, Department of Anesthesiology and Intensive Care Medicine, Health Centre, Intensive Care Unit, Imperial College NHS Trust, London, United Kingdom

AARTI SARWAL, MD, FNCS, FAAN, FCCM
Associate Professor, Neurology, Section Chief, Neurocritical Care Unit, Wake Forest Baptist Medical Center, Winston Salem, North Carolina, USA

EVAN S. SCHWARZ, MD
Associate Professor of Emergency Medicine, Medical Toxicology Division Chief, Washington University School of Medicine, Saint Louis, Missouri, USA

MICHAEL SIRIMATUROS, PharmD, BCNSP, BCCCP, FCCM
Department of Pharmacy, Houston Methodist Hospital, Houston, Texas, USA

MAUDE ST-ONGE, MD, PhD, FRCPC
Assistant Professor, Medical Director of the Centre Antipoison du Québec, CIUSSSCN, Clinician-Scientist for the Population Health, Optimal Health Practice Research Unit, Trauma – Emergency – Critical Care Medicine, CHU de Québec Research Centre,

Intensivist, CHU de Québec – Université Laval, Faculty of Medicine, Université Laval, Centre Antipoison du Québec, Québec, Canada

MICHAEL WASSERMANN, MD
Department of Emergency Medicine, University of New Mexico Health Sciences Center, Albuquerque, New Mexico, USA

Contents

Pharmacokinetic and pharmacodynamic interactions between drugs and the body play a vital role in the therapeutic effects of drugs as well as their toxicity. Toxic effects may evolve from high doses of drugs or from alterations in the absorption, distribution, metabolism, and excretion of those drugs. The effective dose of a drug is influenced by the initial dose, route of administration, drug formulation, and bioavailability. This effective dose, in conjunction with the frequency of dosing, duration of exposure, and pharmacodynamic variability, directly affects the toxicity experienced in the body.

Sympathomimetic drugs comprise a broad category of substances including both illicit and prescribed drugs that have deleterious effects when ingested or abused. The clinical syndromes that result from overstimulation of the sympathetic nervous system by reuptake inhibition of biogenic amines, such as norepinephrine and dopamine, carry significant morbidity. Recognition and awareness of the appropriate supportive measures are required to mitigate life-threatening complications of multiple organ systems. The sympathomimetic toxidrome is recognized by a constellation of symptoms including agitation, hyperthermia, tachycardia, and hypertension, and the primary treatment involves supportive care, including the liberal use of benzodiazepines.

Over the last 2 decades, prescription and nonprescription substance use has significantly increased. In this article, 3 particular drug classes—opioids, sedatives, and hypnotics—are discussed. For each class, a brief history of the agent, a description of relevant pharmacology, the clinical presentation of overdose, the management of specific drug overdoses, and a summary of salient points are presented. The intent is to provide a clinically relevant and comprehensive approach to understanding these potential substance exposures in order to provide a framework for management of opioid, sedative, and hypnotic overdoses.

> A trend in the increasing use of prescription psychoactive drugs (PADs), including antidepressants, antipsychotics, and mood stabilizers, has been reported in the United States and globally. In addition, there has been an increase in the production and usage of illicit PADs and emergence of new psychoactive substances (NPSs) all over the world. PADs pose unique challenges for critical care providers who may encounter toxicology issues due to drug interactions, side effects, or drug overdoses. This article provides a summary of the toxicologic features of commonly used and abused PADs: antidepressants, antipsychotics, mood stabilizers, hallucinogens, NPSs, caffeine, nicotine, and cannabis.

> Acetaminophen is a common medication taken in deliberate self-poisoning and unintentional overdose. It is the commonest cause of severe acute liver injury in Western countries. The optimal management of most acetaminophen poisonings is usually straightforward. Patients who present early should be offered activated charcoal and those at risk of acute liver injury should receive acetylcysteine. This approach ensures survival in most. The acetaminophen nomogram is used to assess the need for treatment in acute immediate-release overdoses with a known time of ingestion. However, scenarios that require different management pathways include modified-release, large/massive, and repeated supratherapeutic ingestions.

> Managing unstable poisoned patients is often associated with clinician cognitive overload. This article summarizes the mechanisms of toxicity; clinical presentations; and the current evidence available for the treatment of cardiovascular drug toxicity due to calcium channel blockers, beta-blockers, cardiac glycosides, and sodium channel blockers. In addition, management approaches are proposed.

> Medications used to treat diabetes mellitus are heterogeneous, with widely differing safety profiles in therapeutic use and in overdose. Insulin overdose may produce severe and prolonged hypoglycemia. Sulfonylurea poisoning should be treated with octreotide, sparing intravenous dextrose where possible. Acute metformin overdose may lead to life-threatening acidosis with elevated lactate concentrations, which may require hemodialysis. Glucagon-like peptide 1 agonists and dipeptidyl peptidase 4 inhibitors are benign in overdose in diabetic patients but may produce profound hypoglycemia in nondiabetic patients. Euglycemic diabetic ketoacidosis may develop in critically ill patients taking sodium-glucose co-transporter 2 inhibitors.

Anticoagulant and antiplatelet drugs target a specific portion of the coagulation cascade or the platelet activation and aggregation pathway. The primary toxicity associated with these agents is hemorrhage. Understanding the pharmacology of these drugs allows the treating clinician to choose the correct antidotal therapy. Reversal agents exist for some of these drugs; however, not all have proven patient-centered outcomes. The anticoagulants covered in this review are vitamin K antagonists, heparins, fondaparinux, hirudin derivatives, argatroban, oral factor Xa antagonists, and dabigatran. The antiplatelet agents reviewed are aspirin, adenosine diphosphate antagonists, dipyridamole, and glycoprotein IIb/IIIa antagonists. Additional notable toxicities are also reviewed.

As the cancer population increases and immunotherapy becomes widely utilized, severe toxicities from these treatments will become more prevalent. In cancer patients, the most common immunotherapies that lead to critical illness are chimeric antigen receptor T cells, monoclonal antibodies, and immune checkpoint inhibitors. Awareness of their toxicities by the intensive care unit team is of extreme importance. A multidisciplinary approach for diagnosis and treatment is recommended. This article reviews the most common toxicities from immunotherapy and offers a therapy-specific and system-based approach for affected patients.

Drug-induced iatrogenic toxicities are common in critically ill patients and have been associated with increased morbidity and mortality. Early recognition and management of iatrogenic toxicities is essential; however, the diagnosis is usually complicated by the underlying critical illness, comorbidities, and administration of multiple medications. This article reviews several types of iatrogenic toxicities associated with medications that are commonly used in critically ill patients. The mechanism of the iatrogenic toxicities, clinical presentation, and diagnosis, as well as management are discussed.

This article reviews the background, metabolism, clinical effects, and treatment of toxic alcohols, specifically ethylene glycol, methanol, diethylene glycol, propylene glycol, and isopropyl alcohol. This article also reviews the importance of an anion gap metabolic acidosis in relation to toxic alcohols and explores both the utility and the limitations of the osmole gap in patient management.

Carbon monoxide is a colorless, odorless, highly toxic gas primarily produced through the incomplete combustion of organic material. Carbon monoxide binds to hemoglobin and other heme molecules, causing tissue hypoxia and oxidative stress. Symptoms of carbon monoxide poisoning can vary from a mild headache to critical illness, which can make diagnosis difficult. When there is concern for possible carbon monoxide poisoning, the diagnosis can be made via blood co-oximetry. The primary treatment for patients with carbon monoxide poisoning is supplemental oxygen, usually delivered via a nonrebreather mask. Hyperbaric oxygen can also be used, but the exact indications are controversial.

Organophosphorus (OP) compounds remain a leading cause of self-poisoning and mortality, especially in South East Asia, China, and Africa. Organophosphorus causes an acute cholinergic syndrome by inhibiting acetylcholinesterase. Atropine remains the mainstay of treatment, but recently some promising therapies are in the pipeline. Oximes are used widely in the management of organophosphorus poisoning, however clinical efficacy remains to be established. Magnesium sulfate, calcium channel blockers (nimodipine), plasma alkalinizing agents, β-2 agonists, nicotinic receptor antagonists, clonidine, and lipid emulsions are promising treatment alternatives. However, large phase III trials are required to establish their efficacy.

Toxic inhalants include various xenobiotics. Irritants cause upper and lower respiratory tract injuries. Highly water-soluble agents injure the upper respiratory tract, while low water-soluble inhalants injure the lower track. Asphyxiants are divided into simple asphyxiants and chemical asphyxiants. Simple asphyxiants displace oxygen, causing hypoxia, while chemical asphyxiants also impair the body's ability to use oxygen. Cyanide is a classic chemical asphyxiant. Treatment includes hydroxocobalamin. Electronic cigarette or vaping use-associated lung injury (EVALI) is a relatively new illness. Patients present with respiratory symptoms and gastrointestinal distress. EVALI appears to be associated with vaping cannabinoids. Treatment is supportive and may include steroids.

CRITICAL CARE CLINICS

CRITICAL CARE CLINICS

FORTHCOMING ISSUES

October 2021
Acute Respiratory Distress Syndrome
Michael Matthay and Kathleen Doctor,
Editors

January 2022
Diagnostic Excellence in the ICU: Thinking
Critically and Masterfully
Rahul Nanchal and Paul Bergl, Editors

April 2022
Undiagnosed and Rare Disease in Critical
Care
... Zimmerman, MD, MACr
Robert M. Kliegman and Brett Bordini,
Editors

RECENT ISSUES

April 2021
Acute Kidney Injury
Dana Y. Fuhrman and John A. Kellum,
Editors

January 2021
Critical Care of the Cancer Patient &
Oncolytic Critical Care
Stephen M. Pastores, Wendy R. Greene
and Maxwell A. Hockstein, Editors

October 2020
Enhanced Recovery in the ICU after Cardiac
Surgery & New Developments in
Cardiopulmonary Resuscitation
Daniel T. Engelman and Clifton W.
Callaway, Editors

SERIES OF RELATED INTEREST

Emergency Medicine Clinics
Available at: www.emed.theclinics.com

THE CLINICS ARE AVAILABLE ONLINE!
Access your subscription at:
www.theclinics.com

Preface

Poisons and Patients

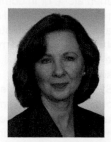

Janice L. Zimmerman, MD, MACP, MCCM
Editor

Critical care providers frequently care for patients who are poisoned under a variety of circumstances and develop a wide range of clinical syndromes. Poisonings may be intentional (eg, suicide, homicide) or unintentional (eg, recreational abuse, medication error). They may involve over-the-counter medications, prescribed outpatient drugs, inpatient drug regimens, illicit substances, or environmental exposures. In the United States, deaths from overdoses reached 70,630 in 2019.[1] Exposures with more serious outcomes (moderate, major, or death) increased 4.61% per year since 2000.[2] Taken together, these data suggest more poisoning patients will require critical care. An increased incidence in intensive care unit (ICU) admissions for overdose and increased death rate related to overdose were documented between 2009 and 2015 in a large US database.[3] While ICU patients with overdose may have more favorable outcomes than other ICU patients, the cost of care is significant.[3,4]

Although the number of potential toxins is large and new drugs continually enter the market, this toxicology issue highlights selected topics relevant for clinicians caring for seriously ill patients. In the sixteenth century, Paracelsus stated that all things are poisons and that only the dose determines toxicity.[5] The interaction of substances and the individual is now known to be much more complex. In their article, Michael Sirimaturos and Annette Lista review pharmacokinetic and pharmacodynamic principles important in toxicology, including drug metabolism, genetic factors, drug interactions, and comorbidities.

Prescription or illicit drugs of abuse account for a large proportion of overdose deaths. While opioids are responsible for the greatest number of deaths, deaths from cocaine and other stimulants are also increasing.[1] A single-center study found 13.1% of ICU admissions were related to illicit drugs.[6] Drs Brown and Pollard review the clinical presentation and management of toxicity from sympathomimetic drugs of abuse, and Dr Azevedo and colleagues provide information on managing overdoses from opioids and other sedative/hypnotic drugs.

Crit Care Clin 37 (2021) xiii–xv
https://doi.org/10.1016/j.ccc.2021.03.015
0749-0704/21/© 2021 Published by Elsevier Inc.

Antidepressants continue to be commonly involved in exposures reported to poison control centers.[2] Dr Prisco and colleagues review the management of toxicity from tricyclic antidepressants and selective serotonin reuptake inhibitors as well as other psychoactive substances used therapeutically and recreationally.

Over-the-counter and prescription drugs are often involved in intentional and unintentional toxicity due to availability in homes. Acetaminophen alone or in combination with other drugs continues to account for a significant number of fatalities and remains the leading cause of acute liver failure in North America, Europe, and Australia. Dr Chiew reviews the approach to a patient with acetaminophen poisoning and modifications to the acetylcysteine antidote regimen that may be needed in special circumstances. Cardiovascular drugs, especially beta-blockers and calcium channel blockers, can cause significant toxicity and death. Dr St-Onge reviews the clinical manifestations of toxicity from cardiovascular drugs and provides structured management approaches. Diabetes is prevalent worldwide, and an increasing number of oral and injectable drugs are available for treatment. Drs Baumgartner and Devgun outline the potential toxic effects of insulins and newer agents along with management. Anticoagulant and antiplatelet drugs are part of the treatment for thrombotic and cardiovascular diseases in hospitalized patients and outpatients. The major toxicity is hemorrhage, and Drs Liss and Mullins review the pharmacology of the different classes of agents and recommendations for reversal.

New drugs often have unique toxicities that are important to recognize and manage. In the field of oncology, use of immunotherapeutic agents, such as chimeric antigen receptor T cells, monoclonal antibodies, and immune checkpoint inhibitors, is increasing. Dr Gutierrez and colleagues review the manifestations and management of the cytokine release syndrome, immune effector cell–associated neurotoxicity syndrome, hypersensitivity reactions, and other life-threatening toxicities of these drugs.

Many drugs are administered to complex critically ill patients, which can result in unintentional toxic effects. Lama Nazer and colleagues review iatrogenic toxicities that can develop in critically ill patients, the difficulty of diagnosis, impact of comorbidities, and therapeutic interventions.

Several articles cover toxicities from nonmedical substances that may cause poisoning by abuse or through accidental exposures. Dr Ross and colleagues outline the management of toxic alcohol poisonings and review the limitations of the osmole gap and anion gap in assessment and management of patients. Dr Chenoweth and colleagues discuss the multiple toxic effects of carbon monoxide exposure, appropriate evaluation, and management, including the controversies of hyperbaric oxygen use. Organophosphorus poisoning is more common in low- and middle-income countries but is associated with significant morbidity and mortality. Dr Aman and colleagues provide information on management with atropine and oximes as well as data on promising new interventions. Dr Schwarz reviews toxicity of inhaled irritants and asphyxiants that may result from occupational and environmental exposures but also from substances that are inhaled recreationally.

Last, I would like to thank the authors for their time, energy, and commitment in writing and revising articles. The work on this issue occurred during recurrent surges in the COVID-19 pandemic when clinicians had unprecedented burdens of physical workloads and emotional stresses. Despite those circumstances, the contributions of the authors make this toxicology issue a valuable resource for clinicians managing poisoned patients.

Janice L. Zimmerman, MD, MACP, MCCM
Baylor College of Medicine
Houston, TX, USA

E-mail address:
drjanicez@gmail.com

REFERENCES

1. Hedegaard H, Miniño AM, Warner M. Drug overdose deaths in the United States, 1999-2019. NCHS Data Brief 2020;(394):1–8. Available at: www.cdc.gov/nchs/data/databriefs/db394-H.pdf.
2. Gummin DD, Mowry JB, Beuhler MC, et al. 2019 annual report of the American Association of Poison Control Centers' National Poison Data System (NPDS): 37th annual report. Clin Toxicol 2020;58:1360–541. Available at: https://piper.filecamp.com/uniq/9ZN62pw4DkShNNNS.pdf.
3. Stevens JP, Wall MJ, Novack L, et al. The critical care crisis of opioid overdoses in the United States. Ann Am Thorac Soc 2017;14:1803–9.
4. Fernando SM, Reardon PM, Ball IM, et al. Outcomes and costs of patients admitted to the intensive care unit due to accidental or intentional poisoning. J Intensive Care Med 2020;35:386–93.
5. Borzelleca JF. Paracelsus: herald of modern toxicology. Toxicol Sci 2000;53:2–4.
6. Westerhausen D, Perkins AJ, Conley J, et al. Burden of substance abuse-related admissions to the medical ICU. Chest 2020;157:61–6.

Pharmacokinetic and Pharmacodynamic Principles for Toxicology

Annette D. Lista, PharmD, BCCCP,
Michael Sirimaturos, PharmD, BCNSP, BCCCP, FCCM*

KEYWORDS

- Pharmacokinetics • Pharmacology • Drug overdose • Toxicology
- Drug-related side effects and adverse reactions

KEY POINTS

- Drug toxicity can be related to multiple factors, including drug overdose, genetics, comorbidities, drug interactions, and additive adverse effects from concomitant therapies.
- Individuals vary in the degree of their response to the same concentration of a single drug, and a given individual may not always respond in the same way to the same drug concentration.
- Understanding the pharmacokinetic and pharmacodynamic characteristics of drugs can help determine the best treatment strategy for drug-related toxicity.

INTRODUCTION

Pharmacokinetics and pharmacodynamics play an essential role in the toxicologic effects of drugs and management of drug toxicity. Pharmacokinetics, more simply described by what the body does to drugs, are characterized by the study of the absorption, distribution, metabolism, and excretion of drugs.[1] Pharmacodynamics, described by what drugs do to the body, are characterized by the relationships between drug concentration and pharmacologic response, which involves receptor binding, post-receptor effects, and chemical interactions. It is important for clinicians to understand that changes in drug effects are infrequently proportional to the change in drug dose or concentration.[2]

The effective dose of a drug is influenced by the initial dose, route of administration, drug formulation, and bioavailability. This effective dose, in conjunction with the frequency of dosing, duration of exposure, and pharmacodynamic variability, directly affects any toxicity experienced in the body (**Fig. 1**). An understanding of

Department of Pharmacy, Houston Methodist Hospital, 6565 Fannin Street, DB1-09, Houston, TX 77030, USA
* Corresponding author.
E-mail address: MWSirimaturos@houstonmethodist.org

Crit Care Clin 37 (2021) 475–486
https://doi.org/10.1016/j.ccc.2021.03.001

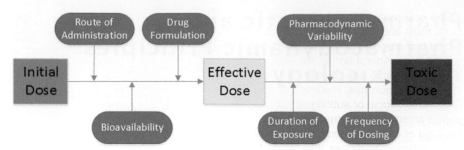

Fig. 1. Essential factors affecting drug accumulation that can lead to toxicity.

pharmacokinetic and pharmacodynamic principles can lead to more accurate interpretations of plasma concentrations and how these relate to the time course of a drug. As a result, clinicians can better estimate the appropriate duration of patient observations and the specific treatments needed to manage toxic effects.

Many specific toxicology interventions aim to alter the pharmacokinetics of the toxin.[3] However, the pharmacokinetic characteristics of drugs taken at toxic levels may differ from the pharmacokinetic characteristics of drugs observed following therapeutic doses. These differences are a result of dose-dependent changes in absorption, distribution, metabolism, elimination, or pharmacologic and pathophysiologic effects of the drug overdose.[4]

Phenytoin toxicity, for example, has influences on both pharmacokinetic and pharmacodynamic principles. Based on pharmacokinetics, the oral formulation of phenytoin is nearly completely absorbed after ingestion. In therapeutic doses, it is rapidly absorbed with peak plasma concentration occurring at 1.5 to 3.0 hours postingestion for immediate-release formulations and 4 to 12 hours for extended-release formulations. However, due to gastrointestinal (GI) motility effects and its poor water solubility, phenytoin absorption can be delayed in oral overdoses with peak concentrations occurring as late as 24 to 48 hours postingestion. Pharmacodynamically, 1% to 5% of phenytoin is excreted unchanged in the urine, and the remainder is metabolized by the hepatic P450 enzyme system, predominantly CYP2C9 and CYP2C19. Phenytoin also induces CYP3A4, which accounts for its numerous drug-drug interactions. At plasma concentrations less than 10 mg/L, the rate of elimination is proportional to the drug concentration. However, saturation of phenytoin metabolism occurs with increasing plasma concentrations greater than 10 mg/L. As a result, the half-life of phenytoin, which is typically 22 hours, increases, but the phenytoin elimination rate remains the same.[5] Therefore, pharmacokinetic and pharmacodynamic principles of drugs under therapeutic conditions may be altered during large ingestions or overdoses requiring prolonged observation for development of toxicity due to increased elimination half-lives and prolonged drug elimination.

DISCUSSION
Absorption

Drug absorption, the movement of a drug from its site of administration into a central compartment, is determined by the drug properties, formulation, and route of administration. Drug formulations (eg, tablets, suppositories, injectables, powders, liquids, gases) are administered via various routes (eg, oral, sublingual, rectal, parenteral, inhalation, insufflation). Regardless of the route of administration, drugs must be absorbed to demonstrate their pharmacologic or toxicologic effects.

The oral route is the most common method of drug administration. A drug given orally must endure a low pH, copious GI secretions, and degrading enzymes. Absorption of oral drugs involves transport across membranes of the epithelial cells in the oral and GI tract. Absorption is affected by differences in pH, surface area of absorption, blood flow to the site of absorption, presence of bile and mucus, and the nature of epithelial membranes. The oral mucosa has a thin epithelium and is rich in vasculature. Therefore, buccal or sublingual administration of drugs (eg, nitroglycerin, tacrolimus) can be an effective alternative route for rapid absorption when the gastric route is inaccessible or compromised. In addition, venous drainage from the mouth directly flows to the superior vena cava, thus bypassing the portal circulation. As a result, a buccal or sublingual drug is protected from rapid intestinal and hepatic first-pass metabolism.

Beyond the oral cavity, the stomach and small intestine are the next primary organs with significant contact with an oral drug. Although the stomach has a relatively large epithelial surface, its thick mucus layer and short transit time limit drug absorption. The small intestine, however, has the largest surface area for drug absorption in the GI tract, and its membranes are more permeable. For these reasons, most drugs are absorbed primarily in the small intestine.[6,7]

Drug formulations and routes of administration play a large role in the absorption of drugs and maintenance of therapeutic or toxic levels. Modified-release formulations (eg, controlled, delayed, extended, sustained-release) are designed to reduce dosing frequency for drugs with a short elimination half-life and duration of effect. These formulations also limit fluctuation in plasma drug concentrations, providing a more uniform therapeutic effect while decreasing the intensity of adverse effects. However, modified-release formulations also can lead to delayed development of symptoms and prolonged toxic effects. Patients should be monitored for a longer duration of time when ingestion of modified-release drug formulations is suspected in overdoses (**Table 1**).[8] In contrast, intravenous formulations of drugs enter the systemic circulation directly. Availability is more rapid and predictable when a drug is given by intravenous injection and the effective dose can be delivered more accurately by a specific dose. In addition to the intravenous route, other common parenteral routes include subcutaneous and intramuscular. Drugs injected subcutaneously or intramuscularly must cross one or more biologic membranes to reach the systemic circulation. This rate of absorption is limited by the area of the absorbing capillary membranes and by the solubility of the substance in the interstitial fluid.

Because absorption is the first pharmacokinetic principle that can lead to toxicity, it is fitting that treatment of potential or known toxicities focuses on decreasing absorption immediately after intoxication. GI decontamination within an hour or two of ingestion is used with some ingestions. This may include gastric lavage to remove a portion of the drug from the GI tract or binding agents (eg, chelators, activated charcoal), which bind or adhere to the drug to prevent absorption. Increasing GI transit may also be considered with the use of cathartics (eg, sorbitol) or whole bowel irrigation (eg, polyethylene glycol electrolyte solutions), but these methods may not effectively decrease absorption and are not routinely recommended. For toxicity caused by cutaneous absorption, removal of the offending agents (eg, patches, chemical soaked clothing) can limit intoxication.

Bioavailability

Bioavailability describes the extent and rate at which an active drug enters the systemic circulation unaltered.[9] Insufficient time for absorption in the GI tract is a common cause of low bioavailability. The time at the absorption site may be inadequate if the drug does not dissolve readily or cannot penetrate the epithelial membrane due to

Table 1
Modified-release oral drug formulations affecting duration of drug toxicity

System	Drug Category	Modified-Release Oral Drug Products
Cardiovascular	Antiarrhythmics	Diltiazem, disopyramide, propafenone, verapamil
	Antihypertensives	Carvedilol, clonidine, felodipine, guanfacine, isosorbide dinitrate/mononitrate, isradipine, metoprolol succinate, nevirapine, nifedipine, nisoldipine, propranolol
	Antilipemics	Colestipol, fenofibric acid, fluvastatin, lovastatin, niacin
	Other	Ranolazine
Endocrine		Glipizide, metformin, prednisone, risedronate
Gastrointestinal		Budesonide, crofelemer, dexlansoprazole, esomeprazole, hyoscyamine, lansoprazole, mesalamine, omeprazole, pancrelipase, pantoprazole, rabeprazole
Genitourinary		Alfuzosin, calcifediol, darifenacin, doxazosin, fesoterodine, mirabegron, oxybutynin, tamsulosin
Hematologic		Aspirin, pentoxifylline
Immunologic		Mycophenolate, tacrolimus, tofacitinib
Infectious diseases		Amoxicillin, ciprofloxacin, clarithromycin, didanosine, doxycycline, minocycline, posaconazole, rifamycin
Musculoskeletal	Analgesics/anti-inflammatories	Acetaminophen, diclofenac, hydrocodone, hydromorphone, gabapentin, morphine, naproxen, oxycodone, oxymorphone, pregabalin, sulfasalazine, tapentadol, tramadol
	Other	Cyclobenzaprine, orphenadrine, pyridostigmine
Neurologic	Anticonvulsants	Carbamazepine, lamotrigine, levetiracetam, oxcarbazepine, topiramate
	Psychotropics	Alprazolam, amantadine, amphetamine/dextroamphetamine salts, bupropion, desvenlafaxine, dexmethylphenidate, divalproex, duloxetine, fluvoxamine, galantamine, levodopa/carbidopa, levomilnacipran, lithium, memantine, methylphenidate, paliperidone, paroxetine, pramipexole, quetiapine, valproic acid, venlafaxine, zolpidem
	Other	Dalfampridine, dimethyl fumarate, ropinirole
Pulmonary		Albuterol, guaifenesin, theophylline, treprostinil, zileuton
Miscellaneous		Cysteamine, potassium chloride

its highly ionized or polar characteristics. This results in a highly variable bioavailability. Orally administered drugs then pass through the intestinal wall before portal circulation to the liver. This first-pass metabolism occurs before a drug reaches the systemic circulation. As a result, drugs may be metabolized before adequate plasma concentrations are reached. Other factors that can affect a drug's bioavailability include age, sex, physical activity, genetic phenotype, stress, GI disorders (eg, malabsorption syndromes), or GI surgery (eg, bariatric surgery) (Table 2).[9,10]

Distribution

Following absorption into the bloodstream or systemic administration, drugs distribute into tissues and organs. Cardiac output, regional blood flow, capillary permeability, and tissue volume all affect the rate of delivery and amount of drug distributed into tissues, which at high levels or doses, can lead to toxicity. The liver, kidneys, brain, and other well-perfused organs receive a large majority of the drug initially, whereas delivery to muscle, most viscera, skin, and fat is limited and slower (Table 3).[7]

Volume of distribution (Vd) is a pharmacokinetic parameter representing the ability of a drug to either remain in the plasma or redistribute to other tissues. A drug with a high Vd (eg, digoxin, meperidine, propofol) can penetrate more tissues, which in turn requires a higher dose of the drug to achieve a given plasma concentration. Vd may be increased due to volume overload from sepsis or surgery, ascites in hepatic disease, or during pregnancy. Conversely, a drug with a low Vd (eg, gentamicin, lithium, phenytoin) tends to remain in the plasma, thereby requiring a lower dose of the drug to achieve a given plasma concentration. Some drugs distribute mostly into fat, others remain in extracellular fluid, and others are bound extensively to specific tissues, which all affect the toxicology profile of a drug.[11] In addition, significant decreases or shifts in the Vd over time from conditions such as dehydration or from use of diuretics can increase drug concentrations and lead to toxicity.

The extent of drug distribution into tissues also depends on the degree of plasma protein and tissue binding. The amount of bound drug in plasma is determined by the drug concentration as well as the affinity and concentration of available binding sites. In the bloodstream, drugs are transported partially in solution as unbound (ie, free drug) and partially reversibly bound to blood components, such as plasma

Table 2		
Changes in bioavailability for special populations		
Special Population	**Mechanism**	**Bioavailability**
Obesity	Reduced expression of gastric drug metabolizing enzymes, greater splanchnic blood flow, altered membrane permeability	↑
Children	Immature development of gastric drug metabolizing enzymes	↑
Elderly	Reduction in gastric acid secretion, reduced gastric emptying, longer gastric transit time	↑
Renal impairment	Impaired first pass metabolism Reduced bile acid excretion	↑ ↓
Hepatic impairment	Impaired first pass metabolism	↑
Pregnancy	Increased gastric pH, diminished intestinal motility Increased gastric pH, diminished gastric motility	↑ ↓

Abbreviations: ↑, increased bioavailability; ↓, decreased bioavailability.

Table 3 Distribution of cardiac output in a 70-kg male individual at rest		
	Blood Flow	
Organs	**Milliliters per Minute**	**% Cardiac Output**
Liver	1700	31
Kidneys	1100	20
Brain	800	14.5
Heart	250	4.5
Skeletal muscle	900	16.4
Fat	250	4.5

proteins. Of the many plasma proteins that can interact with drugs, the most important are albumin, alpha-1 acid glycoprotein, and lipoproteins. Only free drug is available for passive diffusion to extravascular or tissue sites where the pharmacologic effects of the drug occur. Therefore, the unbound drug concentration in systemic circulation typically determines the drug concentration at the active site, which is directly correlated to the efficacy of the drug. Valproic acid, for example, is highly albumin bound (~90%), and the unbound active drug is small in comparison to the total dose. When the fraction of protein binding is altered due to drug-drug interactions or reductions in total serum protein concentrations, a substantial increase in the bioavailable active drug can occur, leading to toxicity. In addition to valproic acid, other highly albumin-bound drugs include amiodarone, calcium, ceftriaxone, naproxen, lorazepam, phenytoin, verapamil, and warfarin.

Drugs also can bind to substances other than proteins. For example, binding may occur when a drug is dispersed into body fat. A large fraction of drug in the body may be bound in this fashion and serve as a reservoir that prolongs the action of the drug in the tissue or at a distant site reached through the circulation. As a result, this tissue binding and drug accumulation can lead to local and prolonged toxicity. Diazepam, for example, is highly lipid-soluble, which increases its Vd and causes the drug to have a relatively short therapeutic effect. Diazepam does not stay in the plasma as long as other benzodiazepines, and over time its concentrations accumulate in fat, which may add to the toxicity (eg, excessive sedation) seen with prolonged use. Metoprolol, propranolol, propofol, and rifampin are also highly lipid-soluble and can have prolonged toxic effects. With regard to poisonings, organophosphates are an example of prolonged toxicity due to the high lipid solubility of the organophosphate compounds (see Sakib Aman and colleagues' article, "Management of Organophosphorus Poisoning: Standard Treatment and Beyond," in this issue).

Blood Brain Barrier

Drugs can also reach the central nervous system (CNS) via brain capillaries and cerebrospinal fluid (CSF). Although the brain is well-perfused, drug penetration can be restricted because of the brain's permeability structure. Highly lipophilic drugs (eg, gabapentin) are more likely to penetrate the CSF and have the potential to cause increased neurologic toxicity (eg, prolonged sedation).

Metabolism

The liver is a major site of drug metabolism with the goal of making the drug easier to excrete. Drugs can be metabolized by oxidation, reduction, hydrolysis, hydration, conjugation, condensation, or isomerization. Although the enzymes involved in metabolism are present in many other tissues throughout the body, these enzymes are primarily concentrated in the liver.[12]

Drug metabolism rates can vary among individuals. Some individuals are rapid metabolizers of drugs, which may cause a lack of therapeutic concentrations in blood and tissues. In contrast, other individuals can be slow metabolizers of drugs, which can result in toxic effects. Individual drug metabolism rates may be influenced by genetic factors, comorbidities (eg, liver disease, heart failure) and drug interactions. Decreased metabolism may be more prevalent in the elderly and can be caused by other factors such as liver failure and hypothermia.[13]

For many drugs, metabolism occurs in 2 phases:

- Phase I reactions involve oxidation, reduction, or hydrolysis of a drug, creating metabolites that are more polar, and thus more easily excreted.
- Phase II reactions involve conjugation by coupling the drug or its metabolites to another molecule, such as glucuronidation. Metabolites formed in synthetic reactions are also more polar and readily excreted by the kidneys and the liver.

The most important enzyme system of phase I metabolism is cytochrome P-450 (CYP450), a family of enzymes that catalyzes the oxidation of many drugs. CYP450 enzymes can be induced or inhibited by many drugs and substances resulting in drug interactions, thereby enhancing the toxicity or reducing the therapeutic effect of another drug. With age, the ability of the liver to metabolize via the CYP450 enzyme system is reduced by $\geq 30\%$ because hepatic volume and blood flow are decreased. Thus, drugs that are metabolized through this system (eg, carbamazepine, fluoxetine, paroxetine, phenobarbital, phenytoin) reach higher levels and have prolonged half-lives in elderly patients. Neonates, on the other hand, have partially developed hepatic enzyme systems and also have difficulty metabolizing many drugs as well.[14]

Glucuronidation is the most common and most important phase II reaction that occurs in the liver enzyme system. Glucuronides are secreted in bile and eliminated in urine. Thus, conjugation increases drug solubility and enhances excretion by the kidneys.

Excretion

Drugs are eliminated from the body either unchanged or as metabolites. The kidney is the most important organ for excreting drugs and their metabolites. Renal excretion of unchanged drugs is a major route of elimination for 25% to 30% of drugs. Renal excretion of drugs and metabolites in the urine involves 3 distinct processes: glomerular filtration, active tubular secretion, and passive tubular reabsorption. The amount of drug entering the tubular lumen by filtration depends on the glomerular filtration rate and the extent of plasma binding of the drug, with only unbound drug being filtered. In the renal tubules, the nonionized forms of weak acids and bases undergo net passive reabsorption. Because the tubular cells are less permeable to the ionized forms of weak electrolytes, passive reabsorption of these substances depend on the pH. When the tubular urine is made more alkaline, weak acids are largely ionized and are excreted more rapidly and to a greater extent. Conversely, acidification of the urine will reduce fractional ionization and excretion of weak acids. Effects of changing urine pH are opposite for weak bases. In the treatment of drug poisoning, the excretion of some drugs may be accelerated by appropriate alkalization or acidification of the urine. For example, treatment of aspirin toxicity includes administration of sodium bicarbonate to manipulate the urinary pH to enhance excretion because aspirin is a weak acid. In addition to the kidneys, the biliary system contributes to excretion when a specific drug is not reabsorbed from the GI tract. Also, excretion of drugs in breast milk is important to remember, as excreted drugs may affect the breastfeeding infant.

Renal drug excretion decreases with age. For example, at age 80, clearance is approximately reduced to half of what it was at age 30. Renal drug excretion may also change with various health conditions. In critically ill patients, kidney injury may temporarily decrease renal drug excretion, which is a major cause of unintentional overdose and toxicity (**Table 4**). In contrast, augmented renal clearance may enhance renal drug excretion, resulting in subtherapeutic plasma concentrations of certain drugs, especially antimicrobials.[15]

Pharmacodynamics

Pharmacodynamics refers to the relationship between the drug concentration at the site of action and the resulting effects, including the time course and intensity of therapeutic and adverse effects. Pharmacodynamics, with pharmacokinetics, helps explain the relationship between the dose and response (**Table 5**).[16]

The pharmacologic response depends on the drug binding to its target. The concentration of the drug at the receptor site influences the effects of the drug. Physiologic changes due to a disorder, a disease, the aging process, or other drugs can affect the pharmacodynamics of a drug. Disorders that affect pharmacodynamic responses include genetic mutations, malnutrition, and myasthenia gravis. These disorders can change receptor binding, alter the level of binding proteins, or decrease receptor sensitivity.

Patients with myasthenia gravis, for example, have a 70% to 90% reduction in the number of acetylcholine receptors (AChR) in neuromuscular junctions. This reduction results from antibodies that attack components of the postsynaptic membrane, such as AChR, impair neuromuscular transmission, and lead to weakness and fatigue of

Table 4 Drug toxicity related to decreased renal drug clearance	
Renal Failure–Associated Drug Toxicity	**Medications**
Bleeding	Direct-acting oral anticoagulants, enoxaparin
Bradycardia	Digoxin, hydrophilic beta-blockers (acebutolol, atenolol, bisoprolol, nadolol)
Hyperkalemia	ACE inhibitors, sulfamethoxazole/trimethoprim
Hypoglycemia	Glyburide, metformin
Hypotension	Hydrophilic beta-blockers (acebutolol, atenolol, bisoprolol, nadolol), digoxin
Hypoventilation	Benzodiazepines, opiates
Nephrotoxicity	ACE inhibitors, allopurinol, aminoglycosides, vancomycin, voriconazole IV
Metabolic acidosis	Lithium, metformin
Ototoxicity	Aminoglycosides, vancomycin
Sedation	Benzodiazepines, gabapentin, opiates
Seizures	Beta-lactam antibiotics
QTc prolongation	Fluconazole, fluoroquinolone antibiotics, metoclopramide

Abbreviations: ACE, angiotensin-converting enzyme; IV, intravenous.

Table 5	
Relationship of pharmacokinetics and pharmacodynamics	
Pharmacokinetics	**Pharmacodynamics**
Drug administered → Drug at site of action	Drug at site of action → Drugs effects
Absorption	Drug interactions
Distribution	Dose-response relationships
Metabolism	Drug-receptor relationships
Excretion	

skeletal muscle. This loss of AChR significantly predisposes patients with myasthenia gravis to disease exacerbation by any drug that impedes neuromuscular transmission. More than 30 drugs have clinical evidence of increasing the risk of respiratory depression in patients with myasthenia gravis (**Table 6**).[17]

Drug Interactions

Drug interactions can be either pharmacokinetic or pharmacodynamic. In a patient with multiple comorbidities requiring several drugs, it may be difficult to identify adverse effects due to drug interactions and to determine whether these are pharmacokinetic, pharmacodynamic, or a combination of drug interactions. Concomitant therapy constitutes optimal treatment of many disease states, including heart failure, hypertension, and cancer. When drugs are used in combination, their effects may be different in comparison to when each drug is administered alone. In addition, the coadministration of prescriptions, nonprescriptions, and supplements can result in significant alterations in the effects of drugs, resulting in toxicity, adverse effects, or inhibiting the therapeutic benefit of the drug.

For example, warfarin is subject to numerous important pharmacokinetic and pharmacodynamic drug interactions. Warfarin has a narrow therapeutic range between inhibition of clot formation and bleeding complications. Increases in dietary vitamin K intake may significantly decrease the pharmacodynamics of warfarin and require adjustments in dosing. Administration of antibiotics can alter the intestinal flora of the patient and reduce the bacterial synthesis of vitamin K, thereby enhancing the

Table 6			
Drug-induced neuromuscular blockade in myasthenia gravis			
	Drug-Induced Neuromuscular Blockade		
	Presynaptic	**Postsynaptic**	**Both**
Mechanism	Presynaptic neuromuscular blockade	Postsynaptic neuromuscular blockade	Postsynaptic neuromuscular transmission blockade by conductance interference	Combination presynaptic and postsynaptic neuromuscular blockade
Drugs	Clindamycin Chloroquine Quinidine	Inhaled anesthetics (ether, halothane) Ketamine Clindamycin Chloroquine Amphetamine	Amantadine	Gentamicin Tobramycin Phenytoin Amitriptyline Barbiturates Haloperidol
Result	Respiratory depression			

therapeutic effect of warfarin. Administration of drugs like amiodarone, fluconazole, metronidazole, or sulfamethoxazole-trimethoprim can cause significant CYP450 inhibitory interactions, which can increase the international normalized ratio (INR) by as much as twofold. Last, concurrent administration of antiplatelets (eg, aspirin, clopidogrel) or nonsteroidal anti-inflammatory drugs (eg, ibuprofen) with warfarin can increase the risk of GI bleeding almost fourfold.

In the elderly, drug pharmacokinetics and pharmacodynamics can be altered, possibly requiring avoidance of specific drugs in that population (eg, amitriptyline, diphenhydramine, paroxetine, zolpidem) or significant alterations in the drug dose or frequency (eg, benzodiazepines, opiates) to safely produce the desired therapeutic effect. Most drugs are primarily studied in younger and middle-aged adults, with minimal literature in children and elderly individuals. Drug interactions always should be considered when unexpected responses to drugs occur, especially toxicity. Understanding the mechanisms for which drug interactions can occur helps prevent them from happening.[18]

Dose-Response Relationships

Regardless of how a drug effect occurs, through binding or chemical interaction, the concentration of the drug at the site of action controls the effect. However, response to concentration may be complex and is often nonlinear. Dose-response, involving the principles of pharmacokinetics and pharmacodynamics, determines the required dose and frequency, as well as the therapeutic index for a drug in a patient. The therapeutic index (TI) is defined as a ratio that compares the blood concentration at which a drug becomes toxic and the concentration at which the drug is effective. The TI helps determine the efficacy and safety of a drug. The larger the TI, the safer the drug. Increasing the dose of a drug with a small TI can increase the likelihood of toxicity of the drug (eg, digoxin, gentamicin, lithium, phenytoin, warfarin). However, these features differ by patient and are affected by patient-related factors, such as pregnancy, age, and organ function.

Drug-Receptor Interactions

Receptors are transmembrane proteins that enable the transfer of chemical signals from outside the cell to inside the cell, as well as within the cell. Receptors allow for cell-cell communication and regulation of many cellular biochemical processes. When the receptor binds to a drug, the state of activation for a receptor is changed. Drugs that bind to a receptor are called ligands. The binding can be specific and reversible. A ligand may activate or inactivate a receptor, and activation of that receptor may increase or decrease cell function. A drug's ability to affect a receptor is related to the drug's affinity to that specific receptor and intrinsic activity. The affinity and activity of a drug are determined by its chemical structure. The pharmacologic effect is also determined by the duration of time that the drug-receptor complex exists.

Receptor Agonists

A receptor agonist is a mimetic of the natural ligand and produces a similar effect as the natural ligand when it binds to the receptor. Agonists activate receptors to produce the desired drug response. Conventional agonists (eg, clonidine, morphine) increase the proportion of activated receptors. Inverse agonists (ie, atropine, diphenhydramine) are agents that bind to the same receptor as an agonist but cause a pharmacologic response opposite to that agonist.

Receptor Antagonists

Receptor antagonists are inhibitors of receptor activity. Antagonists mimic ligands that bind to a receptor and prevent receptor activation by a natural ligand. Receptor antagonists can be classified as reversible or irreversible. Reversible antagonists readily disconnect from their receptor, whereas irreversible antagonists form a stable chemical bond with their receptor. Pseudo-irreversible antagonists slowly disconnect from their receptor over time. Three types of receptor antagonists are described:

- Competitive antagonists (eg, flumazenil, naloxone) bind to the active site of a receptor.
- Noncompetitive antagonists (eg, ketamine) bind to a different site than the active site.
- Uncompetitive antagonists (eg, memantine) differ from noncompetitive antagonists because they require receptor activation by an agonist before they can bind to a separate binding site.

Pharmacodynamic Variability

Individuals vary in the degree of their response to the same concentration of a single drug, and a given individual may not always respond in the same way to the same drug concentration. Drug responsiveness may change because of disease, age, or previous drug administration. Receptors are dynamic, and their concentrations and functions may be upregulated or downregulated by various endogenous and exogenous factors.

SUMMARY

Drug toxicity is multifaceted. Many pharmacokinetic elements play a large role in the toxic effects of drugs including enhanced absorption, varied distribution into tissues, altered metabolism, and decreased excretion. The direct pharmacodynamic effects of drugs at the receptor site also can lead to increased toxicity. A thorough review of the pharmacokinetic and pharmacodynamic properties of a drug should occur before selecting the optimal treatment during toxicologic emergencies.

CLINICS CARE POINTS

- Factors that can affect a drug's bioavailability include age, sex, physical activity, genetic phenotypes, stress, GI disorders (eg, malabsorption syndromes), or GI surgery (eg, bariatric surgery).

- With age, the ability of the liver to metabolize via the CYP450 enzyme system is reduced by ≥30% because hepatic volume and blood flow are decreased.

- In critically ill patients, kidney injury may temporarily decrease renal drug excretion, which is a major cause of unintentional overdose and toxicity.

- Drug interactions (eg, prescriptions, nonprescriptions, supplements) should be considered when unexpected responses to drugs occur, as these interactions can result in significant alterations in the effects of drugs, resulting in toxicity, adverse effects, or inhibiting the therapeutic benefit of the drug.

DISCLOSURE

Nothing to disclose.

REFERENCES

1. Shargel L, Yu A, Wu-Pong S. Introduction to biopharmaceutics and pharmacokinetics. In: Shargel L, Yu ABC, editors. Applied biopharmaceutics and pharmacokinetics. 6th edition. New York: McGraw-Hill; 2012. p. 1–5.
2. Bauer LA. Clinical pharmacokinetic and pharmacodynamic concepts. In: Weitz M, Thomas CM, editors. Applied clinical pharmacokinetics. 3th edition. New York: McGraw-Hill; 2015. p. 1–4.
3. Roberts DM, Buckley NA. Pharmacokinetic considerations in clinical toxicology: clinical applications. Clin Pharmacokinet 2007;46(11):897–939.
4. Sue YJ, Shannon M. Pharmacokinetics of drugs in overdose. Clin Pharmacokinet 1992;23(2):93–105.
5. DiPiro JT, Yee GC, Posey L, et al. Clinical pharmacokinetics and pharmacodynamics. In: DiPiro JT, Yee GC, Posey ML, et al, editors. Pharmacotherapy: a pathophysiologic approach. 11th edition. New York: McGraw-Hill; 2020. p. 38–42.
6. Vertzoni M, Augustijns P, Grimm M, et al. Impact of regional differences along the gastrointestinal tract of healthy adults on oral drug absorption: an UNGAP review. Eur J Pharm Sci 2019;134:153–75.
7. Brunton LL, Hilal-Dandan R, Knollmann BC. Pharmacokinetics: the dynamics of drug absorption, distribution, metabolism, and elimination. In: Brunton LL, Hilal-Dandan R, Knollman BC, editors. Goodman & Gilman's: the pharmacological basis of therapeutics. 13th edition. New York: McGraw-Hill; 2017. p. 1–12.
8. Echaiz TA. Oral dosage forms that should not be crushed 2020. In: Institute for Safe Medication Practices. 2020. Available at: https://www.ismp.org/recommendations/do-not-crush. Accessed January 27, 2021.
9. Price G, Patel DA. Drug bioavailability. In: StatPearls. 2020. Available at: https://www.ncbi.nlm.nih.gov/books/NBK557852/. Accessed November 22, 2020.
10. Elbarbry F. Oral bioavailability in special populations. MOJ Bioequiv Availab 2015;1(3):49–52.
11. Mansoor A, Mahabadi N. Volume of distribution. In: StatPearls. 2020. Available at: https://www.ncbi.nlm.nih.gov/books/NBK545280/. Accessed November 22, 2020.
12. Le J. Drug absorption. In: Merck manual. 2020. Available at: https://www.merckmanuals.com/professional/clinical-pharmacology/pharmacokinetics/overview-of-pharmacokinetics. Accessed November 22, 2020.
13. Patel M, Taskar KS, Zamek-Gliszczynski MJ. Importance of hepatic transporters in clinical disposition of drugs and their metabolites. J Clin Pharmacol 2016;56(Suppl 7):S23–39.
14. Pan G. Roles of hepatic drug transporters in drug disposition and liver toxicity. Adv Exp Med Biol 2019;1141:293–340.
15. Bilbao-Meseguer I, Rodríguez-Gascón A, Barrasa H, et al. Augmented renal clearance in critically ill patients: a systematic review. Clin Pharmacokinet 2018;57(9):1107–21.
16. Spruill WJ, Wade WE, DiPiro JT, et al. Introduction to pharmacokinetics and pharmacodynamics. In: Bloom R, Fogle B, editors. Concepts in clinical pharmacokinetics. 6th edition. Bethesda (MD): ASHP; 2018. p. 1–6.
17. Barrons RW. Drug-induced neuromuscular blockade and myasthenia gravis. Pharmacotherapy 1997;17(6):1220–32.
18. Farinde A. Overview of pharmacodynamics. In: Merck manual. 2020. Available at: https://www.merckmanuals.com/professional/clinical-pharmacology/pharmacodynamics/overview-of-pharmacodynamics. Accessed November 22, 2020.

Drugs of Abuse
Sympathomimetics

Hallie Brown, MD[a], Katherine A. Pollard, MD[a,b],*

KEYWORDS

- Sympathomimetic • Toxidrome • Amphetamine • Methamphetamine • Cathinone
- MDMA • Cocaine

KEY POINTS

- Sympathomimetics are a widely abused drug class with broad clinical implications affecting multiple organ systems.
- The sympathomimetic toxidrome includes tachycardia, hypertension, hyperthermia, and agitation.
- Sympathomimetic overdoses require liberal and aggressive treatment with benzodiazepines.

INTRODUCTION

Sympathomimetic drugs comprise a broad category of plant-based and synthetic substances including illicit and prescribed drugs that have deleterious effects when abused (**Box 1**). The most commonly recognized drugs in this class that often require medical intervention, hospitalization, and critical care are discussed in this article, and clinical implications and treatment approaches are reviewed.

Mechanistically, cocaine, amphetamines, methamphetamines, and cathinones stimulate the sympathetic nervous system (see the section on pathophysiology). The clinical syndromes that result from overstimulation of the sympathetic nervous system carry significant morbidity and require recognition and awareness of appropriate supportive measures to mitigate life-threatening complications. The complications of sympathomimetic overdose affect nearly every organ system (**Table 1**).

BACKGROUND

The use of sympathomimetic and psychoactive stimulant substances has been described for hundreds of years. Although the use of cocaine, derived from the

---

[a] Department of Emergency Medicine, Indiana University School of Medicine, 720 Eskenazi Avenue, Fifth Third Bank Building – Third Floor, Indianapolis, IN 46202, USA; [b] Department of Medicine, Indiana University School of Medicine, Indianapolis, IN, USA
* Corresponding author. Department of Emergency Medicine, Indiana University School of Medicine, 720 Eskenazi Avenue, Fifth Third Bank Building – Third Floor, Indianapolis, IN 46202.
E-mail address: kapollar@iu.edu

Crit Care Clin 37 (2021) 487–499
https://doi.org/10.1016/j.ccc.2021.03.002
0749-0704/21/© 2021 Elsevier Inc. All rights reserved.

criticalcare.theclinics.com

Box 1
Common sympathomimetic drugs

Caffeine

Cathinones
  Butylone
  Mephedrone
  Methedrone
  Methylone

Cocaine
  Free base form ("crack")
  Hydrochloride salt

Ephedrine

Methamphetamine

Methylphenidate

Phentermine

Phenylethylamines
  Amphetamine
  N-methyl-3,4-methylenedioxyamphetamine (MDMA)

Phenylpropanolamine

Pseudoephedrine

Erythroxylon coca plant, was not documented until the nineteenth century, coca leaves were used as early as 1000 BC in native Andean peoples.[1] Although cocaine abuse and intoxication are still prevalent and responsible for a large number of hospitalizations annually, use of amphetamines, methamphetamines, and other synthetic drugs new to the illicit drug market also play a significant role in sympathomimetic intoxication admissions, and require a broad understanding of the sympathomimetic toxidrome.

Amphetamines represent a class of various psychotropic compounds that have been historically abused for their stimulant, euphoric, and hallucinogenic properties. These compounds derive from β-phenylethylamine. Although amphetamines are synthetic drugs, of which amphetamine, methamphetamine, and N-methyl-3,4-methylenedioxyamphetamine (MDMA [ecstasy]) are well-known examples, humans have used natural amphetamines for hundreds of years through the consumption of naturally occurring amphetamines from plants, such as cathinone (khat) from the plant *Catha edulis* and ephedrine from plants in the genus Ephedra. More recently, a new group of amphetamines appeared on the market, comprised of cathinone derivatives and synthetic cathinones (see **Box 1**).[2] "Ecstasy" is a term that was originally applied to tablets containing MDMA. However, over the past decade an increasing number of substances marketed as ecstasy may contain little to no MDMA, but may contain any of its analogues or new psychostimulant substances.[3–5]

EPIDEMIOLOGY

Stimulants, as a drug class, are the second most widely used illicit drugs after cannabis, with more than 68 million past year users globally.[6,7] The annual prevalence of amphetamine use in North America in 2017 was estimated at 2.1%, which is primarily a reflection of use of amphetamines in the United States. The annual prevalence of

Table 1
Complications of sympathomimetic drugs by organ system

Central Nervous System	Cardiovascular	Pulmonary	Gastrointestinal	Renal	Musculoskeletal
Cerebral edema	Acute coronary syndrome	"Crack lung"	Bowel perforation	Acute kidney injury	Rhabdomyolysis
Hyperthermia	Aortic dissection	Pneumonia	Ischemic colitis	Acute renal failure	
Intracranial hemorrhage	Dysrhythmias	Pneumothorax	Mesenteric ischemia	Renal infarct	
Seizures	Hypertensive emergency	Pulmonary edema			
Stroke		Pulmonary hemorrhage			

methamphetamine use has been increasing, and its use has doubled from 2008 to 2017 to 0.6% of the population aged 12 years and older.[8,9] According to the Substance Abuse and Mental Health Services Administration 2018 National Survey on Drug Use and Health, an estimated 5.5 million people used cocaine in the past year, approximately 2.0% of the population.[10]

Overdose deaths attributed to the use of psychostimulants (including methamphetamine) increased in the United States between 2007 and 2017. Within that time period, approximately 85% to 90% of the drug poisoning deaths that were reported under psychostimulants include mention of methamphetamine in the death certificate. Of additional concern is the marked increase in the number of cases involving stimulants and opioids. Overdose deaths attributed to cocaine use have also been increasing; this increase has been largely attributed to deaths involving cocaine and opioids, in particular synthetic opioids.[11]

Out of more than 70,000 deaths from drug overdose in the United States in 2017, nearly 14,000 involved cocaine.[12] Additionally, the opioid epidemic and appearance of fentanyl-laced cocaine have driven a recent increase in the number of cocaine-related deaths; although nonopioid-related cocaine deaths decreased from 1.59 to 0.78 per 100,000 from 2006 to 2015, the rate of death from cocaine-related overdose involving heroin or synthetic opioids, such as fentanyl, has increased from 0.24 to 1.11 per 100,000 from 2010 to 2015.[13,14]

PATHOPHYSIOLOGY

Cocaine and phenylethylamine drugs are snorted, inhaled, injected intravenously or subcutaneously, and ingested orally. The onset of systemic effects depends on routes of exposure (Table 2).[15] Cardiovascular effects of methamphetamine may be detected within 2 minutes and subjective effects within 10 minutes of intravenous administration.[16] Inhalation of methamphetamine reaches peak plasma levels typically 2.5 hours after smoking.[17] Via the nasal route methamphetamine reaches peak plasma concentration after 4 hours.[18] However, peak cardiovascular and subjective effects occur rapidly (within 5–15 minutes). Acute subjective effects diminish over 4 hours, whereas cardiovascular effects tend to remain elevated.[19]

Cocaine has local anesthetic, vasoconstrictive, and sympathomimetic effects; however, the major toxicities of cocaine use result from sympathomimetic effects.[20] Cocaine inhibits the presynaptic reuptake of biogenic amines, such as norepinephrine, dopamine, and serotonin, throughout the body. Systemic effects include tachycardia and hypertension with diffuse vasoconstriction. The central nervous system (CNS) effects are related to excess dopaminergic activity that produces profound euphoria at

Table 2 Routes and onset of common sympathomimetics		
	Drug Route	Onset of Effect
Cocaine	Inhaled	5–10 s
	Intranasal	3–5 min
	Intravenous	10–20 s
	Oral	10–30 min
Methamphetamine	Inhaled	5–10 s
	Intranasal	5–10 s
	Intravenous	2–5 min
	Oral	10–30 min

lower doses and agitation and delirium at higher doses.[21,22] Cocaine also has thrombogenic effects, likely secondary to increases in plasminogen-activator inhibitor activity, platelet count, platelet activation, and platelet aggregation.[23]

Phenylethylamines and their synthetic derivatives also exert stimulant effects by increasing synaptic concentrations of the neurotransmitters norepinephrine, epinephrine, dopamine, and serotonin. This effective increase in neurotransmitter concentration occurs primarily through two mechanisms. First, amphetamines and amphetamine derivatives (including methamphetamine) inhibit monoamine uptake transporters, causing decreased clearance of the neurotransmitters from the neuromuscular synapse and limiting return of neurotransmitters back to the presynaptic neuron. Additionally, they cause release of neurotransmitters from intracellular stores. Increased intracellular release occurs via changes in vesicular pH and inhibition of the vesicular monoamine transport (VMAT2) receptor. VMAT2 is located on the vesicular membrane and is responsible for monoamine uptake into the vesicles for storage.[24,25] As an amphetamine derivative, MDMA not only increases synaptic concentrations of catecholamines, but also causes increased release of serotonin and inhibits its reuptake. Based on similarities in structure, cathinones are thought to have similar mechanisms.[26]

ASSESSMENT

Although history from acutely intoxicated patients is often limited, the sympathomimetic toxidrome is recognized by a constellation of symptoms on presentation (**Box 2**). Patients with sympathomimetic ingestions can have a wide variety of initial presentations ranging from mild agitation to cardiovascular collapse.

Many sympathomimetics may also precipitate hallucinations, psychosis, and seizures, all of which can be seen on initial presentation. Time from ingestion, quantity of substance ingested, and route of ingestion can affect the severity of symptoms present on initial evaluation.

The approach to diagnostic work-up for the acutely intoxicated patient should be broad, with special considerations given to specific clinical manifestations of severe complications (see **Table 1**). Generally, for the undifferentiated intoxicated patient with symptoms of sympathomimetic overdose the following tests are reasonable for initial evaluation: complete blood count, comprehensive metabolic profile, venous blood gas, creatine kinase, electrocardiogram, urinalysis, and urine drug screen. Many commercially available toxicologic drug screens routinely used in the clinical setting do not differentiate among the different sympathomimetics. Although a drug screen may help to confirm an ingestion, the clinical presentation and recognition of a sympathomimetic toxidrome are more useful in the acute setting. Clinicians should also be aware of common over-the-counter and prescribed medications that can cause false-positive results for amphetamines on commercial urine drug screens

Box 2				
Clinical manifestations of sympathomimetic intoxication				
Central Nervous System	**Cardiovascular**	**Pulmonary**	**Renal**	**Other**
Agitation	Tachycardia	Hypoxia	Oliguria	Diaphoresis
Delirium	Hypertension	Tachypnea		Mydriasis
Hyperactivity	Dysrhythmia			
Psychosis				
Hyperthermia				

including bupropion, promethazine, trazodone.[27] Cathinones are not detected on urine toxicology screens.

CLINICAL MANIFESTATIONS AND MANAGEMENT

Clinical features of sympathomimetic overdose affect multiple organ systems, some with devastating and long-lasting complications.

Central Nervous System

Acute sympathomimetic intoxications have multiple CNS manifestations (see **Box 2**) and complications (see **Table 1**). Serotonin syndrome, neuroleptic malignant syndrome, and sympathomimetic overdose have similar toxidromes that are difficult to differentiate (discussed in Evan S. Schwarz's article, "Inhalants," elsewhere in this issue). A history of exposure and review of the patient's medication list is helpful in distinguishing between these conditions. Additionally, the timeline of symptom onset can help differentiate among drug-induced hyperthermic conditions. Neuroleptic malignant syndrome, an idiopathic reaction to dopamine antagonists, is generally defined by a slow onset with symptoms evolving over several days. This is in contrast to the rapid onset of symptoms seen with serotonin syndrome and sympathomimetic overdose. A thorough neuromuscular examination is helpful in differentiating serotonin syndrome and sympathomimetic overdose, because the presence of clonus and hyperreflexia is common in serotonin syndrome and not in sympathomimetic overdoses.[28]

Patients with sympathomimetic intoxication most commonly present with acute agitation that is often severe, and many patients require immediate intervention to limit self-injury. In these patients, the mainstay of treatment is sedation with benzodiazepines. Lorazepam is administered intramuscularly or intravenously, commonly in 2-mg increments until agitation is controlled. Most acute intoxications require repeated dosing. Alternatively, midazolam, 5 mg (intramuscularly or intravenously), is administered.[29] Treatment with antipsychotics, such as haloperidol, is not recommended because of the potential of lowered seizure threshold and prolongation of the QT interval.[30] Seizures are seen in sympathomimetic overdose because of lowered seizure threshold that occurs with acute ingestions. Seizures occur in patients with known seizure disorders and those without who may have a first-time seizure in the setting of a sympathomimetic ingestion.[31] First-line treatment of the actively seizing patient with suspected sympathomimetic overdose is administration of benzodiazepines.

Psychostimulant use, notably cocaine and methamphetamine, raises the risk of acute ischemic and hemorrhagic stroke. This elevated risk is multifactorial and related to acute blood pressure elevation, vasospasm, and thrombogenic platelet effects.[18,32] Chronic cocaine abuse is also associated with accelerated atherosclerosis through repeated endothelial damage, raising stroke risk in chronic users.[33–35] Recent cocaine use has been associated with an increased risk of aneurysmal subarachnoid hemorrhage and higher rates of aneurysm rebleeding, delayed cerebral ischemia, and in-hospital mortality.[14,36–38] Supportive stroke care consistent with management guidelines should be followed in these patients.[39]

Hyperthermia induced by sympathomimetics results from central thermoregulation dysfunction. Heat exposure and increased heat production caused by agitation and motor activity also contribute to the development of hyperthermia.[40] Phenylethylamines activate the hypothalamic-pituitary-thyroid-adrenal axis, with subsequent thermogenesis.[41] Norepinephrine stimulates vascular α_1-adrenoreceptors, causing vasoconstriction and impaired heat dissipation; it also binds to and activates α- and β-adrenoreceptors regulating the activity of thermogenic tissues.[42] Uncontrolled hyperthermia is independently associated with increased morbidity and mortality.[43] Hyperthermia can cause rhabdomyolysis, liver failure, disseminated intravascular coagulation, and multiorgan failure and thus should be treated aggressively.[44,45] Cooling of the hyperthermic patient is accomplished by external or internal means. Regardless of the cooling method used, skin cooling should not be performed too quickly because shivering and vasoconstriction can result, reducing the therapeutic benefit of cooling the hyperthermic patient.[46] In severe cases of hyperthermia with myotonic or hyperkinetic thermogenesis, benzodiazepines or barbiturates may be used for muscle relaxation.[47] Antipyretics do not have a role in hyperthermia therapy in a sympathomimetic intoxication.[33,48,49]

Cardiovascular

Patients with acute sympathomimetic intoxication are at increased risk of multiple cardiovascular complications (see **Table 1**). The hyperadrenergic state stimulates α-adrenoreceptors and β-adrenoreceptors. Cocaine blocks sodium/potassium channels, which induces abnormal, depressed cardiovascular profiles.[50] Dysrhythmias, such as wide complex tachycardias, should be treated with intravenous sodium bicarbonate to overcome the sodium channel blockade.[51] Cocaine and methamphetamine abuse is associated with increased risk of subsequent cardiovascular complications, such as hypertension, coronary spasm, dysrhythmias, myocardial infarction, cardiomyopathy, atherosclerosis, and coronary artery disease (CAD).[16,21,52]

Acute coronary events occur within minutes to hours after cocaine administration. The tachycardia and hypertension induced by cocaine increases myocardial oxygen demand and reduces myocardial oxygen supply by vasoconstriction.[22,53] During acute methamphetamine intoxication, the associated catecholamine surge is associated with longer-term upregulation of the sympathetic axis and myocardial toxicity with impaired cellular metabolism.[54] Electrocardiogram and troponins should be obtained to identify early patterns and markers of cardiac ischemia, and advanced imaging, such as computed tomography angiography, should be considered in the patient with suspected aortic dissection.[55] Patients presenting with cocaine-associated chest pain or acute coronary syndrome (ACS) should be treated similarly to those with traditional ACS as outlined in the American Heart Association guidelines, including aspirin, intravenous nitroglycerin or nitroprusside for uncontrolled hypertension, and cardiology consultation for possible cardiac catheterization and percutaneous coronary intervention when clinical concern for ST-segment elevation myocardial infarction or non–ST-segment elevation myocardial infarction. However, unique to the management of cocaine-associated chest pain and ACS is the early use of intravenous benzodiazepines.[56]

Cocaine induces sympathetic effects on the cardiovascular system by enhanced inotropic and chronotropic effects through increased vasoconstriction. In particular, cocaine induces acute hypertension caused by increased vasoconstriction. Similarly, acute amphetamine toxicity presents with hypertension and tachycardia. In cocaine and phenylethylamine intoxication presenting with significant hypertension, it is important to achieve blockade of α- and β-adrenoreceptors when treating these patients. Otherwise, paradoxic worsening of hypertension may occur because of unopposed α-mediated vasoconstriction.[57] Appropriate first-line antihypertensives include calcium channel blockers (commonly nicardipine), nitrate therapy, and α-antagonists.[15] Data from a 2018 systematic review found that use of β-antagonists in cocaine-related chest pain does not seem to be associated with an increased risk of myocardial infarction or all-cause mortality.[58] If using a β-antagonist, those with partial α-antagonism, such as carvedilol or labetalol, may provide additional benefit for ongoing α-adrenoreceptor suppression. Additionally, in the acute setting of sympathomimetic intoxication, sedation with benzodiazepines should be administered to help decrease overall adrenergic tone.

Patients with long-term methamphetamine use are at risk for CAD. Methamphetamine use is strongly associated with the development of ischemic heart disease and accelerated atherosclerotic CAD.[23,59] Thus, prior history of abuse should be taken into consideration as a risk factor in evaluation of these patients in the acute setting.

Respiratory

Pulmonary complications of sympathomimetic abuse are often related to smoking or snorting of the abused substance (see **Table 1**) and often present with nonspecific dyspnea, cough, or pain. Pulmonary injury has been attributed to increased intrathoracic pressure in relation to vigorous coughing or repeated Valsalva maneuvers, to absorb the maximal amount of drug.[22] Although large and hemodynamically significant pneumothoraces may require tube thoracostomy, smaller pneumothoraces are managed conservatively with supplemental oxygen, serial imaging, and monitoring for progression.[60,61]

In cocaine users, the acute respiratory syndrome of "crack-lung" can consist of fever, hemoptysis, dyspnea, and infiltrate on chest radiographs after free-base cocaine inhalation. This syndrome can also be associated with pulmonary edema, interstitial pneumonia, diffuse alveolar hemorrhage, and eosinophilic infiltration. High temperatures of volatilized cocaine and the presence of impurities and additives, and cocaine-induced local vasoconstriction have been suggested to explain alveolar damage associated with alveolar hemorrhage.[62] Most pulmonary complications associated with sympathomimetic intoxication are treated supportively.

Renal/Metabolic

Acute renal injury from cocaine and phenylethylamine drugs arises from several different mechanisms (see **Table 1**). Acute renal injury associated with cocaine use is caused by vasoconstriction or thrombosis of renal vessels, rhabdomyolysis, severe hypertension, thrombotic microangiopathy, interstitial nephritis, and glomerulonephritis.[52,63] Known adulterants of cocaine, such as levamisole, an antihelminthic agent, have been associated with novel antineutrophil cytoplasmic antibody–associated systemic vasculitis that should also be considered in the work-up for sympathomimetic-related kidney injury.[64] MDMA's toxic effects include hyperthermia, hypotonic hyponatremia, rhabdomyolysis, and cardiovascular collapse.[53] Hyponatremia is a well-reported complication of MDMA use thought to result from several factors including overhydration with water in the setting of drug-induced secretion of vasopressin.[17,65]

Gastrointestinal

Although less common than CNS and cardiovascular complications, cocaine intoxication can cause ischemic injury to the gastrointestinal (GI) tract. Ingested, intravenous, and inhaled cocaine have been associated with bowel ischemia, infarction, and perforation.[52,66–68] Most cases of GI ischemia involve segments of the small bowel, but ischemic colitis can also occur. Gastroduodenal perforations have also been described.[52] Mechanistically, bowel ischemia has been attributed to vasoconstriction and thrombosis of mesenteric vessels.[52] On presentation, patients may present with abdominal pain and/or bloody diarrhea. Peritoneal signs are often present on physical examination. Surgical consultation and preoperative angiography may be helpful to identify occlusion of celiac or mesenteric vessels. Patients may be managed with surgical exploration or nonoperatively with bowel rest and antibiotics.[52]

Musculoskeletal

In the agitated or hyperthermic patient, rhabdomyolysis and acute renal failure should be considered. In the acutely agitated patient, a serum creatine kinase level should be evaluated promptly and should be trended because initial levels may be falsely low in hypovolemic patients. Resuscitation with aggressive intravenous fluids should be initiated even before test results if clinical suspicion is high. The goal in early and aggressive treatment of rhabdomyolysis is to prevent renal tubular damage caused by the nephrotoxic effects of myoglobin and hemoglobin decomposition products by providing aggressive intravenous hydration with crystalloids. Initial boluses of crystalloid (1–2 L or more) should be targeted to achieve hemodynamic stability and a euvolemic state. Continuous infusion of crystalloid is continued at 200 mL/h to 500 mL/h to achieve adequate urine output.[52,69,70] Electrolytes should be monitored frequently to detect abnormalities, especially hyperkalemia. Severe cases of rhabdomyolysis may require early acute dialysis.

OTHER CONSIDERATIONS/POLYSUBSTANCE INGESTIONS

The use of stimulants, including cocaine and methamphetamine, by regular users of opioids is an increasingly common phenomenon. The literature has documented two main combinations: "speedball," in the case of the simultaneous use of cocaine and heroin; and "bombita," in the case of heroin and methamphetamine.[1,71] The clinical presentation varies and may require interventions for opioid overdose (discussed in Cristina Gutierrez and colleagues' article, "Toxicity of Immunotherapeutic Agents," elsewhere in this issue).

The transport, concealment, and routes of ingestion of illicit drugs should also be considered by the clinician caring for patients presenting with acute sympathomimetic toxidromes. The term "body stuffing" refers to drugs that have been consumed rapidly to conceal them. In these cases, individuals are often unsure of how much drug they ingested, or exactly what drugs were in the ingested packages. In these situations, it is also difficult to predict how rapidly the drug will pass through the GI tract or how much will leak from the packaging and be absorbed. The term "body packing" refers to drugs that have been intentionally packaged for ingestion and packaged as such for distribution and smuggling. Both body stuffers and body packers are at risk for a large catecholamine surge given the quantity of drug ingested. Despite this risk, these patients should be managed conservatively with close monitoring and serial imaging. Endoscopic removal should generally not be attempted because of the high risk of rupturing a packet, which could lead to a potentially life-threatening catecholamine surge.[72,73]

CLINICS CARE POINTS

- Individuals with sympathomimetic toxidromes are at risk for significant central nervous system, cardiovascular, and renal complications.
- Aggressive and early use of benzodiazepines for sedation and to diminish adrenergic tone is indicated in acute sympathomimetic overdose.
- Appropriate cooling and mitigation of hyperthermia should be addressed early in the hyperthermic sympathomimetic overdose.

DISCLOSURE

The authors have no financial or commercial conflicts of interest.

REFERENCES

1. Rivera MA, Aufderheide AC, Cartmell LW, et al. Antiquity of coca-leaf chewing in the south central Andes: a 3,000 year archaeological record of coca-leaf chewing from northern Chile. J Psychoactive Drugs 2005;37(4):455–8.
2. Carvalho M, Carmo H, Costa VM, et al. Toxicity of amphetamines: an update. Arch Toxicol 2012;86(8):1167–231, 5.
3. World Drug Report 2017: Market Analysis of Synthetic Drugs–Amphetamine-type Stimulants, New Psychoactive Substances (United Nations publication, Sales No. E.17. XI.10).
4. Favrod-Coune T, Broers B. The health effect of psychostimulants: a literature review. Pharmaceuticals (Basel) 2010;3(7):2333–61.
5. EMCDDA. Recent changes in Europe's MDMA/ecstasy market: Results from an EMCDDA Trendspotter Study, EMCDDA rapid Communication Series. Luxembourg: Publications Office of the European Union; 2016.
6. World Drug Report 2019 (United Nations publication, Sales No. E.19.XI.8).
7. McKetin R, Lubman DI, Baker AL, et al. Dose-related psychotic symptoms in chronic methamphetamine users: evidence from a prospective longitudinal study. JAMA Psychiatry 2013;70(3):319–24.
8. United States, Center for Behavioral Health Statistics and Quality. Results from the 2017 National Survey on drug use and Health: detailed Tables. Rockville (MD): SAMHSA; 2018.
9. Ben-Yehuda O, Siecke N. Crystal methamphetamine: a drug and cardiovascular epidemic. JACC Heart Fail 2018;6:219–21.
10. SAMHSA, Center for Behavioral Health Statistics and Quality, Results from the 2017 National Survey on Drug Use and Health: Detailed Tables (Rockville, Maryland, 2018).
11. DEA, 2018 National Drug Threat Assessment.
12. Kariisa M, Scholl L, Wilson N, et al. Drug overdose deaths involving cocaine and psychostimulants with abuse potential—United States, 2003-2017. MMWR Morb Mortal Wkly Rep 2019;68(17):388–95.
13. McCall Jones C, Baldwin GT, Compton WM. Recent increases in cocaine-related overdose deaths and the role of opioids. Am J Public Health 2017;107(3):430–2.
14. Caplan RA, Zuflacht JP, Barash JA, et al. Neurotoxicology syndromes associated with drugs of abuse. Neurol Clin 2020;38(4):983–96.
15. Greene SL, Kerr F, Braitberg G. Review article: amphetamines and related drugs of abuse. Emerg Med Australas 2008;20(5):391–402.
16. Mendelson J, Jones RT, Upton R, et al. Methamphetamine and ethanol interactions in humans. Clin Pharmacol Ther 1995;57(5):559–68.
17. Perez-Reyes M, White WR, McDonald SA, et al. Clinical effects of daily methamphetamine administration. Clin Neuropharmacol 1991;14(4):352–8.
18. Hart CL, Gunderson EW, Perez A, et al. Acute physiological and behavioral effects of intranasal methamphetamine in humans. Neuropsychopharmacology 2008;33(8):1847–55.
19. Cruickshank CC, Dyer KR. A review of the clinical pharmacology of methamphetamine. Addiction 2009;104(7):1085–99.
20. Goldstein RA, DesLauriers C, Burda AM. Cocaine: history, social implications, and toxicity: a review. Dis Mon 2009;55(1):6–38.

21. Kaye S, McKetin R, Duflou J, et al. Methamphetamine and cardiovascular pathology: a review of the evidence. Addiction 2007;102(8):1204–11.
22. Davies O, Ajayeoba O, Kurian D. Coronary artery spasm: an often overlooked diagnosis. Niger Med J 2014;55(4):356–8.
23. Heesch CM, Wilhelm CR, Ristich J, et al. Cocaine activates platelets and increases the formation of circulating platelet containing microaggregates in humans. Heart 2000;83(6):688–95.
24. Cozzi NV, Sievert MK, Shulgin AT, et al. Inhibition of plasma membrane monoamine transporters by beta-ketoamphetamines. Eur J Pharmacol 1999;381(1):63–9.
25. Torres GE, Gainetdinov RR, Caron MG. Plasma membrane monoamine transporters: structure, regulation and function. Nat Rev Neurosci 2003;4(1):13–25.
26. Schifano F, Albanese A, Fergus S, et al. Mephedrone (4-methylmethcathinone; 'meow meow'): chemical, pharmacological and clinical issues. Psychopharmacology (Berl) 2011;214(3):593–602.
27. Saitman A, Park HD, Fitzgerald RL. False-positive interferences of common urine drug screen immunoassays: a review. J Anal Toxicol 2014;38(7):387–96.
28. Boyer EW, Shannon M. The serotonin syndrome. N Engl J Med 2005;352(11):1112–20 [published correction appears in N Engl J Med. 2007;356(23):2437] [published correction appears in N Engl J Med. 2009 Oct 22;361(17):1714].
29. Nobay F, Simon BC, Levitt MA, et al. A prospective, double-blind, randomized trial of midazolam versus haloperidol versus lorazepam in the chemical restraint of violent and severely agitated patients. Acad Emerg Med 2004;11(7):744–9.
30. Connors NJ, Alsakha A, Larocque A, et al. Antipsychotics for the treatment of sympathomimetic toxicity: a systematic review. Am J Emerg Med 2019;37(10):1880–90.
31. Sanchez-Ramos J. Neurologic complications of psychomotor stimulant abuse. Int Rev Neurobiol 2015;120:131–60.
32. Kaufman MJ, Levin JM, Ross MH, et al. Cocaine-induced cerebral vasoconstriction detected in humans with magnetic resonance angiography. JAMA 1998;279(5):376–80.
33. Bachi K, Mani V, Jeyachandran D, et al. Vascular disease in cocaine addiction. Atherosclerosis 2017;262:154–62. 9.
34. Sordo L, Indave BI, Barrio G, et al. Cocaine use and risk of stroke: a systematic review. Drug Alcohol Depend 2014;142:1–13.
35. Kim ST, Park T. Acute and chronic effects of cocaine on cardiovascular health. Int J Mol Sci 2019;20(3):584.
36. Chang TR, Kowalski RG, Caserta F, et al. Impact of acute cocaine use on aneurysmal subarachnoid hemorrhage. Stroke 2013;44(7):1825–9.
37. Swor DE, Maas MB, Walia SS, et al. Clinical characteristics and outcomes of methamphetamine-associated intracerebral hemorrhage. Neurology 2019;93(1):e1–7.
38. Vosoughi R, Schmidt BJ. Multifocal leukoencephalopathy in cocaine users: a report of two cases and review of the literature. BMC Neurol 2015;15:208.
39. Hemphill JC 3rd, Greenberg SM, Anderson CS, et al. Guidelines for the management of spontaneous intracerebral hemorrhage: a guideline for healthcare professionals from the American Heart Association/American Stroke Association. Stroke 2015;46(7):2032–60.
40. Marzuk PM, Tardiff K, Leon AC, et al. Ambient temperature and mortality from unintentional cocaine overdose. JAMA 1998;279(22):1795–800.

41. Fernandez F, Aguerre S, Mormède P, et al. Influences of the corticotropic axis and sympathetic activity on neurochemical consequences of 3,4-methylenedioxyme-thamphetamine (MDMA) administration in Fischer 344 rats. Eur J Neurosci 2002; 16(4):607–18.

42. Zhao J, Cannon B, Nedergaard J. alpha1-Adrenergic stimulation potentiates the thermogenic action of beta3-adrenoreceptor-generated cAMP in brown fat cells. J Biol Chem 1997;272(52):32847–56.

43. Gowing LR, Henry-Edwards SM, Irvine RJ, et al. The health effects of ecstasy: a literature review. Drug Alcohol Rev 2002;21(1):53–63.

44. Henry JA, Jeffreys KJ, Dawling S. Toxicity and deaths from 3,4-methylenedioxy-methamphetamine ("ecstasy"). Lancet 1992;340(8816):384–7.

45. Hadad E, Rav-Acha M, Heled Y, et al. Heat stroke: a review of cooling methods. Sports Med 2004;34(8):501–11.

46. Matsumoto RR, Seminerio MJ, Turner RC, et al. Methamphetamine-induced toxicity: an updated review on issues related to hyperthermia. Pharmacol Ther 2014;144(1):28–40.

47. Chan TC, Evans SD, Clark RF. Drug-induced hyperthermia. Crit Care Clin 1997; 13(4):785–808.

48. Bernheim HA, Block LH, Atkins E. Fever: pathogenesis, pathophysiology, and purpose. Ann Intern Med 1979;91(2):261–70.

49. Eyer F, Zilker T. Bench-to-bedside review: mechanisms and management of hy-perthermia due to toxicity. Crit Care 2007;11(6):236.

50. Schwartz BG, Rezkalla S, Kloner RA. Cardiovascular effects of cocaine. Circula-tion 2010;122(24):2558–69.

51. Bauman JL, DiDomenico RJ. Cocaine-induced channelopathies: emerging evi-dence on the multiple mechanisms of sudden death. J Cardiovasc Pharmacol Ther 2002;7(3):195–202.

52. Rezkalla SH, Kloner RA. Cocaine-induced acute myocardial infarction. Clin Med Res 2007;5(3):172–6.

53. Pennings EJ, Leccese AP, Wolff FA. Effects of concurrent use of alcohol and cocaine. Addiction 2002;97(7):773–83.

54. Paratz ED, Cunningham NJ, MacIsaac AI. The cardiac complications of metham-phetamines. Heart Lung Circ 2016;25(4):325–32.

55. Kevil CG, Goeders NE, Woolard MD, et al. Methamphetamine use and cardiovas-cular disease. Arterioscler Thromb Vasc Biol 2019;39(9):1739–46.

56. McCord J, Jneid H, Hollander JE, et al. Management of cocaine-associated chest pain and myocardial infarction: a scientific statement from the American Heart Association Acute Cardiac Care Committee of the Council on Clinical Cardiology. Circulation 2008;117(14):1897–907.

57. Lange RA, Cigarroa RG, Flores ED, et al. Potentiation of cocaine-induced coro-nary vasoconstriction by beta-adrenergic blockade. Ann Intern Med 1990; 112(12):897–903.

58. Pham D, Addison D, Kayani W, et al. Outcomes of beta blocker use in cocaine-associated chest pain: a meta-analysis. Emerg Med J 2018;35(9):559–63.

59. Lappin JM, Darke S, Farrell M. Stroke and methamphetamine use in young adults: a review. J Neurol Neurosurg Psychiatry 2017;88(12):1079–91.

60. Zimmerman JL. Cocaine intoxication. Crit Care Clin 2012;28(4):517–26.

61. Perper JA, Van Thiel DH. Respiratory complications of cocaine abuse. Recent Dev Alcohol 1992;10:363–77.

62. Mégarbane B, Chevillard L. The large spectrum of pulmonary complications following illicit drug use: features and mechanisms. Chem Biol Interact 2013; 206(3):444–51.

63. Nzerue CM, Hewan-Lowe K, Riley LJ Jr. Cocaine and the kidney: a synthesis of pathophysiologic and clinical perspectives. Am J Kidney Dis 2000;35(5):783–95.

64. Pendergraft WF 3rd, Herlitz LC, Thornley-Brown D, et al. Nephrotoxic effects of common and emerging drugs of abuse. Clin J Am Soc Nephrol 2014;9(11): 1996–2005 [published correction appears in Clin J Am Soc Nephrol. 2019 Apr 5;14(4):586].

65. Baggott MJ, Garrison KJ, Coyle JR, et al. MDMA Impairs Response to Water Intake in Healthy Volunteers. Adv Pharmacol Sci 2016.

66. Muñiz AE, Evans T. Acute gastrointestinal manifestations associated with use of crack. Am J Emerg Med 2001;19(1):61–3.

67. Linder JD, Mönkemüller KE, Raijman I, et al. Cocaine-associated ischemic colitis. South Med J 2000;93(9):909–13.

68. Feliciano DV, Ojukwu JC, Rozycki GS, et al. The epidemic of cocaine-related juxtapyloric perforations: with a comment on the importance of testing for *Helicobacter pylori*. Ann Surg 1999;229(6):801–6.

69. Richards JR. Rhabdomyolysis and drugs of abuse. J Emerg Med 2000; 19(1):51–6.

70. Bosch X, Poch E, Grau JM. Rhabdomyolysis and acute kidney injury. N Engl J Med 2009;361(1):62–72 [published correction appears in N Engl J Med. 2011 May 19;364(20):1982].

71. Leri F, Bruneau J, Stewart J. Understanding polydrug use: review of heroin and cocaine co-use. Addiction 2003;98(1):7–22.

72. Webb WA. Management of foreign bodies of the upper gastrointestinal tract: update. Gastrointest Endosc 1995;41(1):39–51.

73. Fung BM, Sweetser S, Wong K, et al. Foreign object ingestion and esophageal food impaction: an update and review on endoscopic management. World J Gastrointest Endosc 2019;11(3):174–92.

Drugs of Abuse—Opioids, Sedatives, Hypnotics

Keith Azevedo, MD[a],*, Molly Johnson, MD[b], Michael Wassermann, MD[b], Jessica Evans-Wall, MD[b]

KEYWORDS

• Opioids • Benzodiazepines • Sedatives • Hypnotics • Overdose

KEY POINTS

- Acute opioid overdose primarily manifests with respiratory depression and hypercapnic respiratory acidosis.
- Acute benzodiazepine overdose can often be associated with other agents, namely opiates and alcohol, and can result in respiratory depression, hypotension, and altered mental status.
- The mainstay of therapy for sedative-hypnotic overdoses, both benzodiazepine and non-benzodiazepine classes, is primarily supportive treatment with serial evaluations of respiratory and neurologic status.

INTRODUCTION

Opioids, sedatives, and hypnotics are commonly prescribed and abused medications.[1] In the 2018 Annual Report of the American Association of Poison Control Center's National Poison Data System, both opioids and sedative hypnotics are in the top 5 drug classes most frequently involved in all human exposures. Of these agents, sedatives, hypnotics, and antipsychotics were associated with the most life-threatening outcomes.[2] As a result, the management of unintentional intoxication, intentional overdose, and withdrawal is increasingly relevant for critical care clinicians.

Opioids

History
"If the entire materia medica at our disposal were limited to the choice and use of only one drug, I am sure that a great many, if not the majority, of us would choose opium"—Macht, 1915.[3]

[a] Departments of Emergency and Internal Medicine, University of New Mexico Hospital, MSC11 6025, 1 University of New Mexico, Albuquerque, NM 87131, USA; [b] Department of Emergency Medicine, University of New Mexico Health Sciences Center, MSC11 6025, 1 University of New Mexico, Albuquerque, NM 87131, USA
* Corresponding author.
E-mail address: kazevedo@salud.unm.edu

Crit Care Clin 37 (2021) 501–516
https://doi.org/10.1016/j.ccc.2021.03.003
0749-0704/21/© 2021 Elsevier Inc. All rights reserved.
criticalcare.theclinics.com

The use and misuse of opium-derived substances span 6 millennia of human history. It has been a constant throughout wars, famines, peace, revolutions, colonization, and globalization. The first documented references to opium are from a Sumerian tablet circa 4500 BC and in the ninth century BC in Homer's *The Odyssey*, in which opium is referred to as a drug "to lull all pain and bring forgetfulness of every sorrow."[4] In 371 BC the Greek philosopher and botanist Theophrastus stated that the effects of the poppy were "both blessedly beneficial and occasionally lethal."[5] By the eighth century AD, opium was traded in India and China, and by the thirteenth century, opium had spread throughout Europe. In 1624, the English physician Thomas Sydenham published *Observationes Medicae,* a medical textbook used for over a century, wherein he praised the use of opium in the tincture form of laudanum, a mix of alcohol and powdered opium for the treatment of a myriad of illnesses. As US trade with China and the Middle East intensified during the nineteenth century, opium became widely available to the public. Laudanum was even advertised as the "poor child's nursemaid."[6] With such widespread use, there was concern about the lack of a consistent formula for dosing. In hopes of regulating dosing for safety, a French physician in 1804 isolated morphine and named it for the Greek god of sleep, Morpheus.[4] Frequent accidental overdoses persisted, however, due to minimal regulation and continued dosing inconsistencies.

Because chemists refined the alkaloids of opium and these products remained readily available and inexpensive, death and addiction continued. In 1898, the German company Bayer introduced heroin, named for its ability to make the user feel like a hero. It was not until 1961 that an antagonist, naloxone, was patented.[5]

In recent years, opioid overdose deaths have been increasing. According to the CDC, between October 2018 and October 2019, greater than 47,000 deaths were directly attributed to opioid overdose. Of these, 71% were due to synthetic opioid overdose. Although natural opioid overdose deaths remain stable, synthetic compounds, excluding methadone, represent an increasing percentage of the overall annual deaths.[7] These data demonstrate a need to both more effectively prevent and treat patients experiencing an overdose.

Pharmacology

Papaver somniferum, the opium poppy, is endemic to Turkey and grows well in warm, dry climates. Afghanistan and Mexico are currently the largest producers of opium.[8] Compounds are either opiates, derived from the poppy plant, or opioids that are altered into semisynthetic or fully synthetic compounds.[9] The classification of opioid subtypes is provided in **Table 1**.[10]

Table 1 Classification of opioid types		
Synthetic Opioids	**Semisynthetic Opioids**	**Natural Opioids**
Fentanyl	Oxycodone	Morphine
Carfentanyl	Hydromorphone	Codeine
Acetylfentanyl		
Furanylfentanyl		
Methadone		
Tramadol		
Tapentadol		

There are 3 main opioid receptors: mu-opioid receptor (MOR), delta opioid receptor (DOR), and kappa opioid receptor (KOR). All 3 receptor types are G protein–coupled receptors and are distributed primarily in the central nervous system (CNS), blocking ascending pain signals. However, these receptors are also present in the heart and gastrointestinal tract and have an effect on the immune system.[11,12] Endogenous opioid compounds are known to affect sensations of pain and mood, mostly through the MOR pathway, and exogenous opioid compounds target the same receptors, producing the effects of euphoria and analgesia.[12,13] These same receptors also seem to mediate the addictive nature of opioids.[14] Activating the KOR results in the cessation of pain but can also cause dysphoria. The DOR is thought to play a role in chronic pain.[11] Because these receptors become upregulated with exogenous opioid use, the lack of stimulation can lead to an increase in nociception, making the addictive properties not only the seeking of euphoria but also an escape from pain. **Table 2** outlines the pharmacologic properties of various opioids and opiates.

Clinical presentation and diagnosis of overdose

Because of the mechanism of action of CNS depression, particularly the MOR in the pons, the most severe presentation of opioid overdose is apnea. In more mild overdoses, the respiratory rate is slowed and tidal volumes are often decreased, with reduced response to hypercapnia. Overdose patients seem somnolent, with slowed respirations and miosis. Blood pressure may be lower than baseline with reduction in sympathetic signals. Heart rate may be increased in the setting of hypoxia from reduced minute ventilation.[12,15,16] If numerous agents are ingested, the classic toxidrome may not be present, such as miosis. With prolonged respiratory depression there can be a concomitant decrease in the arterial oxygen partial pressure (Pa_{O_2}), which can result in hypoxia if supplemental oxygen is not administered in a timely fashion.[16] If hypoxia progresses, acute cardiac arrest can occur, as tissue oxygenation becomes increasingly unavailable to meet cellular and metabolic demand.

Management of overdose

Naloxone, a nonselective MOR antagonist, is used to reverse respiratory depression in overdose.[17] Because it nonselectively binds to the MOR receptors, naloxone can precipitate withdrawal while decreasing respiratory depression. The removal of the opioid agonists from their receptors can also cause hyperalgesia, diarrhea, diaphoresis, and dysphoria. Administration of naloxone can occur via intramuscular, intravenous (IV), or intranasal routes. Emergency Medical Services (EMS) providers and general public have access to 2 mg intranasal kits with preloaded syringes and atomizer. Standard IV dosing is 0.4 to 2 mg, with doses being repeated every 2 to 3 minutes as needed. Although it is often impossible to know what was ingested, it may take higher doses of naloxone to reverse synthetic compounds. If a patient is known to be opioid dependent, it may be prudent to start with a lower initial dose (0.1–0.2 mg) and titrate to respiratory effect, so as not to precipitate full withdrawal.[17] Goal in administration is to reverse respiratory depression and not full arousal. In rare cases, pulmonary edema can occur with naloxone administration. Causality research is ongoing to determine if this is due to a higher naloxone dosage. A recent EMS-based study showed an increased risk of pulmonary edema in out-of-hospital administration of naloxone greater than 0.4 mg.[17] The half-life of naloxone is 30 minutes, and most opioids have a longer half-life (see **Table 2**); therefore, naloxone may require repeat dosing or continuous infusion. One-half of the initial dose to resolve respiratory depression can be used as a starting hourly dose for infusion.[17] Patients who have experienced

Table 2
Comparison of opioid and opiate properties

Substance	Mechanism of Action	Time to Plasma Peak	Half-Life	Toxicologic Effects	Elimination	Unique Property
Oxycodone	Full agonist of the mu receptor	1 h	4 h	Central nervous system (CNS) depression	Metabolized in liver, excreted in urine	Half-life increases by 2.5 h if liver impairment
Morphine	Full agonist of the mu receptor	Oral: 1 h IV: 20 m	3 h	CNS depression	Hepatic via conjugation with glucuronic acid, excreted in urine	Numerous metabolic compounds
Heroin	Full agonist of the mu receptor	IV: 5 min	2–6 min	CNS depression	Hepatic via glucuronidation, excreted in urine, metabolized to morphine and 6- acetyl morphine	Prodrug with short half-life; metabolites have longer half life
Hydromorphone	Full agonist of the mu receptor	Oral: 30–60 m IV: 10–20 m	2–3 h	CNS depression	Hepatic via glucuronidation, excreted in urine	Cough suppression via direct action on medulla
Fentanyl	Full agonist of the mu receptor	IM: 7 m IV: immediate	2 h	CNS depression	Hepatic via glucuronidation, excreted in urine	Quick on, quick off
Buprenorphine	Partial agonist of the mu receptor	Sublingual film: 2–3 h	24–42 h	Nausea, constipation, precipitated withdrawal	Hepatic metabolism based on hepatic blood flow	Highest affinity for mu receptor
Methadone	Full agonist of the mu receptor	Oral: 1–7.5 h	8–59 h	CNS depression	Hepatic via glucuronidation, excreted in urine	Prolongs QT Variable and long half-life
Loperamide	Agonist of mu receptor in gut	Oral: 5 h	9–13 h	Antidiarrheal	Hepatic oxidative N-demethylation	Prolongs QT, cardiac dysrhythmias, torsades
Tramadol	Agonist of mu receptors in the CNS	Oral: 2 h, 12 h ER	~6 h IR, ~10 h ER	CNS depression, seizures	Metabolized in liver, excreted in urine	Acts on serotonergic and noradrenergic nociception, whereas its metabolite O-desmethyltramadol acts on the μ-opioid receptor

Tapentadol	Agonist of the mu receptor, norepinephrine reuptake inhibitor	Oral: ~ 1.25 h, ~6 h ER	~4 h IR, ~6 h ER	CNS depression, seizures	Metabolized in liver, excreted in urine	Unlike tramadol, no known active metabolites

Abbreviations: IM, intramuscular; IV, intravenous; IR, immediate release; ER, extended release.

a positive response to naloxone but require repeated bolus doses (up to 10–20 mg) may benefit from a continuous infusion.[17] If respiratory depression is not adequately addressed by naloxone, more invasive means of airway security, such as intubation, need to be considered.

Summary

Given the widespread use of opioids, overdoses are common. The prompt management of overdoses both in the prehospital and intrahospital setting can be lifesaving. As with all recreational drugs, it is helpful to assume that coingestion with other pharmacologic agents is present, keeping in mind that some formulations also contain acetaminophen. The presence of cardiac dysrhythmias suggests overdose with methadone or loperamide, which is often not regarded as a drug of abuse (see **Table 2**). Overall patient management in opioid overdoses should focus on respiratory status with continuous clinical, pulse oximetry, and arterial or end tidal CO 2 monitoring. In addition, because many opiate and opioid compounds have longer half-lives than naloxone, continuous reassessment is imperative and redosing of naloxone may be necessary. Following an overdose, a chest radiograph may demonstrate pulmonary edema, and more advanced airway management, with either noninvasive or invasive ventilation, may be necessary.

Sedative-Hypnotics

Sedatives are inherently designed to calm and mitigate agitation, whereas hypnotics are intended to initiate, sustain, or lengthen sleep. These medications can be broadly classified into benzodiazepines and nonbenzodiazepines. Although benzodiazepine and nonbenzodiazepine sedative-hypnotics share similar benefits, side effects, and risks, nonbenzodiazepine sedative-hypnotics have a chemical structure that is fundamentally dissimilar to benzodiazepines. Specifically, the molecular structure of benzodiazepines is defined by the fusion of a benzene ring and a diazepine ring, hence their name. Because of the extensive number of agents comprising sedatives and hypnotics, the two following sections review benzodiazepines/barbiturates and nonbenzodiazepines.

Benzodiazepines/Barbiturates

History

Since the advent of chlordiazepoxide in the 1960s, the formulation, manufacture, and distribution of various benzodiazepines have exploded. What began as an accidental drug discovery by Leo Sternbach, the Austrian chemist credited with the successful synthesis of chlordiazepoxide, quickly paved the way for the modification and synthesis of additional compounds, including diazepam, flurazepam, nitrazepam, flunitrazepam, clonazepam, and trimethaphan.[18,19] Through the 1960s, chlordiazepoxide remained the most globally prescribed medication until it was replaced by diazepam in 1969.[18] Although diazepam is no longer the world's leading prescription medication, benzodiazepine use is still ubiquitous. A review of the top 200 prescription medications in the United States in 2019 revealed that both alprazolam and clonazepam occupy spots in the top 50 most prescribed medications, with alprazolam occupying position 21 and clonazepam at 34.[20]

Barbiturates are similar in structure and function to benzodiazepines (namely through potentiating the effects of the γ-aminobutyric acid type A [GABA$_A$] receptor) and were first synthesized in the mid-nineteenth century by Johan Adolf Baeyer.[21] Although barbiturates existed for almost 100 years before benzodiazepines, their frequency of use decreased over the past 2 centuries, primarily due to their decreased safety profile when used as a single agent.[22]

Pharmacology

The principal mechanism of action of benzodiazepines and barbiturates is by binding to their respective sites on the alpha subunit of the $GABA_A$ receptor, a ligand-gated chloride channel. In the presence of $GABA_A$, both benzodiazepines and barbiturates potentiate the effect of its binding. The binding of $GABA_A$ to the ligand-gated chloride channel receptor causes a depolarization of the cell membrane. In the presence of benzodiazepine binding, the frequency of chloride channel opening increases, contrasted with barbiturate binding, which results in prolonged duration of chloride channel opening (depolarization) and prolonged inhibition of new action potential generation.[23] The significant mortality associated with regular use and intentional/unintentional overdose of barbiturates is due in large part to the prolonged duration of channel opening and extended refractory period of the cell membrane.[22] Given that most of the benzodiazepines and barbiturates rely on the metabolism of active metabolites through the hepatic cytochrome P450 pathway (CYP3A4 and CYP2C19), individuals with significant liver disease or individuals taking substances that inhibit these pathways are prone to increased toxicity.

Clinical presentation of overdose

Over the last 60 years, outpatient benzodiazepine use continues to be widespread, particularly in the United States. As of 2015, approximately 1 in 20 adults in the United States filled a benzodiazepine prescription during a 1-year period. Furthermore, benzodiazepines' overall use increased with advancing age.[24] A possible reason for the popularity of outpatient benzodiazepine use to treat short-term anxiety, seizures, and withdrawal is the demonstrated safety profile of benzodiazepines, especially when compared with barbiturates. When benzodiazepines are misused, they are rarely misused independently. More commonly, benzodiazepines are considered a "secondary drug of abuse," one taken in order to enhance the effects of other substances.[25] Recent literature suggests that approximately 80% of benzodiazepine abuse coincides with abuse of multiple medications, with opioids being the most common coagent of abuse.[26–29]

Current literature still supports the claim that benzodiazepines, when used alone, have a favorable safety profile, causing relatively mild respiratory depression by predominantly affecting postsynaptic CNS $GABA_A$ receptors. When overdose does occur, the principal symptoms include a range of neurologic impairments including, but not limited to, altered mentation, slurred speech, ataxia, dizziness, impaired thought processes, and overall impairment of cognitive function.[30] Diagnosing an acute benzodiazepine overdose warrants a high index of clinical suspicion. A thorough history and physical examination are of paramount importance in aiding diagnosis, as routine urine drug screening can be less beneficial. Although urine drug screens can provide potential insight into an exposure, these tests should not be relied on, given the propensity of false-positive/false-negative results.[31]

If benzodiazepines are coingested with other substances, acute overdose symptoms are more life-threatening. A patient presenting with prolonged coma, significant respiratory depression, and/or hypotension in the setting of known benzodiazepine use should be assumed to have coingested additional CNS depressants, such as alcohol, opioids, certain antidepressants, neuroleptics, and anticonvulsants, all of which decrease the safety profile of benzodiazepines and are responsible for increased morbidity and mortality.[32,33] In addition, continuous infusions of lorazepam and diazepam have been associated with severe metabolic acidosis due to propylene glycol, which is used as a diluent (see Jennifer A. Ross and colleagues' article, "Toxic Alcohols," in this issue). Typically seen with inpatient treatment of severe alcohol withdrawal, lorazepam and diazepam infusions set at a rate of greater than 1 mg/kg per day may result in severe lactic acidosis, nephrotoxicity, and hyperosmolar states.[34]

Management of overdose and withdrawal

Given the increase of overdose deaths related to benzodiazepines in combination with other substances, clinicians must consider that respiratory depression, hypotension, and coma associated with a suspected acute benzodiazepine intoxication are likely related to polysubstance ingestion. The mainstay of management in an overdose, either alone or in combination with other drugs, is primarily supportive treatment. Although flumazenil can be used as a benzodiazepine antagonist, the duration of its effects is variable and predisposes the acutely intoxicated patient to rebound toxicity once flumazenil has been metabolized.[30] The routine use of flumazenil in benzodiazepine overdose is not recommended, as most instances of intoxication resulting in decreased mental status are associated with coingestion. Flumazenil administration, in the context of undifferentiated coingestions with decreased mental status, can increase seizure risk due to possible ingestion of seizure-potentiating substances, particularly tricyclic antidepressants.[35,36] In addition, flumazenil has been associated with increased cerebral perfusion pressure and is contraindicated in patients with an acute head injury.[37]

In addition to the adverse events associated with benzodiazepine overdose, acute withdrawal symptoms, namely CNS hyperactivity, remain a major area of concern and should be suspected in any patient who abruptly discontinues benzodiazepines after long-term use (typically defined between 6–12 months). Aside from withdrawal symptoms such as anxiety, agitation, and autonomic hyperactivity, the gravest concern is the risk of seizures, as abrupt discontinuation of benzodiazepines effectively unmasks the downregulated state of $GABA_A$ receptors.[32] The time frame for which benzodiazepine withdrawal can occur is largely contingent on whether the patient is taking short-acting or long-acting agents, as defined by their elimination half-life (**Table 3**). Cessation of short-acting benzodiazepines results in withdrawal symptoms within 2 to 3 days and 5 to 10 days for long-acting substances.[30] The mainstay of treatment of acute withdrawal is readministration of the benzodiazepine that was discontinued with the notable exception that alprazolam withdrawal should be treated with clonazepam, which has shown increased efficacy compared with other long-acting benzodiazepines.[38]

Summary

Benzodiazepines and barbiturates have a long history of use and abuse in the twentieth century. Although barbiturates are associated with cardiopulmonary collapse when ingested as a single agent, benzodiazepines are safer due to their limited effect on respiratory depression when used alone. Both benzodiazepines and barbiturates achieve sedative, anxiolytic, and hypnotic effects by binding to the $GABA_A$ receptor. Acute overdose as a single agent is associated with overall impaired cognitive function, slurred speech, and incoordination, whereas overdose combined with other CNS depressants, such as alcohol or opioids, can manifest with life-threatening CNS depression and cardiopulmonary collapse.

Nonbenzodiazepines

In contrast to benzodiazepines, nonbenzodiazepine sedative-hypnotics have a chemical structure inherently dissimilar to benzodiazepines, lacking a benzene or diazepine

Table 3
Drug profiles for commercially available benzodiazepines in the United States[30]

Drug	Time to Peak Effect	Half-life Elimination (h)	Duration of Action (h)	Metabolism of Active Metabolite	Elimination of Inactive Metabolites
Alprazolam	1–2 h	6–12	4–7	CYP3A4	Urine
Midazolam	IV 1–2 min IM 10–15 min PO 0.5–1 h	3–6	IV 2 IM 4–6 PO 4–6	CYP3A4	Urine
Oxazepam	0.3–0.5 h	5–10	3–6	UGT2B15 UGT1A9 UGT2B7	Urine
Triazolam	0.25–0.5 h	2–5	6–7	CYP3A4	Urine
Estazolam	1 h	10–24	<12	CYP3A4	Urine
Lorazepam	IV 5–20 min IM 20–30 min PO 0.5–1 h	9–16	6–8	UGT2B15	Urine
Temazepam	1.5 h	9–12	5–20	CYP3A4 CYP2C19 UGT2B15 UGT2B7	Urine
Chlordiazepoxide	2 h	5–30	5–30	CYP3A4	Urine
Clonazepam	0.3–0.5 h	20–80	<12	CYP3A4	Urine
Clorazepate	1–2 h	48	8–24	CYP3A4 CYP2C19	Urine
Diazepam	IV 1–5 min PO 15–45 min PR 5–45 min	20–50	IV 0.25–1 PO 12–24	CYP3A4 CYP2C19	Urine
Flurazepam	0.5–1 h	2	12	CYP3A4	Urine
Quazepam	0.5–2 h	27–41	12–24	CYP3A4 CYP2C9 CYP2C19	Urine

ring. The benefits, side effects, and risks of these drugs share common characteristics with benzodiazepines. Most nonbenzodiazepine sedative-hypnotics have been designed to treat anxiety and insomnia or to provide sedation.[39] The following sections focus on the more common nonbenzodiazepines that the clinician is likely to encounter in the case of acute toxicity.

History

As a class, nonbenzodiazepine sedative-hypnotics have a vast and complex history in clinical practice. Although all of the substances listed in **Table 4** are still available today, their use and popularity throughout time remains varied. Chloral hydrate, for example, was first discovered in 1832 and is the oldest sedative-hypnotic still available today.[51,52] The remaining substances listed in **Table 4** were synthesized over the course of the mid-to-late twentieth century with a variety of safety profiles. For example, meprobamate, previously sold under the name "Miltown" as an homage to Miltown, New Jersey, was once a common household name, but the abuse profile and synergistic effects with other GABA$_A$ agonists led to strict regulation and decreased frequency of prescription use.[53,54] Nonbenzodiazepine sedative-hypnotics, much as their benzodiazepine counterparts, are rarely dangerous when

Table 4
Nonbenzodiazepine sedative-hypnotics[40–50]

Drug	Mechanism of Action	Time to Peak	Elimination	Half-Life	Toxicologic Effects
Buspirone	Unknown but it has a high affinity for serotonin 5-HT2 receptors and moderate affinity for dopamine D2 receptors, no effect on GABA receptors	40–90 min	Hepatic oxidation; CYP3A4; active metabolite 1-pyrimidinylpiperazine; urine and feces excretion	2–3 h	Sedation, seizures, serotonin syndrome
Carisoprodol	Unknown, central depressant, anxiolytic, sedative	1.5–2 h	Hepatic via CYP2C19; active metabolite meprobamate; urine excretion	2 h	Sedation, coma, cardiovascular collapse, pulmonary edema, myoclonic jerks
Chloral hydrate	CNS depressant unknown mechanism	Onset in 15–30 min Lasts 1–2 h	Hepatic via alcohol dehydrogenase to trichloroethanol, which is an active metabolite eventually metabolized by glucuronidation in the liver; urine excretion	8–12 h	Coma, cardiac instability, ventricular dysrhythmias, sensitivity to catecholamines, GI upset, hemorrhagic gastritis
GHB (sodium oxybate; precursors: γ-butyrolactone and 1,4-butanediol)	GABA$_b$ agonist; GHB-specific receptor agonist	30–60 min	GHB dehydrogenase converts GHB to succinic acid semialdehyde, which is converted to succinic acid and enters Krebs cycle; succinic acid semialdehyde can also be converted to gamma-aminobutyric acid, which is an inhibitory neurotransmitter	20–60 min	Amnesia, sedation, seizure, coma, cardiac and respiratory depression, steep dose-response curve, sudden awakening

Melatonin	Acts on melatonin (MT) receptors 1 and 2 to regulate circadian rhythm	30–60 min	Hepatic via CYP1A2	40–50 min	Sedation, disoriented
Meprobamate	Unknown, central depressant, anxiolytic, sedative	1.5–2 h	Hepatic via CYP2C19; active metabolite meprobamate; urine excretion	10 h	Sedation, coma, cardiovascular collapse, gastric bezoar with prolonged coma
Ramelteon	MT-1 and MT-2 receptor agonist	45 min	Hepatic via CYP1A2, CYP2C and CYP3A4; forms active metabolite (M-II), urine excretion	1–2.6 h	Sedation
Tasimelteon	MT-1 and MT-2 receptor agonist	0.5–3 h	Hepatic via CYP1A2, CYP3A4, urine excretion	1.3 h	Headache
Zaleplon	Acts on α1 benzodiazepine sites on the GABA$_A$ receptor, lacks activity at α2 and peripheral α3	0.7–1.4 h	Hepatic via aldehyde oxidase or CYP3A4, mostly urine and some feces excretion	0.9–1.2 h	Sedation, dyscoordination, headache
Zolpidem	benzodiazepine sites (less muscle relaxation and anticonvulsant activity)	1–2 h	Hepatic via CYP3A4, CYP2C9, CYP1A2, CYP2D6, and CYP2C19, urine and feces excretion	1.4–4.5 h	Sedation, coma, vomiting
Zopiclone		1.5–2 h	Hepatic via CYP3A4 and CYP2C8, mostly urine and some feces excretion	5–6 h	Sedation, methemoglobinemia, hemolytic anemia

taken alone and at the prescribed dose, but their potential for abuse cannot be overstated. To illustrate this point, γ-hydroxybutyrate (GHB) was created as an adjunct during surgery by providing the opportunity to induce reversible coma with a rapid onset of action. It now occupies a space in popular culture as a "club drug," recreationally abused due to its euphoric and hypnotic effects, specifically when coingested with other agents that potentiate its sedative effects, such as ethanol.[55–57]

Pharmacology
Although each medication in this class has a slightly different mechanism of action, the result is modulation of neurotransmitters via dopamine receptors, $GABA_A$ receptors, serotonin receptors, or melatonin receptors with the resulting effect of CNS depression. However, the mechanism of action is not clear for many of these drugs, and therefore, specific mechanisms are described in greater detail in **Table 4**.

Clinical presentation of an overdose
In the event of an overdose, a thorough history and physical examination are crucial, in addition to maintaining a high index of clinical suspicion for an acute toxicologic exposure to nonbenzodiazepine sedative hypnotics, as these substances are not routinely detected on urine toxicology immunoassays. Because CNS depression is a common effect of nonbenzodiazepine sedative-hypnotics in overdose, excessive sedation is common. The primary effects of an acute buspirone overdose are an overall increase in sedation, whereas a few case reports have noted that seizures are a possible, albeit rare, side effect.[58] Given buspirone's effect on the serotonin 1A receptor, there is a theoretic risk of serotonin syndrome, especially when combined with other serotonergic agents.[59] In an acute overdose of carisoprodol and meprobamate symptoms including sedation, coma, cardiovascular collapse, and in rare cases, pulmonary edema and myoclonic jerks have been noted.[60,61] Overdoses with chloral hydrate often occur with coingestion of ethanol, and the overall toxicologic effects include coma, cardiac instability (including ventricular dysrhythmias), decreased cardiac contractility, sensitivity to catecholamines, gastrointestinal issues, and hemorrhagic gastritis.[51] The toxicologic effects of GHB, sodium oxybate, γ-butyrolactone, and 1,4-butanediol include CNS depression, euphoria, seizures, anterograde amnesia, and hypothermia. As discussed with previous medications, effects are amplified with coingestion of other CNS depressants.

Management of overdose
There are no reversal agents for nonbenzodiazepine sedative-hypnotics, and the mainstay of treatment in an acute overdose is primarily aimed at supportive measures while the drug is metabolized. These measures include monitoring the patient's overall hemodynamics, respiratory status, and avoiding drugs that further potentiate the $GABA_A$ receptors, namely benzodiazepines. Several agents within this class deserve further information on management. In a buspirone overdose, close monitoring for the development of seizures or serotonin syndrome is crucial. In the event that generalized tonic-clonic seizures do occur, treatment is aimed at seizure termination with the use of benzodiazepines.[62] Chloral hydrate ingestion management should focus on monitoring respiratory status and hemodynamics. When ventricular dysrhythmias occur, beta-blockers are the preferred first-line agent.[63,64] In a GHB intoxication, patients often spontaneously awaken once excessive levels are metabolized, negating the need for advanced airway management in most of the patients.[65]

Summary
Nonbenzodiazepine sedatives and hypnotics are varied in their structure, function, and potential for abuse. Similar to their benzodiazepine counterparts, nonbenzodiazepines demonstrate the danger of combining multiple agents with other sedative-hypnotics (benzodiazepines, barbiturates), ethanol, and opiates. The mainstay of therapy for sedative-hypnotic overdoses, both benzodiazepine and nonbenzodiazepine classes, is primarily supportive treatment with serial evaluations of respiratory and neurologic status.

OVERALL SUMMARY

Over the course of the last decade, prescription and nonprescription substance use has increased significantly.[1] There are multiple clinical considerations that clinicians must keep in mind when evaluating a potential toxicologic exposure; specifically, the fact that coingestion of multiple drug agents remains a major concern when managing acute intoxication. Policy initiatives aimed at curtailing misuse of these drugs still remain in the relatively early stages of deployment.

In the interim, the critical care clinician should remain vigilant to the toxicologic effects and maintain a high index of suspicion for coingestions. Opioid overdose can be recognized by respiratory depression. It is treated with naloxone titrated to respiratory effect, supportive care, and continuous monitoring. Benzodiazepines, although relatively safe agents when used alone, have the potential for abuse in conjunction with other sedatives, opioids, and hypnotics. This potential cannot be understated. Treatment of benzodiazepine overdose should focus on frequently evaluating the patient's respiratory status with a low threshold for intervention if respiratory decompensation occurs. In the case of nonbenzodiazepine sedative-hypnotics, supportive treatment measures remain the mainstay of managing accidental and nonaccidental exposures.

CLINICS CARE POINTS

- Acute opioid intoxication classically presents with respiratory depression, hypercapnic respiratory acidosis, and miosis.

- An acute opioid overdose is initially treated with naloxone. Standard IV dosing is 0.4 to 2 mg, with doses being repeated every 2 to 3 minutes, as needed. If a patient is known to be opioid-dependent, it may be prudent to start with a lower initial dose (0.1–0.2 mg) and titrate to respiratory effect.

- Sedative-hypnotic intoxication, both benzodiazepine and nonbenzodiazepine classes, presents with altered mentation, slurred speech, ataxia, dizziness, and impaired thought processes.

- The mainstay of therapy for sedative-hypnotic overdoses, both benzodiazepine and nonbenzodiazepine classes, are primarily supportive treatment with serial evaluations of respiratory and neurologic status.

- A high index of clinical suspicion for coingestions must be maintained in the critically ill patient with a suspected toxicologic exposure to either opioids, benzodiazepines, barbiturates, and/or nonbenzodiazepine sedative hypnotics.

DISCLOSURE

The authors declare that they have no relevant commercial, material, or financial interests that relate to the research described in this article.

REFERENCES

1. McHugh RK, Nielsen S, Weiss RD. Prescription drug abuse: from epidemiology to public policy. J Subst Abuse Treat 2015;48:1–7.
2. Gummin DD, Mowry JB, Spyker DA, et al. 2018 annual report of the American association of poison control Centers' National poison data system (NPDS): 36th annual report. Clin Toxicol 2019;57(12):1220–413.
3. Macht D. The history of opium and some of its Preparations and alkaloids. JAMA 1915;LXIV(6):477–81.
4. Gussow L. Toxicology rounds: opium, from ancient sumeria to Paracelsus to kerouac. Emerg Med News 2013;35(4):25.
5. Jones MR, Viswanath O, Peck J, et al. A brief history of the opioid epidemic and strategies for pain medicine. Pain Ther 2018;7(1):13–21.
6. Brownstein MJ. A brief history of opiates, opioid peptides, and opioid receptors. Proc Natl Acad Sci U S A 1993;90(12):5391–3.
7. Wilson N, Kariisa M, Seth P, et al. Drug and opioid-involved overdose deaths - United States, 2017-2018. MMWR Morb Mortal Wkly Rep 2020;69:290–7.
8. International heroin Market. Office of National drug control policy. The Whitehouse President Barak Obama. Available at: https://obamawhitehouse.archives.gov/ondcp/global-heroin-market. Accessed May 6, 2020.
9. Berkowitz BA. The relationship of pharmacokinetics to pharmacological activity: morphine, methadone and naloxone. Clin Pharmacokinet 1976;1(3):219–30.
10. Manuals M. Global medical knowledge 2020. Kenilworth \ (NJ): Merck Manuals; 2016. Available at: http://www.merckmanuals.com/professional/resourcespages/global-medical-knowledge-2020. Accessed December 27, 2020.
11. Pathan H, Williams J. Basic opioid pharmacology: an update. Br J Pain 2012; 6(1):11–6.
12. Valentino RJ, Volkow ND. Untangling the complexity of opioid receptor function. Neuropsychopharmacology 2018;43(13):2514–20.
13. Darcq E, Kieffer BL. Opioid receptors: drivers to addiction? Nat Rev Neurosci 2018;19(8):499–514.
14. Matthes HW, Maldonado R, Simonin F, et al. Loss of morphine-induced analgesia, reward effect and withdrawal symptoms in mice lacking the mu-opioid-receptor gene. Nature 1996;383(6603):819–23.
15. Boom M, Niesters M, Sarton E, et al. Non-analgesic effects of opioids: opioid-induced respiratory depression. Curr Pharm Des 2012;18(37):5994–6004.
16. Sibbald WJ, Fink MP, Messmer KF. Tissue oxygenation in acute medicine (Update in intensive care medicine, jean Louis Vincent, series editor). New York: Springer; 2002.
17. Farkas A, Lynch MJ, Westover R, et al. Pulmonary complications of opioid overdose treated with naloxone. Ann Emerg Med 2020;75(1):39–48.
18. Stossel S. My age of anxiety, fear, hope, dread, and the search for peace of mind. New York: Vintage Books; 2015. p. 193–4.
19. Wick JY. The history of benzodiazepines. Consult Pharm 2013;28(9):538–48.
20. Kane SP. ClinCalc DrugStats Database, Version 20.0. ClinCalc. 2019. Available at: https://clincalc.com/DrugStats. Accessed December 2020.
21. Cozanitis DA. One hundred years of barbiturates and their saint. J R Soc Med 2004;97(12):594–8.
22. Gresham C, LoVecchio F. Barbiturates. In: Tintinalli J, editor. Emergency medicine: a comprehensive study Guide. 9th edition. New York City: McGraw Hill; 2020. p. 1214–5.

23. Hoffman R, Nelson L, Howland M. Antidotes in Depth: benzodiazepines. In: Nelson L, editor. Goldfrank's toxicologic Emergencies. 9th edition. New York City: McGraw Hill; 2011. p. 1109–14.
24. Olfson M, King M, Schoenbaum M. Benzodiazepine use in the United States. JAMA Psychiatry 2015;72(2):136–42.
25. O'Brien CP. Benzodiazepine use, abuse, and dependence. J Clin Psychiatry 2005;66(Suppl 2):28–33.
26. Jones JD, Mogali S, Comer SD. Polydrug abuse: a review of opioid and benzodiazepine combination use. Drug Alcohol Depend 2012;125(1–2):8–18.
27. Jones CM, Mack KA, Paulozzi LJ. Pharmaceutical overdose deaths, United States, 2010. JAMA 2013;309(7):657–9.
28. Gold MS, Miller NS, Stennie K, et al. Epidemiology of benzodiazepine use and dependence. Psychiatr Ann 1995;25:146–8.
29. Jones CM, McAninch JK. Emergency department visits and overdose deaths from combined use of opioids and benzodiazepines. Am J Prev Med 2015; 49(4):493–501.
30. Quan D. Benzodiazepines. In: Tintinalli J, editor. Emergency medicine: a comprehensive study Guide. 9th edition. New York City: McGraw Hill; 2020. p. 1214–5.
31. Algren DA, Christian MR. Buyer beware: Pitfalls in toxicology Laboratory testing. Mo Med 2015;112(3):206–10.
32. Longo LP, Johnson B. Addiction: Part I: benzodiazepines-side effects, abuse risk and alternatives. Am Fam Physician 2000;61(7):2121–8.
33. Soumerai SB, Simoni-Wastila L, Singer C, et al. Lack of relationship between long-term use of benzodiazepines and escalation to high dosages. Psychiatr Serv 2003;54(7):1006–11.
34. Wilson KC, Reardon C, Theodore AC, et al. Propylene glycol toxicity: a severe iatrogenic illness in ICU patients receiving IV benzodiazepines: a case series and pro- spective, observational pilot study. Chest 2005;128:1674.
35. Penninga EI, Graudal N, Ladekarl MB, et al. Adverse events associated with flumazenil treatment for the management of suspected benzodiazepine intoxication: a systematic review with meta-analyses of randomised trials. Basic Clin Pharmacol Toxicol 2016;118:37.
36. Kreshak AA, Cantrell FL, Clark RF, et al. A poison center's ten-year experi- ence with flumazenil administration to acutely poisoned adults. J Emerg Med 2012; 43:677.
37. Hoffman EJ, Warren EW. Flumazenil: a benzodiazepine antagonist. Clin Pharm 1993;12(9):641–56.
38. Ait-Daoud N, Hamby AS, Sharma S, et al. A review of alprazolam use, misuse, and withdrawal. J Addict Med 2018;12:4–10.
39. Richey SM, Krystal AD. Pharmacological advances in the treatment of insomnia. Curr Pharm Des 2011;17:1471.
40. Lexicomp online, carisoprodol. Hudson (OH): UpToDate, Inc.; 2020.
41. Lexicomp online, chloral hydrate. Hudson (OH): UpToDate, Inc.; 2020.
42. Fuhrman B, Zimmerman J, editors. Pediatric critical care. 4th edition. Philadelphia, PA: Elsevier Health; 2011.
43. Lexicomp online, Gamma Hydroxybuytric acid and related compounds. Hudson (OH): UpToDate, Inc.; 2020.
44. Mortezaee K, Khanlarkhani N. Melatonin application in targeting oxidative-induced liver injuries: a review. J Cell Physiol 2018;233(5):4015–32.
45. Andersen LP, Werner MU, Rosenkilde MM, et al. Pharmacokinetics of oral and intravenous melatonin in healthy volunteers. BMC Pharmacol Toxicol 2016;17:8.

46. Lexicomp online, Ramelteon. Hudson (OH): UpToDate, Inc.; 2020.
47. Lexicomp online, Tasimelteon. Hudson (OH): UpToDate, Inc.; 2020.
48. Lexicomp online, Zolpidem. Hudson (OH): UpToDate, Inc.; 2020.
49. Lexicomp online, Zaleplon. Hudson (OH): UpToDate, Inc.; 2020.
50. Lexicomp online, Zopiclone. Hudson (OH): UpToDate, Inc.; 2020.
51. LoVecchio F. Nonbenzodiazepine sedatives. In: Tintinalli J, editor. Emergency medicine: a comprehensive study Guide. 9th edition. New York City: McGraw Hill; 2020. p. 1219–22.
52. Butler TC. The introduction of chloral hydrate into medical Practice. Bull Hist Med 1970;44(2):168–72.
53. CBC Radio. (August 07, 2017)."Miltown: a game-changing drug you've probably never heard of". Retrieved June 12, 2020.
54. Kumar M, Dillon GH, March. Assessment of direct gating and allosteric modulatory effects of meprobamate in recombinant GABA$_A$ receptors. Eur J Pharmacol 2016;775:149–58.
55. Smith KM, Larive LL, Romanelli F. Club drugs: methylenedioxymethamphetamine, flunitrazepam, ketamine hydrochloride, and gamma-hydroxybutyrate. Am J Health Syst Pharm 2002;59:1067–76.
56. Brennan R, Van Hout MC. Gamma-hydroxybutyrate (GHB): a scoping review of pharmacology, toxicology, motives for use, and user groups. J Psychoactive Drugs 2010;46:243–51.
57. O'Connell T, Kaye L, Plosay JJ. 3d Gamma-hydroxybutyrate (GHB): a newer drug of abuse. Am Fam Physician 2000;62:2478–83.
58. Lexicomp online, buspirone. Hudson (OH): UpToDate, Inc; 2020.
59. Boyer EW, Shannon M. The serotonin syndrome. N Engl J Med 2005;352:1112 [Erratum in: N Engl J Med 356: 2437, 2007].
60. Reeves RR, Burke RS, Kose S. Carisoprodol: update on abuse potential and legal status. South Med J 2012;105:619–23.
61. HØiseth G, SØrlid HK, Bramness J. Acute intoxications with carisoprodol. Clin Toxicol (Phila) 2008;46:307.
62. Catalano G, Catalano MC, Hanley PF. Seizures associated with buspirone overdose: case report and literature review. Clin Neuropharmacol 1998;21:347–50.
63. Laurent Y, Wallemacq P, Haufroid V, et al. Electrocardiographic changes with segmental akinesia after chloral hydrate overdose. J Emerg Med 2006;30:179–82.
64. Zahedi A, Grant MH, Wong DT. Successful treatment of chloral hydrate cardiac toxicity with propranolol. Am J Emerg Med 1999;17:490–1.
65. Chin RL, Sporer KA, Cullison B, et al. Clinical course of gamma-hydroxybutyrate overdose. Ann Emerg Med 1998;31:716–22.

Toxicology of Psychoactive Substances

Lara Prisco, MD, MSc, AFRCA, AFFICM[a,b],*, Aarti Sarwal, MD, FNCS, FCCM[c],
Mario Ganau, MD, PhD, MBA, FRCS(Ed), FEBNS[d],
Francesca Rubulotta, MD, PhD, MBA, FRCA, FFICM[e,f]

KEYWORDS

- Psychoactive substances • Antidepressants • Selective serotonin reuptake inhibitors
- antipsychotics • Mood stabilizers • Hallucinogens

KEY POINTS

- Monitoring agencies have reported a significant increase in the introduction, production, and nonmedical use of new psychoactive substances paralleled by increasing use of long-time available psychoactive drugs (PADs) from licit channels as well as illegal manufacturers.
- With increasing antidepressant and antipsychotic use, intensive care providers need to be cognizant of cardiac and neurologic toxicity of these drugs and be able to differentiate the anticholinergic syndrome, serotonin syndrome, tyramine crisis, and neuroleptic malignant syndrome.
- A high index of suspicion with careful attention to history taking is emphasized, given emerging synthetic cannabinoids and new psychoactive substances that may not be detected on conventional drug screens. Mixed ingestions are not infrequent.
- Reducing exposure and supportive care are the cornerstones of management of toxic ingestions of most PADs. Benzodiazepines are the drug of choice for delirium and seizures related to most PADs.
- Extracorporeal treatments (hemodialysis and hemoperfusion) are possible options for hyperammonemia associated with valproic acid toxicity and lithium poisoning.

[a] Neurosciences Intensive Care Unit, Oxford University Hospitals NHS Foundation Trust, John Radcliffe Hospital, Level 1 West Wing, Headley Way, Oxford OX3 9DU, UK; [b] Nuffield Department of Clinical Neurosciences, University of Oxford, John Radcliffe Hospital, Level 6 West Wing, Headley Way, Oxford OX3 9DU, UK; [c] Neurocritical Care Unit, Wake Forest Baptist Medical Center, Medical Center Boulevard, Winston Salem, NC 27157, USA; [d] Neurosciences Department, Oxford University Hospitals NHS Foundation Trust, John Radcliffe Hospital, Level 2 West Wing, Headley Way, Oxford OX3 9DU, UK; [e] Critical Care Program Department of Anesthesia, McGill University, 845 Sherbrooke St W, Montreal, Quebec H3A 0G4, Canada; [f] Department of Anesthesiology and Intensive Care Medicine, Health Centre, Intensive Care Unit, Imperial College NHS Trust, Charing Cross Hospital, Fulham Palace Road, London W6 8RF, UK
* Corresponding author. Neurosciences Intensive Care Unit, Oxford University Hospitals NHS Foundation Trust, John Radcliffe Hospital, Level 1 West Wing, Headley Way, Oxford OX3 9DU, UK.
E-mail address: Lara.prisco@ouh.nhs.uk

Crit Care Clin 37 (2021) 517–541
https://doi.org/10.1016/j.ccc.2021.03.013
0749-0704/21/© 2021 Elsevier Inc. All rights reserved.
criticalcare.theclinics.com

Table 1
Neurotransmitter pathways, major systemic effects, and interfering substances (mimics and blockers)

Neurotransmitter	Effects	Substances
Norepinephrine	↑ Heart rate ↑ Euphoria ↑ Alertness and responsiveness ↑ Pain threshold	Mimics: amphetamines, cocaine, TCAs, SNRIs, MAOIs, LSD, pseudoephedrine, pyridostigmine Blockers: propranolol, clonidine, phentolamine, lithium
Dopamine	↑ Euphoria ↑ Alertness and responsiveness ↓ Hunger	Mimics: amphetamines, cocaine, MAOIs, ergolines Blockers: antipsychotics, tetrabenazine, lithium
Serotonin (5-HT)	↑ Euphoria ↑ Happiness ↑ Pain threshold	Mimics: amphetamines, cocaine, LSD, psychedelics, SSRIs, SNRIs, TCAs, MAOIs, lithium Blockers: AAs, ondansetron
Acetylcholine	↓ Heart rate ↑ Sweat, salivation ↑ Enhanced memory ↑ Muscle tone/contraction	Mimics: nicotine, muscarine, physostigmine, pilocarpine Blockers: benzodiazepines, scopolamine, benztropine, TCAs, AAs
Glutamate	↑ Enhanced learning and memory ↑ Diffuse neuronal depolarization (seizures)	Mimics: none Blockers: phencyclidine, ketamine, dextromethorphan,
γ-aminobutyric acid	↑ Drowsiness ↓ Anxiety ↓ Alertness and responsiveness ↓ Memory ↓ Muscle tone/contraction	Mimics: alcohol, barbiturates, benzodiazepines, GHB, muscimol, lithium Blocker: flumazenil
Cannabinoids	↑ Hunger ↓ Nausea and vomiting ↓ Cognition and memory ↓ Neuroinflammation ↑ Pain threshold	Mimics: tetrahydrocannabinol (marijuana, hashish), nabilone Blocker: rimonabant
Histamine	↑ Alertness and responsiveness ↑ Gastric acid production ↑ Pruritis ↓ Hunger	Mimics: opiates, betahistine Blockers: TCAs, AAs, ranitidine

INTRODUCTION

Health care providers increasingly need to be aware of toxic effects of prescribed and illicit psychoactive drugs (PADs).[1–4] This article reviews the epidemiology, pharmacology, adverse effects, and management of toxicity related to PADs. The neurotransmitter pathways, major systemic effects, and interfering substances (mimics and blockers) for the known licit and illicit PADs are listed in **Table 1**.

EPIDEMIOLOGY OF PSYCHOACTIVE SUBSTANCES

Although typically seen as a disease of the young, the proportion of older adults using PADs and seeking treatment of a PAD-related condition is increasing.[5] Data on gender-based differences in the use of PADs support an increasing prevalence of use in women of all ages, and women seem to be the fastest growing population of substance abusers in the United States.[6-9] Women are more likely to seek treatment of misuse of central nervous system (CNS) depressants.[10,11] Young people in high-income countries tend to use club drugs, such as ecstasy, methamphetamine, cocaine, ketamine, lysergic acid diethylamide (LSD), and γ-hydroxybutyrate (GHB), for recreational experiences, whereas those living in poverty tend to choose PADs for their low price, availability, and ability to rapidly induce a sense of euphoria, such as inhalants (eg, paint thinner, gasoline, paint, correction fluid, and glue).[12]

ANTIDEPRESSANTS

Antidepressants were the drugs prescribed most frequently to young patients (18–44 years) between 2005 and 2008 in the United States and were the third most pre-scribed drugs among patients of all ages.[13] The American Association of Poison Con-trol Centers reported antidepressants to be among the top 5 substances involved in human exposures in 2019, with a 3.9% increase per year in cases with serious out-comes over the past 10 years.[14]

Tricyclic Antidepressants

Pharmacology and use
Newer antidepressants have replaced tricyclic antidepressants (TCAs) in manage-ment of depression, limiting their use to treatment of depression refractory to newer agents. Despite this, there is an increase in TCA overdose–associated hospitalization and lethality, predominantly in patients with chronic pain and neuropsychiatric disor-ders, because of the narrow therapeutic index.[15] The pharmacology of TCAs is shown in **Table 2**.[16,17]

Toxicity
TCA intoxication can be rapidly fatal, with life-threatening dysrhythmias and death occurring within 24 hours of ingestion. The rapid absorption in the gastrointestinal (GI) tract is promoted by alkaline conditions of the small intestine. The ingestion of 10 mg/kg to 20 mg/kg is potentially life-threatening with onset of initial symptoms in 30 minutes to 40 minutes and signs of toxicity becoming clinically apparent within 2 hours.[18] History of coingestion with other medications like acetaminophen, aspirin, and alcohol is frequent and may confound the clinical presentation. Mixed overdose causing delayed gastric emptying may delay onset of symptoms. Initial signs and symptoms are attribut-able to the anticholinergic effects of TCAs: dry mouth, blurred vision, urinary retention, constipation, decreased or absent bowel sounds, dizziness, and vomiting. Plasma con-centrations of TCAs greater than 450 ng/mL can lead to agitation, confusion, memory impairment, and anxiety. Toxicity and death are reported at plasma levels of 2000 ng/mL to 3000 ng/mL with most TCAs; dothiepin levels as low as 1000 ng/mL can be fatal.[19] The most severe cases may present with CNS depression with reduced level of consciousness, hypoventilation, coma, and seizures.[20] Cardiac effects include con-duction abnormalities with prolonged QRS, QT, and PR intervals that can lead to ven-tricular tachycardia, torsades de pointes, and ventricular fibrillation. Hypotension results from a combination of reduced myocardial contractility and reduced systemic vascular resistance due to α-adrenergic blockade.[21] TCA toxicity is worsened by acid-emia, hypotension, hypoxia, and hyperthermia.

Management
Treatment of TCA overdose depends on the severity of symptoms. It is important to assess for evidence of anticholinergic syndrome (**Table 3**), cardiac toxicity, and

Table 2
Antidepressant drugs

Class	Drugs	Mechanism of Action	Medical Use	Pharmacology
TCAs	Dibenzazepines (imipramine, desipramine, clomipramine, trimipramine, lofepramine), dibenzocycloheptadienes (amitriptyline, nortriptyline, protriptyline, butriptyline), dibenzoxepins (doxepin), dibenzothiepines (dosulepin), dibenzoxazepines (amoxapine)	• Norepinephrine reuptake inhibitors • Serotonin reuptake inhibitors • Acetylcholine receptor antagonist (muscarinic) • H1 histamine receptor antagonists	Depressive disorder (refractory to SSRI, SNRI, MAOI), migraine prophylaxis, neuralgic pain, obsessive-compulsive disorder, nocturnal enuresis (children only)	Time to onset of signs of toxicity: 30–40 min for initial symptoms; signs of toxicity clinically apparent within 2 h Half-life: average elimination $t_{1/2}$ ~1 d (up to 3 d for protriptyline) Metabolism: substantial presystemic first-pass metabolism, large volume of distribution, extensive protein binding, metabolized by hepatic cytochrome P450 oxidative enzymes
MAOIs	Isocarboxazid, phenelzine, tranylcypromine, selegiline	• MAOIs	Panic disorder with agoraphobia, depression or anxiety disorders, bulimia, posttraumatic stress disorder, borderline personality disorder, obsessive-compulsive disorder, bipolar depression, Parkinson disease (selegiline), migraine prophylaxis, dysthymia complicated by panic disorder or hysterical dysphoria	Time to onset of signs of toxicity: symptoms slowly apparent within first 24–48 h Half-life: irreversible MAOIs are rapidly absorbed and quickly eliminated, with plasma elimination $t_{1/2}$ 1.5–4 h Metabolism: because of irreversible inhibition of MAO, the physiologic effects of phenelzine, isocarboxazid, and tranylcypromine persist for up to 2–3 wk

| SSRI | Citalopram, escitalopram, fluvoxamine, paroxetine, sertraline | • Serotonin reuptake inhibitors | Depression, panic attacks and panic disorders, anxiety, agoraphobia | Time to onset of signs of toxicity: 1–2 wk
Half-life: elimination half-life is approximately 24 h
Metabolism: good oral absorption, highly protein bound, large volume of distribution (12–97 L/kg), hepatic metabolism to water soluble and less active metabolites |
| SNRI | Atomoxetine, duloxetine, venlafaxine, desvenlafaxine | • Norepinephrine reuptake inhibitors
• Serotonin reuptake inhibitors | Generalized anxiety disorders, social anxiety disorder, panic disorder, agoraphobia | Time to onset of signs of toxicity: 3–6 wk
Half-life: 5–11 h (depending on metabolites half-life)
Metabolism: good oral absorption, large volume of distribution, metabolites might need long time to eliminate |

neurologic toxicity to guide proper management while addressing immediate resuscitation needs.[22] Activated charcoal adsorbs the drug in the GI tract and, therefore, is most effective if given within 1 hour to 2 hours of TCA ingestion. Other decontamination methods (gastric lavage, whole-bowel irrigation, or ipecac-induced emesis) are not recommended.

TCAs are protein-bound and become free in acidic conditions. Increasing arterial or venous pH to greater than or equal to 7.45 significantly reduces available free drug and may ameliorate toxicity. An intravenous sodium bicarbonate (SB) bolus of 1 mEq/kg to 2 mEq/kg followed by infusion using 150 mEq/L diluted in a 5% dextrose solution titrated to blood pH and QRS is recommended in cases of metabolic acidosis along with mild hyperventilation until the QRS falls below 100 milliseconds. The sodium load in SB solutions also helps reverse the sodium channel blocking effects of TCAs and is the treatment of choice to prevent seizures and dysrhythmias. SB should be given in all cases of metabolic acidosis, QRS prolongation (even in the absence of metabolic acidosis), malignant dysrhythmias, hypotension, and cardiac arrest due to TCAs.[23] Hypertonic saline or lipid emulsion can be used in patients not responding to standard therapies.[24]

Continuous cardiac monitoring is essential in TCA overdose, and lidocaine may be used for dysrhythmias if SB load fails with caution to avoid precipitating seizures.[25] Magnesium has been recommended as well given its antiarrhythmic and antiepileptic properties.[26] Class 1a and class 1c agents should not be administered due to sodium channel effects.

Benzodiazepines and propofol are treatments of choice for sedation and treatment of seizures due to TCA -induced central γ-aminobutyric acid (GABA)-A receptor inhibition. Phenytoin should be avoided due to its sodium channel effect. Lacosamide is avoided due to cardiac side effects.

Selective Serotonin Reuptake Inhibitors, Serotonin-Norepinephrine Reuptake Inhibitors, and Monoamine Oxidase Inhibitors

Pharmacology and use

Selective serotonin reuptake inhibitors (SSRIs), serotonin-norepinephrine reuptake inhibitors (SNRIs), and monoamine oxidase inhibitors (MAOIs) are the major agents used in outpatient treatment of depression.[27] Antidepressant use increased from 10.6% to 13.8% between 2009 to 2010 and 2017 to 2018.[28] During 2015% to 2018%, 13.2% of adults in the United States used antidepressants in the past 30 days, with higher use in women and older age groups, and more than 50,000 overdose cases were reported in 2016 with 102 fatalities.[29] Clinical indications, mechanism of action, and pharmacology of SSRIs, SNRIs, and MAOIs are described in **Table 2**.

Toxicity

SSRIs are the first-line antidepressants prescribed most frequently due to decreased toxicity compared with MAOIs and TCAs. The most common toxicity of SSRIs manifests in autonomic instability leading in severe cases to serotonin syndrome (see **Table 3**).[30] Toxicity is enhanced when SSRIs are coingested with other drugs with serotonergic effects. The prognosis generally is favorable, and long-term sequelae rarely are observed in single-agent overdose.

Among the SSRIs, citalopram is associated with the greatest risk of cardiotoxicity (QTc prolongation) and neurotoxicity (seizures); the most frequent symptoms of toxicity are drowsiness, tachycardia, QTc prolongation, decreased level of consciousness, coma, and seizures.[31] Citalopram (>600 mg) and escitalopram (>300 mg) both cause dose-dependent QT prolongation with high risk of torsades de pointes.[32]

Table 3
Comparison of the clinical features of serotonin syndrome, anticholinergic syndrome, neuroleptic malignant syndrome, and malignant hyperthermia

Condition	Serotonin Syndrome	Anticholinergic Syndrome	Neuroleptic Malignant Syndrome	Malignant Hyperthermia
Exposure	Serotonergics (antidepressants, fentanyl, tramadol, linezolid, sumatriptan, ondansetron)	Anticholinergics	Antipsychotics (dopamine antagonists) and dopamine withdrawal	Inhalational anesthetics, depolarizing muscle blockers (succinylcholine)
Onset after exposure	<12 h (25% of cases can develop symptoms after 24 h)	<12 h	24–72 h	0.5–24 h
Resolution after treatment initiation	Within 24 h	Hours to days	Up to 10 d	24–48 h
Temperature	Hyperthermia (>41.1°C)	Hyperthermia (<38.8°C)	Hyperthermia (>41.1°C)	Hyperthermia (up to 46°C)
Cardiorespiratory signs	Hypertension, tachycardia, tachypnea	Hypertension (mild), tachycardia, tachypnea	Hypertension, tachycardia, tachypnea	Hypertension, tachycardia, tachypnea
Pupils	Dilated	Dilated	Normal	Normal
Neuromuscular signs	Neuromuscular hyperactivity, increased tone (lower limbs > upper limbs), tremor, myoclonus	Normal muscle tone	Neuromuscular hypoactivity, diffuse rigidity (lead pipe–like), bradykinesia	Rigor mortis–like rigidity
Reflexes	Hyperreflexia, clonus	Normal	Bradyreflexia	Hyporeflexia
Mental status	Agitation, delirium, coma	hypervigilance, agitation, delirium, hallucinations, mumbling speech, coma	Stupor, mutism, coma	Agitation
Mouth	Sialorrhea	Dry	Sialorrhea	Normal
Skin	Sweaty	Red, hot, dry	Pale, sweaty	Mottled, sweaty
GI signs	Increased bowel sounds	Decreased bowel sounds	Normal or decreased bowel sounds	Decreased bowel sounds

Most SNRIs are well tolerated in overdose and symptoms rarely are severe. Patients may need intensive care unit (ICU) admission in cases of decreased level of consciousness. Venlafaxine, in particular, is associated with increased reports of deaths, dysrhythmias, and seizures compared with other SNRIs.[33]

MAOI toxicity presents as a syndrome of catecholamine excess followed by hypotension, seizures, coma, and death.[34] People taking MAOIs are instructed to avoid excessive ingestion of foods and beverages containing tyramine (cheese, soy sauce, and salami) due to potential of triggering a fatal hypertensive crisis. Use of MAOIs in combination with SSRIs, TCAs, ecstasy, meperidine, tramadol, or dextromethorphan can cause lethal reactions.

Management

The treatment of SSRI and SNRI intoxications is focused on supportive care, discontinuation of all serotonergic agents, and continuous electrocardiogram (ECG) monitoring. Consensus-based guidelines have been developed to guide out-of-hospital management of SSRI overdose.[30,35] Patients with ingestions less than 5 times the therapeutic dose can be monitored at home but patients with mixed overdoses or ones involving greater than 5 times the therapeutic dose should be referred to the hospital. Asymptomatic patients with a normal 12-lead ECG can be discharged after 6 hours to 12 hours of observation. Symptomatic patients with or without abnormal ECG may need an additional 12 hours to 24 hours of monitoring. Several side effects are transient but others may take a few weeks to resolve.

Benzodiazepines are the drugs of choice for management of seizures, agitation, and muscle rigidity (diazepam or lorazepam, 0.1–0.2 mg/kg) associated with serotonin syndrome. Haloperidol and droperidol inhibit sweating and are contraindicated for agitation. Severe toxicity may require aggressive support, including cooling, intubation, ventilation, and neuromuscular paralysis.[36] Muscle rigidity propagates hyperthermia, and uncontrolled fever can trigger seizures and dehydration. Serotonin antagonists like cyproheptadine or chlorpromazine for serotonin syndrome refractory to benzodiazepines have minimal anecdotal evidence. Cyproheptadine, which is available only enterally, is a first-generation antihistaminic with antiserotonergic effects and can be considered for severe serotonin syndrome.[35] Depolarizing muscle relaxants should be avoided in patients with suspected rhabdomyolysis who need intubation and paralysis.

Short acting β-blockers can be used to treat hypertension and tachycardia but should be avoided in cases of predominant MAOI overdose where unopposed α-adrenoreceptor stimulation may exacerbate hypertension. Nitroglycerin and sodium nitroprusside are acceptable options for management of MAOI-related hypertension.

Patients who develop severe serotonin toxicity often require ICU admission.[37] Patients with single-agent intoxication have a good prognosis and recover without complications unless renal failure and refractory hypotension are present. Serotonin syndromes involving MAOIs tend to produce the most severe and prolonged cases. Other differential diagnoses to consider in cases without a clear-cut exposure to serotonergic agents include neuroleptic malignant syndrome (NMS), malignant hyperthermia, anticholinergic toxicity, sympathomimetic toxicity, and infectious causes, such as meningitis and encephalitis (see **Table 3**).

ANTIPSYCHOTICS
Pharmacology and Use

Antipsychotics or neuroleptic drugs are indicated in several neurologic and psychiatric conditions (**Table 4**). Developed in the 1950s, this category accounts for approximately 30 currently available drugs with increasing use in younger age groups and decreasing

Table 4
Antipsychotics and mood stabilizers

	Class	Drugs	Mechanism of Action	Medical Use	Pharmacology
Antipsychotics	TAs	Phenothiazines (chlorpromazine, fluphenazine, perphenazine, thioridazine) thioxanthenes (chlorprothixene) butyrophenones (haloperidol) diphenypbutylpiperidines (pimozide) Dihydroindolones (molindone)	• Dopamine receptor antagonists	Prophylaxis of postoperative nausea and vomiting, schizophrenia, psychosis, Paranoid psychosis	Time to onset: >1 wk (up to 6 wk) Half-life: >100 h Metabolism: high protein binding, hepatic metabolism and renal excretion
	AAs	Aripiprazole, clozapine, iloperidone, olanzapine, paliperidone, quetiapine, risperidone, ziprasidone 77	• Acetylcholine receptor antagonist (muscarinic) • Dopamine receptor antagonists • Norepinephrine reuptake inhibitor (quetiapine) • Serotonin receptor antagonists • H1 histamine receptor antagonists	Schizophrenia, treatment of mania in bipolar disorder	Time to onset: < 1 wk Half-life: 7–12 h Metabolism: hepatic metabolism
Mood stabilizers	Anticonvulsants	Carbamazepine, valproic acid, lamotrigine	Mechanisms of action are not completely elucidated • Sodium channel blocker (lamotrigine) with suppression of glutamate and aspartate release	Epilepsy, neuropathic pain (trigeminal neuralgia, peripheral neuropathy), resistant obsessive disorders, migraine, cluster headaches, affective disorders, bipolar disorders, schizophrenia, borderline personality disorders	Time to onset: 4 h Half-life: 12–30 h Metabolism: hepatic metabolism: some drugs are strong inducers of hepatic enzymes

(continued on next page)

Table 4
(continued)

Class	Drugs	Mechanism of Action	Medical Use	Pharmacology
Mineral	Lithium	• Decreases norepinephrine release • Increases serotonin release • Interference with dopamine signaling • Modulation of glutamate levels • Increases levels of GABA • Inhibition of enzyme inositol monophosphate • Interference with the sodium-potassium pump	Bipolar disorders, depressive disorder refractory to antidepressants, schizophrenic disorders	Time to onset: 7–14 d Half-life: 18–36 h Metabolism: absorbed in the small intestine and renally excreted

use in the elderly with dementia.[38] The toxicity of these drugs is generally high and can vary considerably although death from a pure neuroleptic ingestion is uncommon.[39] Antipsychotics often are classified in 2 groups: typical antipsychotics (TAs), known as first-generation drugs, and atypical antipsychotics (AAs) (see **Table 4**).

Toxicity

The most common side effects of antipsychotics include acute extrapyramidal symptoms, including dystonia, oculogyric crisis, torticollis, acute parkinsonism, akathisia, and other movement disorders.[40] AAs generally are preferred over TAs because of less frequent extrapyramidal side effects, dyskinesia, and withdrawal but chronic use of both AAs and TAs is associated with tardive dyskinesia, parkinsonism, and akathisia. Additional adverse effects include anticholinergic symptoms similar to TCAs (see **Table 3**), seizures, QT interval and QRS prolongation, orthostatic hypotension, hypothermia, sedation, and respiratory depression.

Antipsychotics (TAs more frequently than AAs) also could lead to the development of NMS, a life-threatening condition that affects multiple organ systems and results in significant mortality (see **Table 3**).[41] Patients may develop signs of serious toxicity days after exposure with rigidity, fevers, possible dysrhythmias, status epilepticus, autonomic instability, or coma and may present for intensive care management despite no apparent antecedent exposure. Initiation of high-dose, high-potency antipsychotics or a rapid increase in dose of previously well-tolerated doses can lead to NMS. Although the incidence of NMS is less common with AA use, it can occur when multiple agents are used even if smaller doses. Young men and postpartum women have an unexplained predisposition to NMS. NMS is characterized by fever, confusion, muscle rigidity, and autonomic instability similar to serotonin syndrome and may have forme fruste presentations with delayed onset. Serotonergic agents, carbamazepine, and mixed ingestions of serotonergics and antipsychotics also can cause forme fruste presentations of NMS. Similar symptoms may occur with rapid withdrawal of dopaminergic agents (eg, levodopa/carbidopa). Several clinical decision tools have been proposed for NMS but no single one has gained widespread use.[42] Signs and symptoms of rhabdomyolysis and metabolic acidosis may occur.

Management

The management of NMS centers on supportive care and cessation of the offending agent. There is no specific antidote for antipsychotics. Activated charcoal may be considered in recent acute ingestions, but ileus could hinder this method of GI decontamination. Aggressive hydration with intravenous fluids is recommended in case of hypotension, hyperthermia, or rhabdomyolysis. Norepinephrine is recommended in cases of shock. Epinephrine and dopamine could induce paradoxic hypotension due to simultaneous neuroleptic α-blockade and unopposed β-agonist peripheral vasodilation. Benzodiazepines can be used for most seizures given they are self-limited.[43]

Patients presenting with NMS and worsening hyperthermia must be treated immediately with physical and pharmacologic cooling methods. In cases of severe hyperthermia (core temperatures >40.6°C) and significant muscle rigidity, dantrolene, 1-mg/kg to 2.5-mg/kg initial dose, followed by 1-mg/kg infusion every 6 hours (maximum 10 mg/kg/d) may be considered.[41] Bromocriptine and amantadine are central dopaminergic agonists only available in enteral formulations and can be used to reverse the neuroleptic-induced dopaminergic blockade, although their effect has slow onset (eg, several days). Once NMS resolves, they should be tapered gradually to avoid rebound episodes of dopamine withdrawal mimicking NMS. Parkinson patients or patients on long-term dopamine agonists (eg, metoclopramide) could develop NMS on sudden withdrawal of their dopaminergic therapy.[44] In these cases, levodopa/carbidopa, bromocriptine, and/or amantadine should be supplemented urgently.[45] Anecdotal reports of refractory NMS cases treated with pulse steroid therapy have shown to reduce the illness duration and improve symptoms.[46]

MOOD STABILIZERS
Pharmacology and Use

Mood stabilizers include some antipsychotics, anticonvulsants (lamotrigine, valproic acid, and carbamazepine, which have similar toxicology profiles), and lithium (the classic mood stabilizer).[47] The mechanisms of action and therapeutic action are reviewed in **Table 4**. Mood-stabilizers often are used in combination, and carbamazepine cointoxication is more than 2-fold as fatal compared with lithium, which is notable for its narrow therapeutic index. The safest and most efficient combination appears to be valproic acid plus lithium.[48]

Toxicity

Carbamazepine and lamotrigine have systemic and neurologic side effects. Systemic effects include nausea, vomiting, diarrhea, hyponatremia, pruritis, and rash, whereas the neurologic effects include headache, dizziness, blurry vision or diplopia, tremor, stupor, and drowsiness. Acute valproate toxicity manifests with lethargy whereas the chronic use of valproic acid causes weight gain, GI disturbances, alopecia, tremor, and easy bruising. Approximately 5% to 10% of patients develop self-resolving transaminitis. More severe forms of valproic acid toxicity include encephalopathy secondary to hyperammonemia, hepatotoxicity, and acute pancreatitis.[49]

Acute intoxication with lithium presents with GI symptoms (nausea, diarrhea, vomiting, and cramps), neuromuscular signs (tremor, dystonia, hyperreflexia, and ataxia), and rarely cardiac effects, such as T-wave flattening, sinus node dysfunction, and QT prolongation, which often are reversible.[50] The therapeutic range of lithium concentration is 0.5 mmol/L to 1.0 mmol/L, and levels may increase in renal failure or elderly patients. Chronic intoxication is more challenging to treat and is precipitated by impaired kidney function and hypovolemia. Symptoms are primarily neurologic (altered mental status, coma, seizures), and severely intoxicated patients may present with the syndrome of irreversible lithium-effectuated neurotoxicity (SILENT), characterized by cognitive dysfunction, cerebellar dysfunction, brainstem dysfunction, extrapyramidal motor symptoms, myopathy, nystagmus, and sometimes loss of vision.[51] This syndrome is a rare but important sequela of lithium toxicity that can persist despite normalization of levels. Lithium is a potent renal toxin causing nephrogenic diabetes insipidus, chronic tubulointerstitial nephritis, renal tubular acidosis, and nephrotic syndrome. Endocrine disorders, such as hypothyroidism and myxedema, can occur in cases of chronic toxicity.[52] It is important to recognize that acute on chronic toxicity of lithium can develop in patients taking daily lithium in settings of dehydration, drug interactions, or changes in renal function.[53]

Management

Management of carbamazepine toxicity includes supportive care, addressing airway protection, and close cardiac monitoring.[54] Activated charcoal (repeated dose of 1 g/kg each, every 2–4 hours) can be used if patients are able to protect their airway with aspiration precautions. It can be given even after 2 hours if extended-release preparations are ingested. Whole-bowel irrigation after ingestion of modified-release carbamazepine may be considered (adults and adolescents, 1.5–2 L/ h, and small children, 0.5 L/h, of polyethylene glycol electrolyte lavage solution), but evidence of improved outcomes is lacking.

SB should be administered when the QRS complex is longer than 100 milliseconds. Given the high fatality rate, up to 13%, an aggressive treatment plan may require charcoal hemoperfusion, hemodialysis, intravenous lipid emulsion, and/or multiple doses of activated charcoal.[55] Seizures can be controlled with benzodiazepines or propofol, depending on severity and patient's intubation status.

Treatment of patients with valproic acid toxicity also mainly is supportive.[56] Levocarnitine may be used for hyperammonemia by loading 100 mg/kg intravenously followed by 50 mg/kg every 8 hours. Naloxone has been anecdotally reported to reverse the CNS depression from valproate although the effect is not universal.[57] Hemodialysis and hemoperfusion may be indicated for severe cases with hyperammonemia.[58]

It is important to admit patients with suspected acute lithium intoxication with significant symptoms regardless of the plasma levels of lithium. Lithium is an intracellular ion similar to potassium so serum levels do not reflect the total body load. Because most lithium formulations are sustained release, serial levels are necessary to assess for ongoing absorption. The treatment of acute lithium toxicity may include GI decontamination with gastric lavage or whole-bowel irrigation if ingestion occurred within 1 hour. Activated charcoal does not adsorb lithium and is not recommended unless there is suspicion of a mixed ingestion.[59] Volume resuscitation is necessary in the management of lithium intoxication with a goal to restore glomerular filtration rate, normalize urine output, and enhance lithium clearance.[60] Extracorporeal treatment is recommended in severe lithium poisoning and in situations with lithium levels greater than 4.0 mEq/L with impaired renal function or presence of neurologic or cardiac side effects irrespective of levels. Patients who receive chronic lithium therapy should be admitted if plasma levels are higher than 2.0 mEq/L, and those who present with severe neurotoxicity require extracorporeal renal support and ICU admission.[61] The Extracorporeal Treatments In Poisoning workgroup (https://www.extrip-workgroup.org) has specific recommendation on use of extracorporeal treatment in lithium poisoning. Extracorporeal treatment is continued for a minimum of 6 hours until there is a clinical improvement or the lithium levels fall below 1.0 mEq/L, with monitoring of serum levels every 12 hours for possibility of lithium rebound from redistribution or ongoing absorption. Hemodialysis is the most efficient extracorporeal treatment, but continuous renal replacement is an acceptable alternative.

HALLUCINOGENS
Pharmacology and Use

Hallucinogens comprise a unique group of substances that are used to induce hallucinations and cause alteration of thought and emotion. Natural hallucinogens can be found in plants and mushrooms and continue to be used worldwide for religious and recreational purposes.

Hallucinogens can be classified according to chemical family (**Table 5**).[62] Use of ketamine as a dissociative hallucinogen also is increasing with illicit access being sourced from veterinary offices.

Toxicity

Most patients presenting with hallucinogen intoxication have a history of recent exposure, but mixed use of hallucinogens with drugs, such as acetaminophen, caffeine,

Table 5
Hallucinogens

Class	Drugs	Mechanism of Action	Medical Use	Pharmacology
Psychedelics	Tryptamines Psilocybin and psilocin (mushrooms), bufotenin (toads), DMT (plants)	• Serotonin receptor partial agonist (5-HT2)	None Psilocybin and LSD have been investigated in the treatment of cluster headache	Time to onset: 20–30 min Half-life: 1 h Metabolism: metabolized by several pathways, including monoamine oxidase, limiting the oral bioavailability of some compounds
	Ergolines LSD, lysergic acid amide (plants)	• Serotonin receptor agonist • Dopamine receptor partial agonist • Norepinephrine receptor agonist		Time to onset: 3–4 h (depending on the route of administration) Half-life: 6–24 h Metabolism: extensively metabolized by the liver, predominantly via hydrolysis
	Phenethylamines Mescaline (peyote cactus), 2C-series drugs (2C-B, 2C-I, 2C-C, 2C-T-7), 3C-E, 4-MTA, PMA, DO-series drugs (DOC, DOB, DOI, DOM)	• Serotonin receptor agonist		Time to onset: >1 h (up to 24 h) Half-life: 5–10 min Metabolism: urinary excretion of the main metabolite, phenylacetic acid
Dissociative drugs	Phencyclidine, dextromethorphan, ketamine	• NMDA receptor antagonist • Sigma-1 receptor agonist	Anesthesia	Time to onset: 2–60 min Half-life: 6 h – 3 d Metabolism: complex active metabolites
Deliriants	Scopolamine and atropine (plants), diphenhydramine, dimenhydrinate	• Acetylcholine receptor antagonist (muscarinic)	Multiple legitimate uses (anesthesia, resuscitation, cardiology, ophthalmology, etc.)	Time to onset: 1–5 min Half-life: 2–9.5 h Metabolism: destroyed by enzymatic hydrolysis, particularly in the liver, with

Substance	Mechanism	Effects	Pharmacokinetics
Salvinorin A (*Salvia divinorum*)	• Selective agonist of the kappa opioid receptor	Similar to some pain relief medications (pentazocine)	13% to 50% excreted unchanged in the urine Time to onset: rapid when smoked (40 s) Half-life: 8 min Metabolism: quick metabolism in the GI tract
Muscimol (amanita muscaria)	• GABA-A agonist	Research only	Time to onset: 30–120 min Half-life: 5–10 h Metabolism: urinary excretion

barbiturates, antipsychotics, or other pharmaceuticals is common.[63] Although mushrooms containing psilocybin are recognizable, other hallucinogenic mushrooms (*Amanita muscaria*) look similar to poisonous ones (*Amanita phalloides*) and may be ingested by mistake causing severe hepatotoxicity.

Patients present with a wide range of behaviors that tend to fluctuate from a calm euphoric state to one of extreme agitation and aggressiveness. An accurate history may be difficult and often depends on circumstantial evidence.[64] Delayed GI effects (nausea and vomiting) can present after 6 hours from ingestion of hallucinogenic mushrooms. Most agents once ingested or inhaled have a predictable duration of effect. N,N-Dimethyltryptamine (DMT) has onset of action in a few seconds and duration of effects less than 60 minutes. The effects of methylenedioxy-methamphetamine last for 4 hours to 8 hours, and LSD can be active for more than 12 hours. General features of hallucinogen intoxication include altered sensorium, tachypnea, tachycardia, and mild to moderate hypertension. Hyperthermia is not a characteristic feature of mild toxicity with single-substance hallucinogens; if present, fever should trigger suspicion of polysubstance intoxication, serotonin syndrome, or anticholinergic syndrome.[65] Marked mydriasis is seen in tryptamine or LSD use. Phencyclidine and ketamine can produce horizontal, vertical, or rotatory nystagmus. Muscle tremors and fasciculation are characteristic of phenylethylamine use, whereas muscular rigidity, hyperreflexia of the lower extremities, and clonus are features of serotonin syndrome (LSD, psilocybin, and mescaline).[62] GI alterations are common with mescaline and DMT.

Management

Due to altered behavior, patients with acute hallucinogen intoxication should be placed in a calm and relaxed environment. If this is not sufficient, physical restraints and sedatives may be required. Most patients who present without medical complications do well with sedatives and reassurance.[64] The first line of sedatives includes benzodiazepines. Haloperidol or droperidol could be considered in addition to benzodiazepines but can cause QT prolongation and torsades de pointes, seizures, or temperature dysregulation.[66] AAs are contraindicated because they can precipitate serotonin syndrome.

A thorough physical examination should pay attention to traumatic injuries, cardiac dysrhythmias, and hyperthermia. Hyperthermia and agitation following ingestion of hallucinogens are life-threatening emergencies and should be managed aggressively. Phencyclidine and new hallucinogens also act as stimulants, causing severe hyperthermia and diffuse muscle fasciculations. Rapid cooling is recommended, and patients may require neuromuscular paralysis. Patients should be given intravenous fluids and observed for the development of rhabdomyolysis.

OTHER COMMONLY USED LICIT PSYCHOACTIVE SUBSTANCES
Caffeine

Popular beverages, such as coffee, tea, soda, and energy drinks, contain caffeine. According to the Mayo Clinic, the maximum recommended amount of caffeine is 400 mg per day for healthy adults (100 mg/d for adolescents and <200 mg/d for pregnant women). The exact amount of caffeine that can lead to overdose is difficult to establish due to its unpredictable half-life (**Table 6**).[67] A caffeine overdose can be life-threatening, but most people notice only some unpleasant symptoms that are self-resolving when the substance is metabolized. Diagnosis can be difficult. Symptoms of acute severe intoxication include anxiety, hallucinations, irritability, uncontrollable muscle movements, vomiting and diarrhea, seizures, and, in extreme cases, status epilepticus, chest pain, and dysrhythmias.[67] Chronic use of high doses of caffeine could lead to hormonal imbalances.

Table 6
Other psychoactive drugs

Drug	Mechanism of Action	Medical Use	Pharmacology
Caffeine (coffee, tea, other plants)	• Adenosine receptor antagonist • MAOI	Headache	Time to onset: 10 min Half-life: from 1.5 h to 9.5 h Metabolism: metabolized by the cytochrome P450 enzyme
Nicotine (tobacco)	• Nicotinic acetylcholine receptor agonist	Nicotine addiction	Time to onset: 20 s Half-life: 1–2 h Metabolism: metabolized to N-oxide, product of the hepatic oxidation by cytochrome P450
Cannabis (tetrahydrocannabinol)	• Cannabinoid receptor partial agonist	Chemotherapy-induced nausea and vomiting, neuropathic pain, sleep disorders, epilepsy	Time to onset: smoking onset in minutes, orally slow onset Half-life: 12–36 h (longer for frequent users) Metabolism: cytochrome P450 enzyme

Nicotine

Nicotine poisoning is rare with traditional tobacco-containing cigarettes and cigars. It has become more frequent in recent years due to increasing availability of alternative products, such as e-cigarettes and pure liquid nicotine, that are more likely to cause poisoning.[68] There also is a worrisome increase in intoxications involving children.[69] Consuming a few e-cigarettes at once could be fatal, given that 30 mg to 60 mg of nicotine is considered lethal in adults.[68] Adults who are not used to nicotine and try vaping for the first time are at higher risk of poisoning compared with others who have smoked cigarettes before. Rarely, exposure can occur from skin contact and ingestion. Another population at risk includes workers involved with nicotine-based products (tobacco plants and harvesting fields).

Nicotine primarily effects the heart and CNS, regardless of the amount ingested or inhaled. Symptoms typically last an hour or 1 after a mild overdose and up to 24 hours for severe poisoning and include dizziness, abdominal pain, sialorrhea, tachypnea, tachycardia, hypertension, headache, and confusion. More severe symptoms include diarrhea, hypoventilation, bradycardia, hypotension, stupor, weakness, uncontrollable muscle movements, and seizures.[70]

Cannabis and Synthetic Cannabinoids

The easy availability of cannabis and synthetic cannabinoids and the associated perception of a low risk of harm makes these among the most common substances used by adolescents often with other substances. Cannabis and synthetic cannabinoids usually are smoked (inhaled). Ingestion of cannabis in health supplements and edible forms is increasing.

Approximately 6% of the world population uses cannabis with reported incidence of 15.3% use in the United States, making it the most common PAD.[71,72] Legalization of cannabis for recreational use has caused a noteworthy decline in the amount of cannabis herb seized globally.[8,73]

All synthetic cannabinoids can cause severe agitation, hallucinations, delusions, paranoia, and schizophrenic behaviors. In severe intoxication, patients can show severe agitation, panic attacks, tremor, seizures, and tachycardia. Cannabinoids adulterated with brodifacoum may present with signs and symptoms of coagulopathy.[74] Diagnosis of intoxication usually is made using urine drug screens for cannabis but synthetic cannabinoids are not detected.[75]

Management

Treatment of caffeine intoxication focuses on increasing elimination from the blood while preventing or treating dysrhythmias. If patients present within an hour of ingestion, activated charcoal can be used. Continuous cardiac monitoring and ongoing neurologic assessment are required. The treatment of cannabis or synthetic cannabinoid intoxication may include the use of benzodiazepines for sedation as well as ventilator support in case of respiratory depression or decreased level of consciousness.

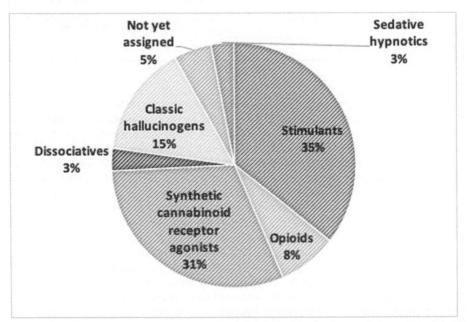

Fig. 1. NPSs by effect group, up to December 2019. (Adapted from World Drug Report 2020 (United Nations publication, Sales No. E.20.XI.6).[8]) Permission to share content from UNODC documents (from United Nations publication, Sales No. E.20.XI.6[8]): "This publication may be reproduced in whole or in part and in any form for educational or non-profit purposes without special permission from the copyright holder, provided acknowledgement of the source is made. The United Nations Office on Drugs and Crime (UNODC) would appreciate receiving a copy of any publication that uses this publication as a source"

Table 7
Toxicology and management strategies for neurologic symptoms

Drug Class	Neurologic Symptoms of Toxicity	Management Strategies Focused on Neurologic Symptoms
TCAs	• Agitation, confusion, memory impairment, and anxiety • CNS depression with reduced level of consciousness, hypoventilation, coma and seizures	• Increasing arterial pH to ≥7.45 with SB • Lipid emulsion in refractory cases • Benzodiazepines and propofol for seizures; avoid phenytoin and lacosamide
SSRIs, SNRIs, and MAOIs	• Neuromuscular excitation, autonomic instability–Hunter criteria • Altered level of consciousness and coma • Serotonin syndrome in case of serotonergic agents • Fatal hypertensive crisis in adrenergic agents	• Muscle relaxants to target rigidity and hyperthermia • Benzodiazepines for management of seizures, agitation and muscle rigidity (diazepam or lorazepam, 0.1–0.2 mg/kg) • Butyrophenones (eg, haloperidol) and droperidol worsen hyperthermia and are contraindicated • Cyproheptadine or chlorpromazine may be considered for symptoms refractory to benzodiazepines • Avoid depolarizing muscle relaxant drugs
Antipsychotics	• Acute extrapyramidal symptoms • Seizures and status epilepticus • Tardive dyskinesia • NMS	• Benzodiazepines (eg, lorazepam, midazolam) for treatment of seizures • NMS–dantrolene sodium (1–10 mg/kg) for muscle rigidity and fever in severe cases Bromocriptine and amantadine for less severe cases • Pulse steroid therapy for refractory cases
Carbamazepine and lamotrigine	• Headache, dizziness, blurry vision or diplopia, tremor, stupor, drowsiness, seizures	• Charcoal hemoperfusion, hemodialysis, intravenous lipid emulsion and multiple doses activated charcoal • Benzodiazepine for seizure control
Valproate	• Tremors, agitation, miosis • Hyperammonemia causing stupor, coma, or death	• L-carnitine for hyperammonemia • Hemodialysis and hemoperfusion for refractory cases
Lithium	• Tremor, dystonia, hyperreflexia, ataxia, confusion, lethargy, seizure • SILENT	• Intravenous fluids to restore renal perfusion • Hemodialysis for removing lithium
Hallucinogens	• Altered sensorium • Marked mydriasis in tryptamine or lysergic acid use	• Benzodiazepines for agitation and seizures • Avoid AAs

(continued on next page)

Table 7
(continued)

Drug Class	Neurologic Symptoms of Toxicity	Management Strategies Focused on Neurologic Symptoms
	• Horizontal, vertical, or rotatory nystagmus with phencyclidine • Life-threatening hyperthermia and agitation	• Aggressive cooling
Caffeine	• Anxiety, hallucinations, irritability, uncontrollable muscle movements • Seizures and status epilepticus	Supportive care Benzodiazepines for agitation and seizures
Nicotine	• Headache, confusion, stupor • Weakness, uncontrollable muscle movements • Seizures	Supportive care Benzodiazepines for agitation and seizures
Cannabis	• Severe agitation, hallucinations, delusions, paranoia, schizophrenic behaviors	Benzodiazepines for agitation and seizures
NPSs	• Seizures, agitation, aggressiveness, and acute psychosis	Supportive care Benzodiazepines for agitation and seizures

NEW PSYCHOACTIVE SUBSTANCES

New psychoactive substances (NPSs), also known as legal highs, bath salts, or research chemicals, have been synthesized for decades but are increasingly popular in the illicit drug market, with more than 500 NPS formulations identified on the market each year. A majority of NPSs identified by United Nations Office on Drugs and Crime monitors are stimulants, cannabinoid receptor agonists, and classic hallucinogens (**Fig. 1**).[8] NPSs in general have not replaced traditional drugs on a larger scale but NPSs with opioid-like effects have been associated with fatalities, and injectable NPSs have been associated with high-risk administration practices.[76]

Globally, the large number of emerging NPSs poses a significant risk to public health and a challenge to drug policy processes. NPS users frequently are hospitalized with severe intoxications. Safety data on many NPSs are limited, and details on long-term adverse effects and risks still are unknown, making both prevention and treatment challenging. Known side effects of NPSs include seizures, agitation, aggressiveness, and acute psychosis. Additionally, impurities or compounds added to stabilize formulations may have high risk of complex and unpredictable severe side effects. Deaths associated with NPSs often are caused by polysubstance use.[76] **Table 7** summarizes the neurologic toxicity and targeted management for PADs and NPSs.

DISCUSSION

In recent years, there have been important changes in the PAD markets. There is increased production and use of NPSs, ongoing use of available PADs, and a rise in the nonmedical use of prescription drugs obtained from licit channels or illegally manufactured. In addition, many substances sold as alleged medicines are being directed for nonmedical use through illicit channels.

Similar to the 2008 economic crisis, reports suggest that the COVID-19 pandemic is shifting trends in PAD trafficking, consumption patterns, and shift in preferred substance of abuse based on accessibility and availability.[8,77] Cannabis use may have increased since the first lockdown measures.[8] Monitoring, reporting, information sharing, early warning, and risk awareness are essential to prepare the response to the emerging health threat associated with PAD use.

CLINICS CARE POINTS

- SB is the mainstay of therapy for severe TCA toxicity by alkalinization effect as well sodium load to reverse the sodium channel blocking effect of TCAs.
- Benzodiazepines are the mainstay of seizure management in most overdose-related seizures due to psychoactive substances.
- Early recognition, discontinuation of drugs, and supportive care are central to managing serotonin syndrome and NMS. Dantrolene should be considered in hyperthermia related to NMS.
- Extracorporeal treatments should be considered in lithium toxicity and severe valproate toxicity
- Symptomatic management of agitation in most hallucinogen ingestions involves careful use of sedatives.

DISCLOSURE

Lara Prisco is a Doctoral Research Fellow (NIHR300741) funded by the National Institute for Health Research (NIHR). The views expressed in this publication are those of the author(s) and not necessarily those of the NIHR, NHS or the UK Department of Health and Social Care.

REFERENCES

1. Rhee TG, Olfson M, Nierenberg AA, et al. 20-year trends in the pharmacologic treatment of bipolar disorder by psychiatrists in outpatient care settings. Am J Psychiatry 2020;177(8):706–15.
2. Yu Z, Zhang J, Zheng Y, et al. Trends in antidepressant use and expenditure in six major cities in China from 2013 to 2018. Front Psychiatry 2020;11:551.
3. Wesselhoeft R, Jensen PB, Talati A, et al. Trends in antidepressant use among children and adolescents: a Scandinavian drug utilization study. Acta Psychiatr Scand 2020;141(1):34–42.
4. Madras BK. The growing problem of new psychoactive substances (NPS). Curr Topbehav Neurosci 2017;32:1–18.
5. Lloyd SL, Striley CW. Marijuana use among adults 50 years or older in the 21st Century. Gerontol Geriatr Med 2018;4. 2333721418781668.
6. Carrasco-Garrido P, Jiménez-Trujillo I, Hernández-Barrera V, et al. Gender differences in the nonmedical use of psychoactive medications in the school population- national trends and related factors. BMC Pediatr 2019;19(1):362.
7. Ait-Daoud N, Blevins D, Khanna S, et al. Women and addiction: an update. Med Clin North Am 2019;103(4):699–711.
8. World drug report 2020. United Nations. 2020. Available at: https://wdr.unodc.org/wdr2020/. Accessed Jan 21,2021.
9. NIDA. Sex and gender differences in substance use. National Institute on Drug Abuse website; 2020. Available at: https://www.drugabuse.gov/publications/research-reports/substance-use-in-women/sex-gender-differences-in-substance-use. Accessed February 9, 2021.
10. Treatment Episode Data Set (TEDS): 2004-2014, National admissions to substance abuse treatment Services. U.S. Department Health & Human Services. Substance Abuse and Mental Health Services Administration, Center for Behavioral Health Statistics and Quality. 2016. Available at: https://www.samhsa.gov/data/report/treatment-episode-data-set-teds-2004-2014-national-admissions-substance-abuse-treatment. Accessed January 21, 2021.
11. Women and depression: Discovering Hope. National Institute of Mental Health Science Writing, Press & Dissemination Branch. Available at: http://www.nimh.nih.gov. Accessed Date Jan 21, 2020.
12. Lipari RN. Understanding adolescent inhalant use. In: Center for behavioral health Statistics and Quality SAaMHSA. The CBHSQ report. 2017.
13. Pratt LA, Brody DJ, Gu Q. Antidepressant use in persons aged 12 and over: United States, 2005-2008. In: NCHS data brief. 2011. p. 76.
14. Gummin DD, Mowry JB, Beuhler MC, et al. 2019 Annual report of the American association of poison control centers' national poison data system (NPDS): 37th annual report. Clin Toxicol 2020;58(12):1360–541.
15. Methling M, Krumbiegel F, Hartwig S, et al. Toxicological findings in suicides - frequency of antidepressant and antipsychotic substances. Forensic Sci Med Pathol 2019;15(1):23–30.

16. Gillman PK. Tricyclic antidepressant pharmacology and therapeutic drug interactions updated. Br J Pharmacol 2007;151(6):737–48.
17. Schatzberg AF, Nemeroff CB, editors. The American psychiatric publishing Textbook of psychopharmacology. 5th edition. Washington, DC: American Psychiatric Association Publishing; 2017.
18. Jarvis MR. Clinical pharmacokinetics of tricyclic antidepressant overdose. Psychopharmacol Bull 1991;27(4):541–50.
19. Schulz M1, Schmoldt A. Therapeutic and toxic blood concentrations of more than 800 drugs and other xenobiotics. Die Pharmazie 2003;58(7):447–74.
20. Hill T, Coupland C, Morriss R, et al. Antidepressant use and risk of epilepsy and seizures in people aged 20 to 64 years: cohort study using a primary care database. BMC Psychiatry 2015;15(1):315.
21. Judge BS, Rentmeester LL. Antidepressant overdose-induced seizures. Neurol Clin 2011;29(3):565–80.
22. Body R, Bartram T, Azam F, et al. Guidelines in Emergency Medicine Network (GEMNet): guideline for the management of tricyclic antidepressant overdose. Emerg Med J 2011;28(4):347–68.
23. Pierog JE, Kane KE, Kane BG, et al. Tricyclic antidepressant toxicity treated with massive sodium bicarbonate. Am J Emerg Med 2009;27(9):1168.e3.
24. McKinney PE, Rasmussen R. Reversal of severe tricyclic antidepressant-induced cardiotoxicity with intravenous hypertonic saline solution. Ann Emerg Med 2003; 42(1):20–4.
25. Yekehtaz H, Farokhnia M, Akhondzadeh S. Cardiovascular considerations in antidepressant therapy: an evidence-based review. J Tehran Heart Cent 2013;8(4):169–76.
26. Emamhadi M, Mostafazadeh B, Hassanijirdehi M. Tricyclic antidepressant poisoning treated by magnesium sulfate: a randomized, clinical trial. Drug Chem Toxicol 2012;35(3):300–3.
27. Linde K, Kriston L, Rücker G, et al. Efficacy and acceptability of pharmacological treatments for depressive disorders in primary care: systematic review and network meta-analysis. Ann Fam Med 2015;13(1):69–79.
28. Brody DJGQ. Antidepressant use among adults: United States, 2015–2018. In: NCHS data brief. 2020.
29. Gummin DD, Mowry JB, Spyker DA, et al. 2016 Annual report of the American association of poison control centers' national poison data system (NPDS): 34th annual report. Clin Toxicol 2017;55(10):1072–252.
30. Nelson LS, Erdman AR, Booze LL, et al. Selective serotonin reuptake inhibitor poisoning: an evidence-based consensus guideline for out-of-hospital management. Clin Toxicol 2007;45(4):315–32.
31. Jimmink A, Caminada K, Hunfeld NG, et al. Clinical toxicology of citalopram after acute intoxication with the sole drug or in combination with other drugs: overview of 26 cases. Ther Drug Monit 2008;30(3):365–71.
32. van Gorp F, Whyte IM, Isbister GK. Clinical and ECG effects of escitalopram overdose. Ann Emerg Med 2009;54(3):404–8.
33. Vo KT, Merriman AJ, Wang RC. Seizure in venlafaxine overdose: a 10-year retrospective review of the California poison control system. Clin Toxicol 2020;58(10):984–90.
34. Nelson JC, Spyker DA. Morbidity and mortality associated with medications used in the treatment of depression: an analysis of cases reported to U.S. poison control centers, 2000-2014. Am J Psychiatry 2017;174(5):438–50.
35. Wang RZ, Vashistha V, Kaur S, et al. Serotonin syndrome: preventing, recognizing, and treating it. Clevel Clin J Med 2016;83(11):810–6.

36. Eyer F, Zilker T. Bench-to-bedside review: mechanisms and management of hyperthermia due to toxicity. Crit Care 2007;11:236.
37. Pedavally S, Fugate JE, Rabinstein AA. Serotonin syndrome in the intensive care unit: clinical presentations and precipitating medications. Neurocrit Care 2014; 21(1):108–13.
38. Højlund M, Pottegård A, Johnsen E, et al. Trends in utilization and dosing of antipsychotic drugs in Scandinavia: comparison of 2006 and 2016. Br J Clin Pharmacol 2019;85(7):1598–606.
39. Pillinger T, McCutcheon RA, Vano L, et al. Comparative effects of 18 antipsychotics on metabolic function in patients with schizophrenia, predictors of metabolic dysregulation, and association with psychopathology: a systematic review and network meta-analysis. Lancet Psychiatry 2020;7(1):64–77.
40. Stroup TS, Gray N. Management of common adverse effects of antipsychotic medications. World Psychiatry 2018;17(3):341–56.
41. Oruch R, Pryme IF, Engelsen BA, et al. Neuroleptic malignant syndrome: an easily overlooked neurologic emergency. Neuropsychiatr Dis Treat 2017;13:161–75.
42. Tse L, Barr AM, Scarapicchia V, et al. Neuroleptic malignant syndrome: a review from a clinically oriented perspective. Curr Neuropharmacol 2015;13(3):395–406.
43. Cobaugh DJ, Erdman AR, Booze LL, et al. Atypical antipsychotic medication poisoning: an evidence-based consensus guideline for out-of-hospital management. Clin Toxicol 2007;45(8):918–42.
44. Berman BD. Neuroleptic malignant syndrome: a review for neurohospitalists. Neurohospitalist 2011;1(1):41–7.
45. Frucht SJ. Treatment of movement disorder emergencies. Neurotherapeutics 2014;11(1):208–12.
46. Sato Y, Asoh T, Metoki N, et al. Efficacy of methylprednisolone pulse therapy on neuroleptic malignant syndrome in Parkinson's disease. J Neurol Neurosurg Psychiatry 2003;74(5):574–6.
47. Hawton AEF, Galit G, Deborah C, et al. Relative toxicity of mood stabilisers and antipsychotics: case fatality and fatal toxicity associated with self-poisoning. BMC Psychiatry 2018;18(1):1–8.
48. Freeman MP, Stoll AL. Mood stabilizer combinations: a review of safety and efficacy. Am J Psychiatry 1998;155(1):12–21.
49. Sztajnkrycer MD. Valproic acid toxicity: overview and management. J Toxicol Clin Toxicol 2002;40(6):789–801.
50. Oruch R, Elderbi MA, Khattab HA, et al. Lithium: a review of pharmacology, clinical uses, and toxicity. Eur J Pharmacol 2014;740:464–73.
51. Adityanjee, Munshi KR, Thampy A. The syndrome of irreversible lithium-effectuated neurotoxicity. Clin Neuropharmacol 2005;28(1):38–49.
52. Ng YW, Tiu SC, Choi KL, et al. Use of lithium in the treatment of thyrotoxicosis. Hong Kong Med J 2006;12(4):254–9.
53. Baird-Gunning J, Lea-Henry T, Hoegberg LCG, et al. Lithium poisoning. J Intensive Care Med 2017;32(4):249–63.
54. Spiller HA. Management of carbamazepine overdose. Pediatr Emerg care 2001; 17(6):452–6.
55. Ghannoum M, Yates C, Galvao TF, et al. Extracorporeal treatment for carbamazepine poisoning: systematic review and recommendations from the EXTRIP workgroup. Clin Toxicol 2014;52(10):993–1004.
56. Manoguerra AS, Erdman AR, Woolf AD, et al. Valproic acid poisoning: an evidence-based consensus guideline for out-of-hospital management. Clin Toxicol 2008;46(7):661–76.

57. Thanacoody HKR. Chronic valproic acid intoxication: reversal by naloxone. Emerg Med J 2007;24(9):677–8.
58. Ghannoum M, Laliberté M, Nolin TD, et al. Extracorporeal treatment for valproic acid poisoning: systematic review and recommendations from the EXTRIP workgroup. Clin Toxicol 2015;53(5):454–65.
59. Bretaudeau Deguigne M, Hamel JF, Boels D, et al. Lithium poisoning: the value of early digestive tract decontamination. Clin Toxicol 2013;51(4):243–8.
60. McKnight RF, Adida M, Budge K, et al. Lithium toxicity profile: a systematic review and meta-analysis. Lancet 2012;379(9817):721–8.
61. Decker BS, Goldfarb DS, Dargan PI, et al. Extracorporeal treatment for lithium poisoning: systematic review and recommendations from the EXTRIP Workgroup. Clin J Am Soc Nephrol 2015;10(5):875–87, 64.
62. Hill SL, Thomas SH. Clinical toxicology of newer recreational drugs. Clinl Toxicol 2011;49(8):705–19.
63. Hardaway R, Schweitzer J, Suzuki J. Hallucinogen use disorders. Child Adolesc Psychiatr Clin N Am 2016;25(3):489–96.
64. Hantson, Frédéric J, Karim J, et al. Management of pharmaceutical and recreational drug poisoning. Ann Intensive Care 2020;10(1):1–30.
65. Simon LV, Keenaghan M. Serotonin syndrome. In: StatPearls. . Treasure Island, FL: StatPearls Publishing; 2020.
66. Ghuran A, Nolan J. Recreational drug misuse: issues for the cardiologist. Heart 2000;83(6):627–33.
67. Murray A, Traylor J. Caffeine toxicity. In: StatPearls. . Treasure Island, FL: StatPearls Publishing; 2020.
68. Mayer B. How much nicotine kills a human? Tracing back the generally accepted lethal dose to dubious self-experiments in the nineteenth century. Arch Toxicol 2014;88(1):5–7.
69. Quail MT. Nicotine toxicity: protecting children from e-cigarette exposure. Nursing 2020;50(1):44–8.
70. Shao XM, Fang ZT. Severe acute toxicity of inhaled nicotine and e-cigarettes: seizures and cardiac arrhythmia. Chest 2020;157(3):506–8.
71. World drug report 2020. United Nations office on drugs and Crime. https://www.unodc.org/. Accessed January 18, 2021.
72. Gummin DD, Mowry JB, Spyker DA, et al. 2018 Annual report of the American association of poison control centers' national poison data system (NPDS): 36th annual report. Clin Toxicol 2019;57(12):1220–413.
73. Lewis B, Fleeger T, Judge B, et al. Acute toxicity associated with cannabis edibles following decriminalization of marijuana in Michigan. Am J Emerg Med 2020.
74. Chan A, Adashek M, Kang J, et al. Disseminated intravascular coagulopathy secondary to unintentional brodifacoum poisoning via synthetic marijuana. J Hematol 2019;8(1):40–3.
75. Schmid Y, Scholz I, Mueller L, et al. Emergency department presentations related to acute toxicity following recreational use of cannabis products in Switzerland. Drug Alcohol Depend 2020;206:107726. https://doi.org/10.1016/j.drugalcdep.2019.107726.
76. Shafi A, Berry AJ, Sumnall H, et al. New psychoactive substances: a review and updates. Ther Adv Psychopharmacol 2020;10. 2045125320967197.
77. Vittadini G, Beghi M, Mezzanzanica M, et al. Use of psychotropic drugs in Lombardy in time of economic crisis (2007-2011): a population-based study of adult employees. Psychiatry Res 2014;220(1–2):615–22.

Acetaminophen Poisoning

Angela L. Chiew, PhD, FACEM[a],*, Nicholas A. Buckley, MD, FRACP[b]

KEYWORDS

- Acetaminophen • Poisoning • Acetylcysteine • Hepatotoxicity • Acute liver injury

KEY POINTS

- Acetaminophen is a common cause of poisoning and acute liver injury.
- Patients at risk of acute liver injury should receive acetylcysteine, which ensures survival in most patients.
- The acetaminophen nomogram assesses the need for treatment in acute immediate-release acetaminophen ingestions with a known time of ingestion. It has not been validated for use in other scenarios.
- Cases that require a different management pathway include modified-release acetaminophen overdoses, large/massive overdoses, and repeated supratherapeutic ingestions.
- Those at increased risk of acute liver injury are patients' receiving acetylcysteine more than 8 hours after acetaminophen ingestion, with high initial acetaminophen concentrations, with glutathione depletion (ie, malnutrition), or with underlying liver disease.

INTRODUCTION

Acetaminophen is a commonly used analgesic and antipyretic agent and in recommended therapeutic doses, is safe in healthy individuals. Because of wide availability and minimal cost, acetaminophen is the most common medication taken in deliberate self-poisoning and unintentional overdose in many countries.[1,2] Acetaminophen toxicity is the leading cause of acute liver failure (ALF) in North America, Europe, and Australia.[3,4]

WHY IS ACETAMINOPHEN TOXIC?

Acetaminophen is mainly metabolized into two nontoxic metabolites, sulfate (~30%) and glucuronide (~55%) conjugates.[5] A highly reactive toxic metabolite, N-acetyl-p-benzoquinone imine (NAPQI), is also formed by cytochromes P-450 2E1 and 3A4. The small amounts of NAPQI produced after therapeutic doses are detoxified by glutathione-dependent reactions to two nontoxic metabolites, mercapturic acid and

a Clinical Toxicology Unit, Prince of Wales Hospital, Barker Street, Randwick, New South Wales 2031, Australia; b Pharmacology and Biomedical Informatics and Digital Health, Faculty of Medicine and Health, University of Sydney, Camperdown, New South Wales 2050, Australia
* Corresponding author.
E-mail address: angela.chiew@health.nsw.gov.au

Crit Care Clin 37 (2021) 543–561
https://doi.org/10.1016/j.ccc.2021.03.005
criticalcare.theclinics.com

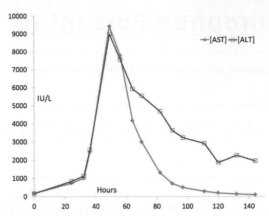

Fig. 1. Time course of AST and ALT concentrations in an actual patient treated for acetaminophen overdose. After the peak concentrations, the AST concentrations decline more rapidly than the ALT concentrations. (*From* McGovern AJ, Vitkovitsky IV, Jones DL, Mullins ME. Can AST/ALT ratio indicate recovery after acute paracetamol poisoning? Clin Toxicol (Phila). 2015;53(3):164-167.; with permission.[13])

cysteine conjugates (~4% each).[5] Glutathione is essential in the metabolism of NAPQI and covalently binds in a 1:1 ratio.[6] NAPQI is responsible for the hepatocellular injury that occurs with acetaminophen toxicity. Once glutathione is depleted, NAPQI can no longer be detoxified and covalently binds to critical cellular proteins.[7] It is hypothesized that this results in loss of activity/function of critical proteins and eventually causes hepatic cell death. In animals, hepatic necrosis is observed once glutathione is depleted by approximately 70%.[8]

TOXIC DOSE AND EFFECTS OF ACETAMINOPHEN

Acetaminophen in therapeutic doses (for adults 500–1000 mg, three to four times per day) has few adverse effects. However, overdose can result in acute liver injury (ALI), hepatotoxicity (defined as an alanine transaminase [ALT] or aspartate transaminase [AST] >1000 U/L), ALF, and death. In general, a single dose of more than 10 g or 150 to 200 mg/kg of acetaminophen carries a risk of ALI[9]; however, smaller doses may also cause ALI.[10] The aminotransferases (ALT/AST) are traditionally measured to monitor for ALI. Elevation following acetaminophen overdose is a latent event that may not occur until 24 hours after the overdose. Most patients who develop ALI recover.[11] Peak hepatic aminotransferase concentrations occur a variable number of days after acute ingestion, but typically within 3 to 4 days (**Fig. 1**).[12,13] Peak AST and ALT concentrations may be in the tens of thousands.[13] A minority develop ALF, characterized by acidemia, encephalopathy, and coagulopathy.[14]

Before an effective antidote was developed, the morbidity following acetaminophen overdose was high; 89% of people developed hepatotoxicity if they had an initial concentration greater than the high-risk 300 mg/L at 4-hour nomogram line, and 28% if the level was between the 200 mg/L and 300 mg/L at 4-hour nomogram lines (**Fig. 2**).[15] Before acetylcysteine was introduced, the mortality rate was approximately 5% in untreated patients with an initial acetaminophen concentration greater than the 200 mg/L at 4-hour nomogram line.[16] Since its introduction in the 1980s the mortality rate has fallen to approximately 0.4%.[17]

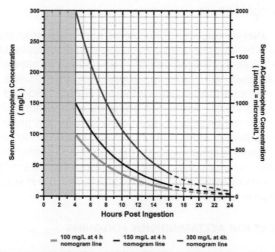

Fig. 2. Thresholds used on acetaminophen treatment nomograms. The 100 mg/L at 4 hours (*green line*) nomogram line, treatment threshold used by the United Kingdom. The 150 mg/L at 4 hours (*blue line*) nomogram line, treatment threshold used by many countries including but not exclusively the United States, Canada, Australia, New Zealand, and Singapore. The 300 mg/L at 4 hours (*red line*), "double" the standard treatment nomogram line (used to indicate increased doses of acetylcysteine required in some countries). *Dotted lines* show extrapolation to 24 hours but lines are not generally validated beyond 15 to 16 hours.

Massive ingestions, resulting in extremely high serum acetaminophen concentrations (ie, >800 mg/L [5000 μmol/L]), may be associated with early coma and lactic acidosis.[18] This is secondary to a direct mitochondrial effect, rather than ALI. These patients have a good prognosis with supportive care and adequate early antidote treatment.[18]

ASSESSMENT OF ACETAMINOPHEN POISONING

The management of acetaminophen poisoning depends on an accurate risk assessment. The key elements to ascertain are:

- Dose and time of ingestion
- Type of ingestion, that is, acute (deliberate) versus repeated supratherapeutic ingestion (RSTI)
- Preparation ingested, that is, immediate-release versus modified-release
- Laboratory results that guide antidote use, that is, initial acetaminophen and aminotransaminase concentrations
- Clinical and laboratory features to monitor for ALI or ALF (late) that is, aminotransaminases, hepatic encephalopathy, blood glucose, arterial/venous blood gases, coagulation profile, renal function, and phosphate

The risk assessment guides treatment interventions required, particularly decontamination and antidote administration. Acetaminophen concentration is a good surrogate marker early postingestion, indicating the potential for ALI. However, clinical or biochemical evidence of ALI may not be apparent for up to 24 hours after acute overdose.

ACETAMINOPHEN NOMOGRAM

Acetaminophen guidelines vary worldwide; some administer acetylcysteine in all who ingest a toxic dose, whereas most use one of several acetaminophen treatment nomograms to guide antidote administration.[19–21] The optimum treatment threshold also varies among guidelines with different nomogram cutoffs used worldwide (see **Fig. 2**). The acetaminophen treatment nomogram is only validated for use in acute immediate-release ingestions, within 4 to 16 hours of ingestion (extrapolated to 24 hours) and where an accurate time of ingestion is known.[16] In particular, acetaminophen concentrations taken before 4 hours postingestion cannot be interpreted on the acetaminophen treatment nomogram. There are many scenarios where the acetaminophen treatment nomogram should not be relied on to determine need for treatment, including ingestions of modified-release tablets, RSTI, and staggered ingestions (overdoses not taken at a single timepoint).

SPECIFIC TREATMENT FOR ACETAMINOPHEN POISONING
Decontamination

Gastrointestinal decontamination is performed in the poisoned patient to decrease the amount of toxin absorbed from the gastrointestinal tract and can involve such modalities as gastric lavage, activated charcoal, or whole-bowel irrigation. The evidence for activated charcoal following acetaminophen ingestion is predominantly from observational and human volunteer studies.[22] Only one small (n = 60) randomized controlled trial compared activated charcoal, gastric lavage, and ipecacuanha. It showed these interventions may reduce the absorption of acetaminophen if commenced within 1 to 2 hours of ingestion; however, the clinical benefit was unclear.[23] Healthy volunteer studies have shown that activated charcoal administered within 2 hours of ingestion reduces the absorption of acetaminophen.[24,25] Observational studies in poisoned patients have demonstrated that those receiving activated charcoal within 2 hours of ingestion are less likely to have an acetaminophen concentration greater than the treatment nomogram line and hence have a decreased need for acetylcysteine compared with those who have no decontamination.[9,26] In an observational study of "massive" acetaminophen ingestion of greater than or equal to 40 g of immediate-release acetaminophen, activated charcoal within 4 hours of ingestion was shown to significantly lower the initial acetaminophen concentration with a reduction in the risk of hepatotoxicity.[27]

The time in which activated charcoal administration is recommended varies between less than 1 or 2 hours postingestion.[19,28] Given the low risk and current evidence, it is reasonable to offer activated charcoal within 2 hours of ingestion in awake and alert patients who have ingested a toxic dose of acetaminophen.[9] In those who ingest large doses of acetaminophen or modified-release preparations the benefits of charcoal may extend beyond 2 hours,[27] and thus some guidelines recommend activated charcoal for immediate-release ingestions of greater than or equal to 30 g up to 4 hours postingestion. Repeated doses may be considered in those with evidence of ongoing absorption or double acetaminophen peaks; most commonly this is modified-release ingestions and/or those who coingest agents that slow gut motility (ie, anticholinergic agents or opioids).[19]

Antidotes

Several antidotes that replenish glutathione and detoxify NAPQI were evaluated in the 1970s, including methionine, cysteine, cysteamine, and dimercaprol.[22] Acetylcysteine is by far the most widely used antidote for acetaminophen toxicity. Cysteamine and methionine were shown in small randomized trials to decrease hepatotoxicity.[29,30] However, cysteamine was associated with severe headache, nausea, and vomiting in nearly all patients, whereas methionine is only available as an oral preparation.[29,30]

Acetylcysteine is a precursor that is hydrolyzed intracellularly to cysteine, which is the rate-limiting factor in replenishing glutathione[31] and thus it stimulates glutathione synthesis.[32] Acetylcysteine also supplies thiol groups, which can directly bind with NAPQI in hepatocytes and enhances nontoxic sulfate conjugation.[33] Prescott and colleagues,[16] in an observational study, reported intravenous acetylcysteine first-line was more effective than cysteamine and methionine and *"noticeably free of adverse effects"*. Since that study, acetylcysteine has been accepted as an antidote for acetaminophen overdose in the intravenous dosing regimen proposed by Prescott and colleagues[16] or a longer 72-hour oral regimen.

Neither the oral nor intravenous regimen was subject to a randomized controlled trial, or the optimum regimen established by dose ranging studies. Instead, acetylcysteine is usually given using the dose calculated by Prescott and colleagues,[16] with a single standard dosage based on weight. This regimen was remarkably effective but had several issues, including that the infusion schedule is complex and can result in errors, and adverse effects are common.[34] Furthermore, the standard 300 mg/kg over 21-hour acetylcysteine regimen assumes that "one size fits all." Recent research has aimed to decrease adverse effects and tailor acetylcysteine dose and duration to match the patient's risk.

The traditional intravenous three-bag acetylcysteine dosage regimen, although efficacious in most patients, frequently causes adverse effects, such as rash, nausea and vomiting, angioedema, tachycardia, bronchospasm, and hypotension.[34,35] The reported rates of adverse effects range widely from 8.5% to 77% depending on study methodology.[34] Various novel acetylcysteine regimens (**Table 1**) have been studied (**Fig. 3**, see **Table 1**). The two-bag and Scottish and Newcastle Anti-emetic Pre-treatment for Paracetamol Poisoning (SNAP) 12-hour regimens all lengthen the duration of the loading dose, with the aim to decrease the incidence of infusion reactions.[36–38]

The SNAP 12-hour regimen and the two-bag regimen (see **Table 1**) have much lower rates of adverse effects compared with the traditional three-bag regimen.[36–38] It is more difficult to establish equivalent efficacy. The high efficacy of all acetylcysteine regimens means large numbers of patients are required to demonstrate noninferiority, and hence a randomized controlled trial is unlikely to eventuate. Both regimens have now been adopted for use clinically, which has allowed observational studies to compare outcomes of thousands of acetaminophen-poisoned patients[19,38,39] and these have so far shown similar efficacy (noninferiority) to the traditional three-bag regimen.[39,40] Major limitations of the evidence for both new regimens are insufficient data on modified-release overdoses and those with very high acetaminophen concentrations.

There is also a one-bag infusion, which uses a standardized dose of acetylcysteine (ie, 30 g of acetylcysteine in 1 L) with programable pumps that alter the infusion rate.[41] These proposed regimens administer 150 mg/kg over 1-hour loading dose and then varying subsequent infusions of 10, 12.5, 14, or 15 mg/kg/h depending on the protocol.[41–44] The aims of these regimens are to simplify acetylcysteine administration and reduce administration errors; however, study numbers have been small.

Oral acetylcysteine has been used in the United States for more than 30 years (see **Table 1**). However, intravenous acetylcysteine is now used in 90% of cases.[2] The efficacy of oral and intravenous acetylcysteine is similar.[45,46] The oral regimen is administered over 72 hours; however, some abbreviate this regimen (≤48 hours) according to acetaminophen and aminotransferase concentrations and international normalized

Table 1
Traditional and modified acetylcysteine regimens, dose, duration, and cumulative dose (standard course and "massive" ingestions)

Acetylcysteine Regimen	Dose	Duration	Cumulative Dose (mg/kg), Standard Course	Cumulative Dose (mg/kg), "Massive"[a] Ingestion
Intravenous regimens				
Traditional 3-step regimen	1/ 200 mg/kg over 15–60 min 2/ 50 mg/kg over 4 h 3/ 100 mg/kg over 16 h	20.25–21 h	300 mg/kg	400 mg/kg (dose of third infusion increased to 200 mg/kg)
2-step regimen (2-bag infusion)	1/ 200 mg/kg over 4 h 2/ 100 mg/kg over 16 h	20 h	300 mg/kg	400 mg/kg (dose of second infusion increased to 200 mg/kg)
SNAP 12-h regimen	1/ 100 mg/kg over 2 h 2/ 200 mg/kg over 10 h	12 h	300 mg/kg over 12 h	500 mg/kg (22 h) (second infusion repeated)
2-step regimen: single bag infusion	1/ 150 mg/kg over 1 h 2/ 10–15 mg/kg/h for 20 h	20 h	350–450 mg/kg	350–450 mg/kg (no change in regimen)
Oral regimen				
Oral acetylcysteine regimen	1/ 140 mg/kg over 1 h 2/ 70 mg/kg over 1 h every 4 h for 17 doses	72 h	490 mg/kg over 20 h 1330 mg/kg over 72 h	490 mg/kg over 20 h 1330 mg/kg over 72 h (no change in regimen)

Abbreviation: SNAP, Scottish and Newcastle Anti-emetic Pre-treatment for Paracetamol Poisoning.
   [a] No standardized definition but typically defined as those with an initial acetaminophen concentration greater than the 300 mg/L at 4-hour nomogram line.

ratio (INR).[47] Nausea and vomiting occur in up to a third of patients.[46] Oral doses are repeated if vomiting occurs within an hour of administration; ongoing vomiting is an indication to switch to intravenous treatment.

TREATMENT MODIFICATION
High Initial Acetaminophen Concentrations

The dose of acetylcysteine received is based on patient weight, rather than the acetaminophen body burden (ie, dose ingested or initial acetaminophen concentration). Logically, the dosage should be based on estimated NAPQI production from the ingested dose.[8,48] For most ingestions 300 mg/kg over 20 hours intravenously is demonstrably adequate. However, it is likely some patients have an insufficient dose or duration, whereas many more are receiving too much or for too long. Those with very high initial acetaminophen concentrations are at increased risk of ALI regardless of time to treatment.[27,49,50] This risk is mitigated by activated charcoal in those

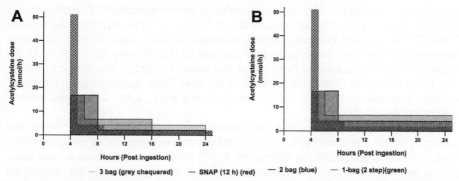

Fig. 3. Comparison of intravenous acetylcysteine regimens in (A) standard acetaminophen ingestions and (B) "massive[a]" ingestions. Comparison of traditional (3-bag) (*checkered*), Scottish and Newcastle Anti-emetic Pre-treatment for Paracetamol Poisoning (SNAP) 12-hour (*red*), 2-bag (*blue*), and 1-bag (2 step) infusion (*green*). Note for "massive" ingestions 2-bag regimen the second infusion dose was doubled and for the 12-hour SNAP regimen the second infusion was repeated. [a]No standardized definition but typically defined as those with an initial acetaminophen concentration greater than the 300 mg/L at 4-hour nomogram line.

presenting within 4 hours of ingestion or increased acetylcysteine dose in those with initial acetaminophen concentrations greater than double the 150 mg/L at 4-hour nomogram line.[27] The optimum acetylcysteine dosing regimen to prevent ALI is unknown. However, the risk is reduced in those with an initial acetaminophen concentration of greater than double the 150 mg/L at 4-hour nomogram line if the final infusion of the traditional or two-bag regimen is increased to 200 mg/kg over 16 hours.[19,27] However, the one-bag infusion, oral regimen, or SNAP 12-hour regimen continued to 20 hours (by repeating 200 mg/kg over 10-hour infusion) routinely administer higher doses of acetylcysteine (see **Fig. 3**, **Table 1**).

Some authors have theorized based on NAPQI conversion rates that even higher doses of acetylcysteine may be required for some patients. For example, those with extremely high acetaminophen concentrations more than triple and quadruple the nomogram line perhaps should receive triple and quadruple doses of acetylcysteine.[8,48] These proposals for simple multiples according to the nomogram are based on "educated" assumptions rather than evidence and assume that pharmacokinetic parameters remain much the same despite the massive ingestions.

Extended/Modified Release

Modified-release acetaminophen formulations differ significantly between countries with (at least) two different formulations. In Australia, Europe, and Asia the common modified-release acetaminophen formulation contains 665 mg of acetaminophen of which 69% is slow-release and 31% immediate-release in a bilayer tablet. In the United States an extended-release formulation contains 650 mg of acetaminophen in a 50:50 ratio of immediate to extended release. Management guidelines for these preparations were initially based on data from volunteer studies and extrapolation of immediate-release overdose guidelines.

Both products have been subject to simulated human volunteer studies of supra-therapeutic (subtoxic) doses of acetaminophen (75 mg/kg).[51–54] The two human volunteer studies of the US product showed differing results despite similar methods.[51,52] One found a lower area under the curve (AUC) and peak concentration

(Cmax) when compared with immediate-release acetaminophen.[52] The other found the AUC to be similar for both preparations.[51] Both studies reported the time to Cmax (Tmax) was not delayed with the extended-release preparation. This finding contrasts with the two human volunteer studies of the 665-mg (69% SR; 31% IR) modified-release preparation. Both found the modified-release preparation to have a reduced AUC and Cmax and a significantly later Tmax approximately 2.8 hours versus approximately 1.3 hours when compared with immediate-release acetaminophen.[53,54]

Overdose data of extended-release acetaminophen from the United States are limited; however, there are case reports of initial nontoxic acetaminophen concentrations that later cross above the nomogram line.[55] Thus, the usual single 4-hour acetaminophen concentration is inadequate for risk assessment. An additional concentration at least 4 to 6 hours after the first may detect such patients, and indicate the need for (delayed) treatment.[55]

This approach was initially adopted in some countries treating the modified-release 665 mg (69% SR; 31% IR) preparation[56]; however, patients developed ALI despite standard treatment protocols.[57–59] Some were found to have erratic acetaminophen pharmacokinetics with persistently high concentrations and double peaks.[57,58] Activated charcoal and increased acetylcysteine did not substantially mitigate the risk of ALI.[58] The optimum management for this preparation is still unknown; the current approach is to treat based on dose ingested rather than acetaminophen concentration.[19,57] All toxic ingestions receive a full course of acetylcysteine and large overdoses greater than or equal to 30 g receive increased acetylcysteine.[19]

Repeated Supratherapeutic Acetaminophen Ingestion

RSTI of acetaminophen, also referred to in some literature as chronic or staggered ingestion, is a significant cause of acetaminophen-related morbidity and mortality. It typically involves patients ingesting multiple doses for therapeutic purposes. Staggered or multiple ingestion may refer to an acute ingestion over more than 1 to 2 hours for the purpose of deliberate self-harm. There is no single agreed on definition, with varying dose and timing thresholds used. Dosing thresholds proposed include any supratherapeutic ingestions over hours or days, or are based on dose ingested per day (ie, $\geq$75 mg/kg per 24 hours, $\geq$10 g or 200 mg/kg [whichever is less] in 24 hours, or $\geq$12 g or 300 mg/kg [whichever is less] over a single 48-hour period), or are based on dose (greater than or equal to a daily therapeutic dose) and symptoms of possible liver injury (ie, vomiting, nausea, or abdominal pain).[19–21,60] Regardless of the exact term accidental, staggered, RSTI, and chronic overdoses who present to hospital when symptoms develop have a high rate of hepatotoxicity.[61] The delay in presentation and hence delay in antidotal treatment is a likely contributor.

Risk assessment is guided by symptoms and biochemistry. Minor subclinical elevations of serum ALT/AST are common with prolonged therapy.[62] Hepatotoxicity has been reported at doses within the therapeutic range and in some cases less. Some patients are likely to have increased risk caused by glutathione depletion or CYP450 induction.[63] Clinical risk factors include pregnancy; prolonged fasting; malnutrition; chronic alcohol use; febrile illness; and chronic use of CYP450-inducing drugs, such as carbamazepine.[63,64]

The acetaminophen treatment nomogram is not useful for RSTI (or staggered/multiple ingestions). Management in some protocols is based on dose ingested, symptoms of ALI, acetaminophen concentration, and ALT or AST. Patients presenting with an ALT less than 50 U/L and an acetaminophen concentration less than 20 mg/

L are at very low risk of developing hepatotoxicity.[60,65] Those who develop ALI commonly have an elevated ALT or AST greater than 50 U/L on presentation.[65] Based on this evidence, many countries recommend initiating acetylcysteine only in those with increased acetaminophen concentration or ALT/AST.[19,21,60] In contrast others recommend treating everyone.[20,66]

Extracorporeal Removal

In the initial management of acetaminophen poisoning, extracorporeal treatment (ECTR) is rarely indicated for the removal of acetaminophen. This should not be confused with dialysis as a supportive measure in the context of ALF. An international consensus guideline recommends ECTR for acetaminophen removal in those with signs of early mitochondrial failure (ie, early coma, elevated lactate concentration, and metabolic acidosis) and an acetaminophen concentration greater than 900 mg/L (5960 μmol/L).[67] The rationale was that standard acetylcysteine regimens may be insufficient to prevent ALI in this setting.[67] However, increased doses of acetylcysteine alone may be sufficient to prevent ALI.[8,48] If used, intermittent hemodialysis (IHD) has a much higher clearance (extraction ratio of ~50%–60%) than continuous renal-replacement therapy and is the preferred modality.[67]

Acetylcysteine is dialyzable, and this also varies according to the ECTR modality. Up to 25% of acetylcysteine is extracted by continuous renal-replacement therapy and up to 50% with IHD. Hence, acetylcysteine doses need to be doubled for patients on IHD.[68]

Early Risk Stratification

The aminotransferases are the current biomarkers usually used to indicate ALI; however, they are slow to rise. An ALT or AST at 24 hours postingestion is often performed to exclude an evolving ALI because it may not be elevated earlier. Ideally risk stratification methods would identify those at higher risk of developing ALI much earlier, and thus provide an opportunity to augment standard treatment protocols. There are many proposed risk stratification tools (**Table 2**) that may be superior in stratifying risk of ALI at presentation, but none have progressed into widespread use.

Currently, patient history, the initial acetaminophen concentration, and aminotransaminases guide most acetylcysteine treatment decisions.[19–21] The acetaminophen ratio (the initial acetaminophen concentration/the nomogram line acetaminophen concentration), is currently used to guide increased acetylcysteine doses in some centers.[19,48] Several modifications to these traditional strategies (acetaminophen-aminotransferase multiplication product; psi parameter; and a combination of initial acetaminophen ratio, ALT, and time to treatment) have been shown to predict outcome better in cohort studies (see **Table 2**)[69–74] The advantage of these tools is that they could easily be integrated into current management protocols because they use available tests. Possible uses for these risk stratification tools would be to guide shorter courses or ongoing need for acetylcysteine in RSTI.[65,71] Future studies should examine the temporal profile and optimal window of these risk stratification tools to predict ALI and whether routine use could improve patient outcomes.

Acute Liver Injury

Acetaminophen is a common cause of ALF. A study from the United States found the prevalence of ALI among patients admitted for acetaminophen overdose was 7.2%, with 10% of these developing severe liver failure.[75,76] Early symptoms of ALI include nausea, vomiting, abdominal pain, and right upper quadrant tenderness. The most important risk factor is the extent of delay beyond 8 hours for acetylcysteine to be

Table 2
Traditional strategies and modifications to these strategies for stratification of acute liver injury in acetaminophen poisoning

Biomarker	Description	Pros	Cons	Use/Proposed Use
Traditional strategies				
ALT and/or AST	Hepatic injury biomarker	Widely available Rapid to perform	Not liver or acetaminophen specific Can remain normal for up to 24 h	Current hepatic biomarker
Acetaminophen concentration vs nomogram)[15,16]	Acetaminophen specific	Widely available Rapid to perform Guides acetylcysteine treatment in acute ingestion	Does not indicate liver injury Limited usefulness in RSTI or unknown time of ingestion Can be undetectable in late presenters (>24 h)	Used to indicate need for treatment
Modifications to these strategies (highly feasible, but less commonly used in practice)				
Acetaminophen-aminotransferase multiplication product[65,70–72]	Multiplication of acetaminophen concentration × greater value of AST or ALT	Does not rely on knowing time since ingestion Can be used regardless of preparation or type of ingestion	Has not yet been integrated into treatment protocols	Cutoff values proposed: 1500 mg/L × U/L (10,000 µmol/L × IU/L) and 10,000 mg/L × U/L (66,000 µmol/L × IU/L) Could be used to guide management (eg, when to discontinue or intensify treatment)
Acetaminophen ratio/ nomogram zone[8,19,27,48–50]	Ratio of the acetaminophen concentration compared with the North American (150 mg at 4 h) nomogram line	Uses readily available data: the initial acetaminophen concentration and the acetaminophen nomogram	Can only be used in acute ingestions with a known time of ingestion	Currently used by the Australian and New Zealand acetaminophen guidelines to guide increased acetylcysteine dose Higher acetaminophen ratios may require even larger acetylcysteine doses

AST/ALT ratio[11-13]	Serial measurements examining AST/ALT ratio	Uses serial measurements of ALT and AST, which are readily available	Requires serial testing AST/ALT ratio has yet to be validated in a large dataset or used in clinical protocols to guide need for transfer to a liver unit or identify the sickest patients	AST/ALT typically rise in 1:1 ratio except in the sickest patients An AST/ALT ratio >2 in the absence of rhabdomyolysis may indicate a worse prognosis
Half-life/nomogram line crossing[86,87]	Repeat acetaminophen concentrations	Uses readily available test to identify high-risk patients High-risk patients are those that cross into higher zones and low-risk are those who cross into a lower zone	Not commonly integrated into treatment protocols	Longer acetaminophen half-life correlates with increasing liver injury Proposed that nomogram line/zone crossing could be used to guide treatment
Psi parameter/psi nomogram[69,72]	Pharmacokinetic-derived model using acetaminophen concentration and time to treatment	Uses readily available data to help predict risk of ALI	Requires data to be entered into an equation and can only be used in acute ingestions of known time Equation based on assumptions, such as time to deplete intrahepatic glutathione of 6 h, patients with early acetylcysteine treatment and lower acetaminophen concentrations are unlikely to develop hepatotoxicity	Rarely used clinically to predict patients at low or high risk of hepatotoxicity

(continued on next page)

Table 2
(continued)

Biomarker	Description	Pros	Cons	Use/Proposed Use
Acetaminophen ratio, ALT, and time to treatment[73]	Risk prediction model using acetaminophen ratio, ALT, and time to treatment	Uses readily available data to help predict risk of ALI	Model still requires further development for clinicians to use Requires validation in other acetaminophen overdose datasets	Initial acetaminophen ratio improved prediction of hepatotoxicity and INR ≥2, when used with current known risk factors of initial ALT and time to presentation

> **Box 1**
> **Criteria Adopted in King's College Hospital for Liver Transplantation in Fulminant Hepatic Failure Acetaminophen Criteria**
>
> King's College Criteria
>   pH <7.30 (irrespective of grade of encephalopathy) after fluid resuscitation
>   OR
>   Prothrombin time >100 seconds (INR >6.5) and serum creatinine greater than 300 μmol/L in patients with grade III or IV encephalopathy
>
> Modified King's College Criteria
>   Criteria as above
>   OR
>   Arterial lactate concentration greater than 3.5 mmol/L after early resuscitation (4 hours)
>   OR
>   pH <7.3 OR lactate >3.0 mmol/L after fluid resuscitation (12 hours after admission)

commenced. Other risk factors include a high initial acetaminophen concentration, hepatitis C, nonalcoholic fatty liver disease, alcoholic liver disease, age older than 40 years, and malnutrition.[50,76,77]

Management of acetaminophen ALI involves prolonged acetylcysteine infusion typically at a dose of 100 mg/kg over 16 hours. The length of treatment varies among guidelines but is determined by clinical and biochemical parameters including clinical improvement, decline in aminotransaminases, low or undetectable acetaminophen concentration, and INR typically lower than 1.3 to 2.0.[19,39]

Most patients recover following acetaminophen overdose with a small number developing severe ALI, hepatic encephalopathy, and consequently ALF.[78] Since the late-1980s, survival from acetaminophen-induced ALF has markedly improved because of improvements in intensive care treatment, earlier illness recognition, and use of emergency orthotopic liver transplantation (OLT) in those expected to die.[79] Over this same period, transplant-free survival in those with acetaminophen-induced ALF has improved to nearly 70%.[3,80] However, in those who develop irreversible liver damage, the ultimate treatment is OLT. The decision to transplant involves balancing the risks associated with delaying listing for transplant against the potential for spontaneous recovery with medical treatment alone, the risks of surgery, the scarcity of donor organs, and the requirement for lifelong immunosuppression.[81] Various criteria have been proposed to determine which patients with ALF should be referred for OLT. The most widely used are the King's College Criteria (KCC) or modified KCC (**Box 1**).[14,82] The KCC have good negative predictive value but many who meet these criteria are too medically unwell for transplant.[81,83] Furthermore, survival rates of patients who met KCC from centers other than King's College are much higher than the 13% initially reported,[14,83] with some centers reporting a survival rate without transplant of 50% or greater.[79,80] Criteria for OLT that have a much higher positive predictive value (for death without transplant) are required.[83] Alternatives or adjuncts to the KCC include lactate, phosphate (a marker of liver regeneration),[84] INR, Sequential Organ Failure Assessment,[85] or novel hepatic biomarkers.

SUMMARY

Acetaminophen is a common drug taken in overdose and a common cause of ALI. Most patients make a full recovery with antidotal treatment and good supportive care. However, acetaminophen poisoning is still a significant cause of morbidity because of its wide availability. Future research should focus on optimal acetylcysteine doses for high- and low-risk patients and more accurate criteria to predict death in those with ALF. Despite acetaminophen being one of the most common poisonings, there is a lack of national guidelines/recommendations in the United States (and many other countries). The simple standardized management used for many decades may have made these seem unnecessary. The rapid recent increase in the amount and complexity of evidence to guide treatment means it may now be warranted to have a coordinated strategy to translate new evidence into practice.

CLINICS CARE POINTS

- Patients at risk of ALI should receive intravenous acetylcysteine.

- The acetaminophen nomogram is used to assess the need for treatment in acute immediate-release acetaminophen ingestions with a known time of ingestion and is not validated in other scenarios.

- Activated charcoal within 2 hours of an acute acetaminophen ingestion decreases acetaminophen absorption and the need for antidote treatment.

- The traditional three-bag intravenous acetylcysteine dosage regimen (300 mg/kg over 21 hours), although efficacious in most patients, is associated with a high rate of adverse effects. Newer regimens, such as the SNAP 12-hour regimen and the two-bag acetylcysteine regimen, have a decreased rate of adverse reactions with similar efficacy (noninferiority).

- Patients with very high initial acetaminophen concentrations are at increased risk of ALI regardless of time to treatment. This risk is mitigated by activated charcoal in those presenting within 4 hours of ingestion or increased acetylcysteine dose in those with initial acetaminophen concentrations greater than double the 150 mg/L at 4-hour nomogram line.

- Most patients recover following acetaminophen overdose with a small number developing severe ALF. Over the past decade there has been a vast improvement in transplant-free survival in those with ALF secondary to acetaminophen.

DISCLOSURE

The authors have no financial or other conflicts of interest relevant to this article to disclose.

REFERENCES

1. Cairns RBJ, Wylie CE, Dawson AH, et al. Paracetamol poisoning in Australia, 2004-2017: an analysis of overdose frequency, overdose size, liver injury and deaths. Med J Aust 2019;211(5):218–23.
2. Gummin DD, Mowry JB, Spyker DA, et al. 2018 annual report of the American Association of Poison Control Centers' National Poison Data System (NPDS): 36th annual report. Clin Toxicol (Phila) 2019;57(12):1220–413.
3. Reuben A, Tillman H, Fontana RJ, et al. Outcomes in adults with acute liver failure between 1998 and 2013: an observational cohort study. Ann Intern Med 2016; 164(11):724–32.
4. Lancaster EM, Hiatt JR, Zarrinpar A. Acetaminophen hepatotoxicity: an updated review. Arch Toxicol 2015;89(2):193–9.
5. Prescott LF. Kinetics and metabolism of paracetamol and phenacetin. Br J Clin Pharmacol 1980;10(Suppl 2):291s–8s.

6. Jones AL. Mechanism of action and value of N-acetylcysteine in the treatment of early and late acetaminophen poisoning: a critical review. Clin Toxicol (Phila) 1998;36(4):277–85.

7. Mitchell JR, Jollow DJ, Potter WZ, et al. Acetaminophen-induced hepatic necrosis: role of drug metabolism. J Pharmacol Exp Ther 1973;187(1):185–94.

8. Rumack BH, Bateman DN. Acetaminophen and acetylcysteine dose and duration: past, present and future. Clin Toxicol (Phila) 2012;50(2):91–8.

9. Buckley NA, Whyte IM, O'Connell DL, et al. Activated charcoal reduces the need for N-acetylcysteine treatment after acetaminophen (paracetamol) overdose. Clin Toxicol (Phila) 1999;37(6):753–7.

10. Kwan D, Bartle WR, Walker SE. Abnormal serum transaminases following therapeutic doses of acetaminophen in the absence of known risk factors. Dig Dis Sci 1995;40(9):1951–5.

11. Curtis RM, Sivilotti ML. A descriptive analysis of aspartate and alanine aminotransferase rise and fall following acetaminophen overdose. Clin Toxicol (Phila) 2015;53(9):849–55.

12. Green TJ, Sivilotti ML, Langmann C, et al. When do the aminotransferases rise after acute acetaminophen overdose? Clin Toxicol (Phila) 2010;48(8):787–92.

13. McGovern AJ, Vitkovitsky IV, Jones DL, et al. Can AST/ALT ratio indicate recovery after acute paracetamol poisoning? Clin Toxicol (Phila) 2015;53(3):164–7.

14. O'Grady JG, Alexander GJ, Hayllar KM, et al. Early indicators of prognosis in fulminant hepatic failure. Gastroenterology 1989;97(2):439–45.

15. Prescott LF, Park J, Ballantyne A, et al. Treatment of paracetamol (acetaminophen) poisoning with N-acetylcysteine. Lancet 1977;2(8035):432–4.

16. Prescott LF, Illingworth RN, Critchley JA, et al. Intravenous N-acetylcysteine: the treatment of choice for paracetamol poisoning. Br Med J 1979;2(6198):1097–100.

17. Gunnell D, Hawton K, Murray V, et al. Use of paracetamol for suicide and non-fatal poisoning in the UK and France: are restrictions on availability justified? J Epidemiol Community Health 1997;51(2):175–9.

18. Shah AD, Wood DM, Dargan PI. Understanding lactic acidosis in paracetamol (acetaminophen) poisoning. Br J Clin Pharmacol 2011;71(1):20–8.

19. Chiew AL, Reith D, Pomerleau A, et al. Updated guidelines for the management of paracetamol poisoning in Australia and New Zealand. Med J Aust 2020;212(4): 175–83.

20. Dalhoff K, Andersen J, Clemmensen O, et al. Treatment of paracetamol poisoning: a new guideline. Rational Pharmacotherapy No. 2. 2013. Available at: https://www.sst.dk/da/udgivelser/2013/rationel-farmakoterapi-2-2013/behan dling-af-paracetamolforgiftning–en-ny-guideline. Accessed November 3, 2020.

21. Ministry of Health, Singapore. Management of poisoning. 2011. Available at: https://www.moh.gov.sg/docs/librariesprovider4/guidelines/management-of-pois oning—summary-card.pdf. Accessed November 3, 2020.

22. Chiew AL, Gluud C, Brok J, et al. Interventions for paracetamol (acetaminophen) overdose. Cochrane Database Syst Rev 2018;2:CD003328.

23. Underhill TJ, Greene MK, Dove AF. A comparison of the efficacy of gastric lavage, ipecacuanha and activated charcoal in the emergency management of paracetamol overdose. Arch Acad Emerg Med 1990;7(3):148–54.

24. Yeates PJ, Thomas SH. Effectiveness of delayed activated charcoal administration in simulated paracetamol (acetaminophen) overdose. Br J Clin Pharmacol 2000;49(1):11–4.

25. Christophersen AB, Levin D, Hoegberg LCG, et al. Activated charcoal alone or after gastric lavage: a simulated large paracetamol intoxication. Br J Clin Pharmacol 2002;53(3):312–7.

26. Duffull SB, Isbister GK. Predicting the requirement for N-acetylcysteine in paracetamol poisoning from reported dose. Clin Toxicol (Phila) 2013;51(8):772–6.

27. Chiew AL, Isbister GK, Kirby KA, et al. Massive paracetamol overdose: an observational study of the effect of activated charcoal and increased acetylcysteine dose(ATOM-2). Clin Toxicol (Phila) 2017;55(10):1055–65.

28. Agrawal S. Acetaminophen toxicity.[updated 2020 sep 15]. In: StatPearls [Internet]. Treasure Island(FL): StatPearls Publishing; 2020. Available at: https://www.ncbi.nlm.nih.gov/books/NBK441917/. Accessed November 1, 2020.

29. Douglas AP, Hamlyn AN, James O. Controlled trial of cysteamine in treatment of acute paracetamol (acetaminophen) poisoning. Lancet 1976;1(7951):111–5.

30. Hamlyn AN, Lesna M, Record CO, et al. Methionine and cysteamine in paracetamol (acetaminophen) overdose, prospective controlled trial of early therapy. J Int Med Res 1981;9(3):226–31.

31. Olsson B, Johansson M, Gabrielsson J, et al. Pharmacokinetics and bioavailability of reduced and oxidized N-acetylcysteine. Eur J Clin Pharmacol 1988; 34(1):77–82.

32. Prescott LF, Donovan JW, Jarvie DR, et al. The disposition and kinetics of intravenous N-acetylcysteine in patients with paracetamol overdosage. Eur J Clin Pharmacol 1989;37(5):501–6.

33. Buckpitt AR, Rollins DE, Mitchell JR. Varying effects of sulfhydryl nucleophiles on acetaminophen oxidation and sulfhydryl adduct formation. Biochem Pharmacol 1979;28(19):2941–6.

34. Chiew AL, Isbister GK, Duffull SB, et al. Evidence for the changing regimens of acetylcysteine. Br J Clin Pharmacol 2016;81(3):471–81.

35. Sandilands EA, Bateman DN. Adverse reactions associated with acetylcysteine. Clin Toxicol (Phila) 2009;47(2):81–8.

36. Bateman DN, Dear JW, Thanacoody HK, et al. Reduction of adverse effects from intravenous acetylcysteine treatment for paracetamol poisoning: a randomised controlled trial. Lancet 2014;383(9918):697–704.

37. Wong A, Graudins A. Simplification of the standard three-bag intravenous acetylcysteine regimen for paracetamol poisoning results in a lower incidence of adverse drug reactions. Clin Toxicol (Phila) 2016;54(2):115–9.

38. Schmidt LE, Rasmussen DN, Petersen TS, et al. Fewer adverse effects associated with a modified two-bag intravenous acetylcysteine protocol compared to traditional three-bag regimen in paracetamol overdose. Clin Toxicol (Phila) 2018;56(11):1128–34.

39. Pettie JM, Caparrotta TM, Hunter RW, et al. Safety and efficacy of the SNAP 12-hour acetylcysteine regimen for the treatment of paracetamol overdose. EClinicalMedicine 2019;11:11–7.

40. Wong A, Isbister G, McNulty R, et al. Efficacy of a two-bag acetylcysteine regimen to treat paracetamol overdose (2NAC study). EClinicalMedicine 2020; 20:100288.

41. Michael E, Mullins MY, O'Grady L, et al. Adverse reactions in patients treated with the one-bag method of N-acetylcysteine for acetaminophen ingestion. Toxicol Commun 2020;4(1):49–54.

42. Johnson MT, McCammon CA, Mullins ME, et al. Evaluation of a simplified N-acetylcysteine dosing regimen for the treatment of acetaminophen toxicity. Ann Pharmacother 2011;45(6):713–20.

43. Oakley E, Robinson J, Deasy C. Using 0.45% saline solution and a modified dosing regimen for infusing N-acetylcysteine in children with paracetamol poisoning. Emerg Med Australas 2011;23(1):63–7.

44. Pauley KA, Sandritter TL, Lowry JA, et al. Evaluation of an alternative intravenous N-acetylcysteine regimen in pediatric patients. J Pediatr Pharmacol Ther 2015; 20(3):178–85.

45. Green JL, Heard KJ, Reynolds KM, et al. Oral and intravenous acetylcysteine for treatment of acetaminophen toxicity: a systematic review and meta-analysis. West J Emerg Med 2013;14(3):218–26.

46. Buckley NA, Whyte IM, O'Connell DL, et al. Oral or intravenous N-acetylcysteine: which is the treatment of choice for acetaminophen (paracetamol) poisoning? Clin Toxicol (Phila) 1999;37(6):759–67.

47. Betten DP, Burner EE, Thomas SC, et al. A retrospective evaluation of shortened-duration oral N-acetylcysteine for the treatment of acetaminophen poisoning. J Med Toxicol 2009;5(4):183–90.

48. Hendrickson RG. What is the most appropriate dose of N-acetylcysteine after massive acetaminophen overdose? Clin Toxicol (Phila) 2019;57(8):686–91.

49. Marks DJB, Dargan PI, Archer JRH, et al. Outcomes from massive paracetamol overdose: a retrospective observational study. Br J Clin Pharmacol 2017;83(6): 1263–72.

50. Cairney DG, Beckwith HK, Al-Hourani K, et al. Plasma paracetamol concentration at hospital presentation has a dose-dependent relationship with liver injury despite prompt treatment with intravenous acetylcysteine. Clin Toxicol (Phila) 2016;54(5):405–10.

51. Stork CM, Rees S, Howland MA, et al. Pharmacokinetics of extended relief vs regular release Tylenol in simulated human overdose. Clin Toxicol (Phila) 1996;34(2): 157–62.

52. Douglas DR, Sholar JB, Smilkstein MJ. A pharmacokinetic comparison of acetaminophen products (Tylenol Extended Relief vs regular Tylenol). Acad Emerg Med 1996;3(8):740–4.

53. Chiew A, Day P, Salonikas C, et al. The comparative pharmacokinetics of modified-release and immediate-release paracetamol in a simulated overdose model. Emerg Med Australas 2010;22(6):548–55.

54. Tan C, Graudins A. Comparative pharmacokinetics of Panadol extend and immediate-release paracetamol in a simulated overdose model. Emerg Med Australas 2006;18(4):398–403.

55. Cetaruk EW, Dart RC, Hurlbut KM, et al. Tylenol extended relief overdose. Ann Emerg Med 1997;30(1):104–8.

56. Chiew AL, Fountain JS, Graudins A, et al. Guidelines for the management of paracetamol poisoning in Australia and New Zealand. Med J Aust 2015;203(5):215–8.

57. Salmonson H, Sjoberg G, Brogren J. The standard treatment protocol for paracetamol poisoning may be inadequate following overdose with modified release formulation: a pharmacokinetic and clinical analysis of 53 cases. Clin Toxicol (Phila) 2018;56(1):63–8.

58. Chiew AL, Isbister GK, Page CB, et al. Modified release paracetamol overdose: a prospective observational study (ATOM-3). Clin Toxicol (Phila) 2018;56(9):810–9.

59. Graudins A, Chiew A, Chan B. Overdose with modified-release paracetamol results in delayed and prolonged absorption of paracetamol. Intern Med J 2010; 40(1):72–6.

60. Daly FF, O'Malley GF, Heard K, et al. Prospective evaluation of repeated supratherapeutic acetaminophen (paracetamol) ingestion. Ann Emerg Med 2004; 44(4):393–8.
61. Craig DG, Bates CM, Davidson JS, et al. Staggered overdose pattern and delay to hospital presentation are associated with adverse outcomes following paracetamol-induced hepatotoxicity. Br J Clin Pharmacol 2012;73(2):285–94.
62. Watkins PB, Kaplowitz N, Slattery JT, et al. Aminotransferase elevations in healthy adults receiving 4 grams of acetaminophen daily: a randomized controlled trial. JAMA 2006;296(1):87–93.
63. Caparrotta TM, Antoine DJ, Dear JW. Are some people at increased risk of paracetamol-induced liver injury? A critical review of the literature. Eur J Clin Pharmacol 2018;74(2):147–60.
64. Kalsi SS, Dargan PI, Waring WS, et al. A review of the evidence concerning hepatic glutathione depletion and susceptibility to hepatotoxicity after paracetamol overdose. Open Access Emerg Med 2011;3:87–96.
65. Egan H, Isbister GK, Robinson J, et al. Retrospective evaluation of repeated supratherapeutic ingestion of paracetamol. Clin Toxicol (Phila) 2019;57(8): 703–11.
66. BMJ Publishing Group. BMJ best practice: paracetamol overdose in adults 2020. Available at: https://bestpractice.bmj.com.acs.hcn.com.au/topics/en-gb/ 3000110. Accessed December 3, 2020.
67. Gosselin S, Juurlink DN, Kielstein JT, et al. Extracorporeal treatment for acetaminophen poisoning: recommendations from the EXTRIP workgroup. Clin Toxicol (Phila) 2014;52(8):856–67.
68. Hernandez SH, Howland M, Schiano TD, et al. The pharmacokinetics and extracorporeal removal of N-acetylcysteine during renal replacement therapies. Clin Toxicol (Phila) 2015;53(10):941–9.
69. Sivilotti ML, Good AM, Yarema MC, et al. A new predictor of toxicity following acetaminophen overdose based on pretreatment exposure. Clin Toxicol (Phila) 2005;43(4):229–34.
70. Sivilotti ML, Green TJ, Langmann C, et al. Multiplying the serum aminotransferase by the acetaminophen concentration to predict toxicity following overdose. Clin Toxicol (Phila) 2010;48(8):793–9.
71. Wong A, Sivilotti ML, Dargan PI, et al. External validation of the paracetamol-aminotransferase multiplication product to predict hepatotoxicity from paracetamol overdose. Clin Toxicol (Phila) 2015;53(8):807–14.
72. Chomchai S, Chomchai C. Predicting acute acetaminophen hepatotoxicity with acetaminophen-aminotransferase multiplication product and the Psi parameter. Clin Toxicol (Phila) 2014;52(5):506–11.
73. Chiew AL, James LP, Isbister GK, et al. Early acetaminophen-protein adducts predict hepatotoxicity following overdose (ATOM-5). J Hepatol 2020;72(3): 450–62.
74. Sivilotti ML, Yarema MC, Juurlink DN, et al. A risk quantification instrument for acute acetaminophen overdose patients treated with N-acetylcysteine. Ann Emerg Med 2005;46(3):263–71.
75. Blieden M, Paramore LC, Shah D, et al. A perspective on the epidemiology of acetaminophen exposure and toxicity in the United States. Expert Rev Clin Pharmacol 2014;7(3):341–8.
76. Nguyen GC, Sam J, Thuluvath PJ. Hepatitis C is a predictor of acute liver injury among hospitalizations for acetaminophen overdose in the United States: a nationwide analysis. Hepatology 2008;48(4):1336–41.

77. Rotundo L, Pyrsopoulos N. Liver injury induced by paracetamol and challenges associated with intentional and unintentional use. World J Hepatol 2020;12(4): 125–36.
78. Craig DG, Bates CM, Davidson JS, et al. Overdose pattern and outcome in paracetamol-induced acute severe hepatotoxicity. Br J Clin Pharmacol 2011; 71(2):273–82.
79. Bernal W, Hyyrylainen A, Gera A, et al. Lessons from look-back in acute liver failure? A single centre experience of 3300 patients. J Hepatol 2013;59(1):74–80.
80. Hey P, Hanrahan TP, Sinclair M, et al. Epidemiology and outcomes of acute liver failure in Australia. World J Hepatol 2019;11(7):586–95.
81. Craig DG, Ford AC, Hayes PC, et al. Systematic review: prognostic tests of paracetamol-induced acute liver failure. Aliment Pharmacol Ther 2010;31(10): 1064–76.
82. Bernal W, Donaldson N, Wyncoll D, et al. Blood lactate as an early predictor of outcome in paracetamol-induced acute liver failure: a cohort study. Lancet 2002;359(9306):558–63.
83. Ding GKA, Buckley NA. Evidence and consequences of spectrum bias in studies of criteria for liver transplant in paracetamol hepatotoxicity. QJM 2008;101(9): 723–9.
84. Schmidt LE, Dalhoff K. Serum phosphate is an early predictor of outcome in severe acetaminophen-induced hepatotoxicity. Hepatology 2002;36(3):659–65.
85. Cholongitas E, Theocharidou E, Vasianopoulou P, et al. Comparison of the sequential organ failure assessment score with the King's College Hospital criteria and the model for end-stage liver disease score for the prognosis of acetaminophen-induced acute liver failure. Liver Transpl 2012;18(4):405–12.
86. Schiodt FV, Ott P, Christensen E, et al. The value of plasma acetaminophen half-life in antidote-treated acetaminophen overdosage. Clin Pharmacol Ther 2002; 71(4):221–5.
87. Mutsaers A, Green JP, Sivilotti MLA, et al. Changing nomogram risk zone classification with serial testing after acute acetaminophen overdose: a retrospective database analysis. Clin Toxicol (Phila) 2019;57(6):380–6.

Cardiovascular Drug Toxicity

Maude St-Onge, MD, PhD, FRCPC

KEYWORDS

- Cardiotoxicants • Cardiotoxic • Calcium channel blockers • Beta-blockers
- Cardiac glycosides • Overdose • Poisoning • Intoxication

KEY POINTS

- Treatment algorithms are outlined for calcium channel blocker and beta-blocker poisonings.
- Two different approaches are suggested for management of cardiac glycoside toxicity depending on whether the patient presents with an acute overdose or chronic toxicity.
- A treatment approach is proposed for sodium channel blocker poisoning, although supportive evidence is sparse.

INTRODUCTION

Nature of the Problem

Cardiovascular drugs are among the substances most frequently involved in human poisoning exposures. As per the American Association of Poison Control Centers' National Poison Data System,[1] cases with serious outcomes increased significantly from 2000 to 2016. These exposures have been associated with many fatalities in single-substance poisonings in 2016 involving calcium channel blockers (CCBs; 3.2%), beta-blockers (BBs; 1.85%), and miscellaneous cardiovascular drugs (3.54%).

While managing these unstable patients, clinicians often report cognitive overload related in part to the significant amount of data requiring processing.[2] Better knowledge of cardiovascular drug toxicity and an integrated, structured approach to manage these patients are key to improving outcomes. To this end, the Centre Antipoison du Québec has developed a checklist to help clinicians manage unstable poisoned patients.[3]

The current article focuses on the specific interventions related to toxicity of CCBs, BBs, cardiac glycosides, and sodium channel blockers.

Definitions, Pharmacology, and Clinical Manifestations

The Vaughan Williams classification of antidysrhythmic agents includes 4 classes.[4,5] (**Fig. 1**). The first class includes sodium channel blockers with moderate prolongation

CIUSSSCN, Optimal Health Practice Research Unit, Trauma – Emergency – Critical Care Medicine, CHU de Québec Research Centre, CHU de Québec – Université Laval, Faculty of Medicine, Université Laval, Centre Antipoison du Québec, 1270 Chemin Sainte-Foy, Pavillon Jeffrey-Hale, 3e étage, Québec G1S 2M4, Canada
E-mail address: maude.st-onge@fmed.ulaval.ca

Crit Care Clin 37 (2021) 563–576
https://doi.org/10.1016/j.ccc.2021.03.006
0749-0704/21/Crown Copyright © 2021 Published by Elsevier Inc. All rights reserved.

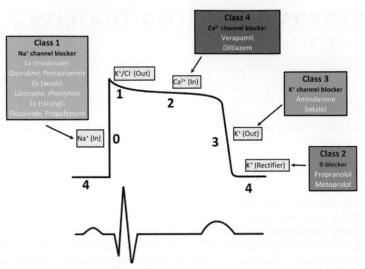

Fig. 1. Drugs affecting the cardiac action potential. (*From* Sundjaja JH, Makaryus AN. Diso-pyramide. 2020 Sep 10. In: StatPearls [Internet]. Treasure Island (FL): StatPearls Publishing; 2021 Jan–. PMID: 32491366; with permission.)

of conduction and repolarization (eg, quinidine, procainamide); minimal effect on conduction and repolarization (eg, lidocaine); or marked prolongation of conduction (eg, flecainide, propafenone). The second class contains BBs (eg, propranolol and atenolol). The third class, not discussed in this article, includes drugs involving a prolongation of repolarization (eg, amiodarone). The fourth class contains CCBs recognized to have an effect on myocardial conduction (eg, verapamil, diltiazem). Some add a fifth class with potential nodal action (eg, digoxin).

CCBs include dihydropyridines, such as amlodipine, and non-dihydropyridines, such as diltiazem or verapamil. At therapeutic doses, dihydropyridines preferentially block calcium channels in vascular smooth muscle, which may result in tachycardia from reflex sympathetic activation.[6] However, in dihydropyridine overdoses, cases presenting with bradycardia, often secondary to loss of selectivity, have been reported.[7] In addition, non-dihydropyridines block calcium channels in cardiac cells, inhibiting the effect of both sinoatrial and atrioventricular nodal tissue.[6]

Therefore, CCB-poisoned patients often present with hypotension and bradycardia from peripheral vasodilation and decreased myocardial contraction. In addition, they can present with hypotension and reflex tachycardia in some cases of dihydropyridine overdoses. When myocardial cells are involved, atrioventricular conduction abnormalities, idioventricular rhythms, complete heart block, and junctional escape rhythms have been observed.[8] CCB-poisoned patients can also present with hyperglycemia, primarily due to the blockade of pancreatic calcium channels and insulin resistance at the cellular level. One retrospective study emphasized that the median peak serum glucose concentrations correlate with the severity of verapamil or diltiazem poisonings.[9]

BBs can be distinguished by their relative affinity for β1 and β2 receptors, intrinsic sympathomimetic activity, blockade of α receptors, differences in lipid solubility, and capacity to induce vasodilatation. First-generation BBs (eg, nadolol, pindolol, propranolol) are nonselective. Second-generation BBs (eg, acebutolol, atenolol, bisoprolol, esmolol, metoprolol) are β1 selective. Third-generation BBs (eg, carvedilol, labetalol) have additional cardiovascular properties (especially vasodilation).[6] Furthermore,

BBs decrease contractility and conduction by blocking β1 receptors. Blockers of β2 receptors increase peripheral vascular resistance, an effect that is opposed in third-generation BBs by their vasodilation effect.

BBs occasionally cause hypoglycemia by interference with glycogenolysis and gluconeogenesis.[10] Moreover, despite the variable myriad of pharmacodynamic actions, BB-poisoned patients always present with at least a decrease in myocardial contraction. Acebutolol, carvedilol, and propranolol inhibit fast sodium channels, which can result in QRS widening in overdoses. Being highly lipid soluble, propranolol is also associated with seizures. Acebutolol and sotalol can prolong QTc and may cause torsades de pointes in overdoses.[10]

Cardiac steroids (digoxin and digitoxin) increase myocardial contraction by increasing intracellular calcium. This effect is indirectly caused by the inhibition of the plasma membrane Na+/K+ ATPase, an enzyme that actively pumps sodium out of and potassium into a cell. By pumping out sodium, this enzyme slightly reduces the gradient across the myocyte membrane, reducing the driving force of calcium (**Fig. 2**). Cardiac steroids have vagotonic and sympatholytic effects. A shorter action potential is observed even at therapeutic levels, which explains the risk of various dysrhythmias in overdoses, except those involving rapid conduction through the sinoatrial and atrioventricular nodes.[6]

Based on the Digitalis Investigation Group (DIG) trial, a serum digoxin concentration of 1.5 nmol/L (1.2 μ g/L) or higher was associated with a hazard ratio (HR) of 1.16 (95% CI, 0.96 – 1.39) when compared with the placebo (HR 1). In contrast, the HR was 0.80 (95% CI, 0.68 – 0.94) for serum digoxin concentrations of 0.6–1 nmol/L (0.5 – 0.8 μ g/L).[11]

In acute toxicity, the first clinical effects are typically nausea, vomiting, abdominal pain, bradycardia, and hypotension. Weakness, lethargy, and confusion also can be observed. In chronic toxicity, similar symptomatology can occur with a more insidious onset. Visual disturbances such as aberrations of color vision (eg, yellow halos around lights) are more typical of chronic toxicity.[12] In acute toxicity, hyperkalemia has important prognostic implications because it reflects how much Na+/K+ ATPase is

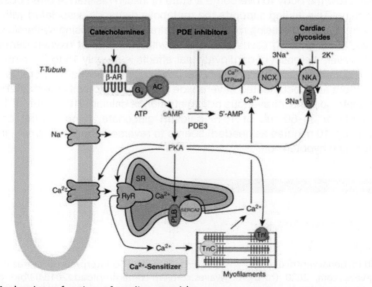

Fig. 2. Mechanism of action of cardiac steroids.

inhibited.[13] In chronic toxicity, hyperkalemia is more often the result of other problems, such as renal failure.[14] Scooping of the ST segment on the electrocardiogram (ECG) mainly occurs with therapeutic use. In toxicity, within all possible dysrhythmias (with the exception of rapidly conducted supraventricular tachydysrhythmias), bidirectional ventricular tachycardia is nearly diagnostic, although not frequent (**Fig. 3**).[15]

Other antidysrhythmics include agents with sodium channel blockade effect. The extent of sodium channel blockade depends on heart rate and membrane potential, as well as drug-specific physicochemical characteristics.[6] Class 1A sodium channel blockers (eg, procainamide, quinidine, disopyramide) have a slow-to-intermediate recovery rate. Class 1B blockers (eg, lidocaine, mexiletine, phenytoin) have a fast rate of recovery. On the other hand, Class 1C blockers (eg, flecainide, propafenone) have a slow recovery rate. Blockade of the sodium channel leads to a delay in the fast influx of sodium, which decreases the slope of Phase 0 of action potential and widens the QRS complex (**Fig. 4**).[16]

Sodium channel blockade manifests as QRS widening with right ventricular delay (shown on the ECG by a prominent R wave in aVR and deep S wave in Lead 1) but can present with different morphologies (**Fig. 5**).

In addition, some antidysrhythmic overdoses will present with a prolonged QTc or torsades de pointes, which reflect a potassium channel blockade (not discussed in this article).

CURRENT EVIDENCE FOR MANAGEMENT INTERVENTIONS
Calcium Channel Blockers

A systematic review conducted in 2014 summarized the existing evidence of the treatment options for CCB poisonings.[17] The risk of bias was high for all interventions, and the quality of evidence was low to very low.

High-dose regular insulin (bolus of 1 unit/kg, followed by an infusion of 0.5 to 2.0 units/kg per hour that can be increased up to 10 units/kg per hour) was associated with improved hemodynamic parameters and lower mortality, but at the risk for both hypoglycemia and hypokalemia. Insulin stimulates glucose entry into myocardial cells, and high doses allow the body to overcome a state of insulin resistance often observed in CCB poisoning. This finding supports the metabolic demands associated with cardiogenic shock, thereby increasing myocardial contractility, decreasing systemic vascular resistances, and improving tissue perfusion[18] with economy of oxygen demand and work.[19] However, the onset of cardiovascular effects is roughly 15 to 30 minutes.[19]

Calcium, dopamine, and norepinephrine improved hemodynamic parameters and survival without any documented severe side effects. By increasing extracellular calcium concentration, the intravenous administration of calcium (10–20 mL of 10% calcium chloride or 30–60 mL of 10% calcium gluconate, if no central access is available, every 10 minutes as needed) seems to reverse negative inotropy, impaired conduction, and hypotension.[8]

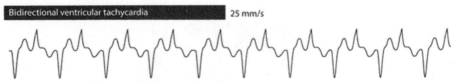

Fig. 3. Bidirectional ventricular tachycardia. (*From* Clinical ECG Interpretation, Araz Rawshani, www.ecgwaves.com, 2020 (https://ecgwaves.com/wp-content/uploads/2016/09/bidirectional_VT.jpg); with permission.)

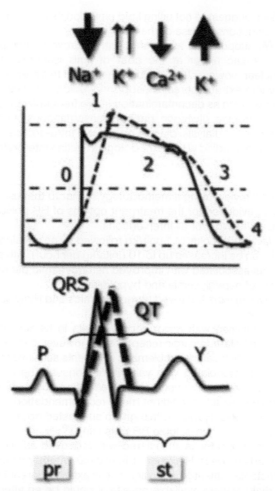

Fig. 4. Sodium channel blockade. (Yates C, Manini AF. Utility of the electrocardiogram in drug overdose and poisoning: theoretical considerations and clinical implications. Curr Cardiol Rev (2012) 8:137-151.)

Lipid emulsion was associated with improved hemodynamic parameters and survival in animal models of intravenous verapamil poisoning but not in models of oral verapamil poisoning. An international expert consensus specifically evaluating the

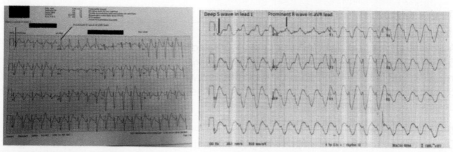

Fig. 5. ECG with manifestations of sodium channel blockade.

uses of lipid emulsion suggested not using lipid emulsion as a first-line therapy but did not make recommendations in case of therapy failure.[20]

Extracorporeal life support was associated with improved survival in patients with severe shock or cardiac arrest at the cost of limb ischemia, thrombosis, and bleeding.[17] It is unclear, however, if it would be beneficial to transport an unstable patient to a facility where extracorporeal life support would be available.

Other interventions, such as decontamination (more frequently the administration of activated charcoal), atropine, glucagon, pacing (transcutaneous or intravenous), levosimendan, hemoperfusion, dialysis, plasma exchange, intra-aortic balloon pump, and the Impella device were studied with methodologies limiting interpretation of results.[17]

Beta-Blockers

In 2020, a systematic review using a methodology similar to that used for CCBs summarized the existing evidence for the treatment options of BB poisonings.[21] In addition, the risk of bias was high for all interventions.

High-dose regular insulin (bolus of 1 unit/kg followed by an infusion of 0.5–2.0 units/kg per hour, which can be increased up to 10 units/kg per hour) with a rationale similar to that for CCBs was associated with improved hemodynamic parameters and lower mortality, at the risk of hypoglycemia and hypokalemia.[21]

Inotropes and vasopressors improved hemodynamics and likely survival in case series and animal studies.[21]

Glucagon was associated with minor improvements in hemodynamics, potentially through bypassing the beta-adrenergic receptor site. However, it is also associated with nausea and vomiting, which can be problematic in patients sensitive to vagal stimuli.[22]

Lipid emulsion was associated with various responses. The international expert consensus specifically evaluating uses of lipid emulsion suggested not to use lipid emulsion as a first-line therapy but did not make recommendations in case of therapy failure for lipid-soluble BBs. However, this group suggested not to use lipid emulsion therapy in all cases of non–lipid-soluble BB poisoning.[20]

Extracorporeal life support was associated with improved survival in patients with severe shock or cardiac arrest. However, it is unclear whether it would be beneficial to transport an unstable patient to a facility where extracorporeal life support would be available.[21] If dialysis were available on-site, it could be an alternative to remove water-soluble BBs, such as atenolol or sotalol, even though no survival or hemodynamic benefit has been established.[21]

Other interventions, such as decontamination (more frequently the administration of activated charcoal), atropine, calcium, and pacing (transcutaneous or intravenous) were studied with methodologies limiting interpretation of results. Levosimendan and amrinone did not seem to yield any benefits.[21]

Cardiac Glycosides

Decontamination

Administration of activated charcoal is associated with a decrease in digoxin levels.[23] Some evidence suggests that digitoxin and digoxin are recirculated enterohepatically, implying that both late and possibly repeated activated charcoal administration (1 g/kg of body weight every 2–4 hours for up to 4 doses) are beneficial in reducing serum concentrations.[12]

Digoxin-Fab

Digoxin-Fab is a monovalent immunoglobulin with an affinity 100 to 1000 times higher for Na+/K+ ATPase than digoxin. Most vials of digoxin-Fab (38–40 mg of Fab) bind approximately 0.5 mg of digoxin within only a few minutes. Digoxin-Fab is removed by both renal clearance and hepatic metabolism.[24] A review published in 2014 reported response rate variations from 80% to 90% to as low as 50%, but the studies used different thresholds to administer the antidote.[24] Moreover, few studies have carefully measured free and bound digoxin concentrations before and after the use of digoxin-Fab. Therefore, there are no current data to establish the lowest effective digoxin-Fab dosing regimen for acute toxicity.

In a prospective chronic toxicity study, 131 patients with elevated digoxin concentration or presenting signs or symptoms of toxicity did not show a mortality benefit with the administration of digoxin-Fab.[25] However, in a similar cohort, the administration of 1 to 2 vials bound all free digoxin with a moderate improvement in heart rate and potassium, suggesting bradydysrhythmia and hyperkalemia may arise from other comorbidities.[26]

Sodium Channel Blockers

Sodium bicarbonate
The exact mechanism by which sodium bicarbonate acts to reverse sodium channel blockade has not been fully elucidated. In general, an increase in sodium concentration and a change in pH may be responsible for the clinical effects that have been mainly documented in animal studies and case reports.[27] In addition, a survey of American Poison Center medical directors found that 71% of directors recommended bolus dosing (1–2 mEq/kg), followed by infusion, and 24% of directors recommended a bolus dose alone.[28] A bolus is more likely to act on extracellular sodium concentration, whereas an infusion is more likely to act on serum pH. Evidence supporting bolus use has been mainly based on animal studies and case reports.[27]

Hypertonic saline
To increase extracellular sodium concentration, the use of hypertonic saline (7.5% saline) also has been studied in animals.[29,30] The evidence for this practice is sparse but gives an alternative in case of contraindications to sodium bicarbonate.

Lipid emulsion
Bupivacaine is a local anesthetic for which results support the efficacy of lipid emulsion. In addition, an international expert consensus[20] recommended its use in case of cardiac arrest due to bupivacaine, failure of other therapies, or as part of other treatment modalities for life-threatening toxicity. For other local anesthetics such as lidocaine (Class I antidysrhythmic), this group suggested lipid emulsion if other therapies failed to control the condition. They did not make recommendations for nonlocal anesthetic antidysrhythmics of first class considering the sparse evidence, although they did suggest not using lipid emulsion as a first-line therapy.

Extracorporeal life support
Cases of extracorporeal life support use have been reported in the management of sodium channel blocker poisonings, mainly in the context of flecainide overdoses.[31–33]

Clinical Relevance of Interventions

Calcium channel blockers
Based on the evidence reported in the systematic review,[17] a workgroup of experts involved in the care of poisoned patients developed evidence-based recommendations to guide the in-hospital management of CCB poisoning.[34] For first-line therapy, they recommended the use of intravenous calcium, high-dose regular insulin, and norepinephrine and/or epinephrine, depending on the type of shock with which the

patient is presenting. In patients refractory to first-line treatments still showing evidence of myocardial dysfunction, high-dose regular insulin can be increased up to 10 U/kg per hour. The algorithm in **Fig. 6** details this suggested approach.[17]

Few options are available for patients poisoned with dihydropyridines presenting with vasoplegic shock. Some may be tempted to use methylene blue, which is believed to treat shock through inhibition of guanylyl cyclase in the nitric oxide pathway. This may make sense for substances increasing nitric oxide such as amlodipine. However, a systematic review of its use for drug-induced shock could not identify a potential benefit of this therapy.[35] Although there have been compelling cases describing improved hemodynamics following the administration of methylene blue, there have also been several cases without observed change. Furthermore, most cases for which lipid emulsion had been administered first did not respond to subsequent administration of methylene blue.[35]

Beta-blockers
Based on previous work regarding CCBs and the results of a more recent systematic review published in 2020, the CCB poisoning management algorithm has been adapted for BB poisoning by the Centre Antipoison du Québec (**Fig. 7**).[36]

Cardiac glycosides
Many drug interactions (eg, verapamil, diltiazem, amiodarone, carvedilol, propafenone, spironolactone, quinidine, macrolides) can exacerbate toxicity of cardiac glycosides and be in part responsible for the development of chronic toxicity. In most cases, the involvement of a pharmacist can be key. A tight control on electrolytes is also important because hypokalemia, hypomagnesemia, and hypercalcemia increase the incidence and severity of intoxication.[37]

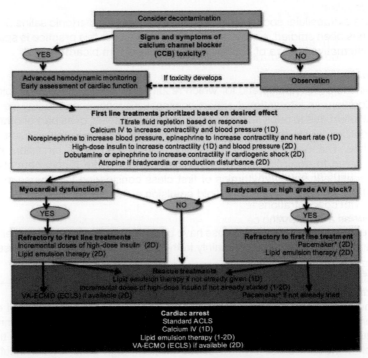

Fig. 6. Algorithm for the management of CCB poisoning.[17]

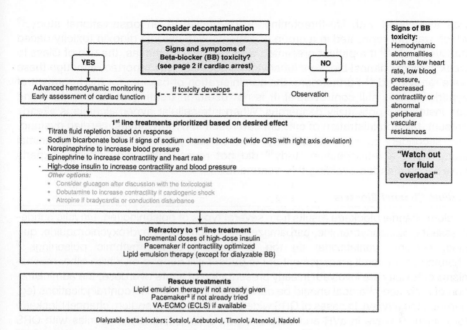

Fig. 7. Algorithm for the management of BB poisoning.[36] [a]In the absence of myocardial dysfunction.

In *acute overdose*, the administration of activated charcoal should be considered if there are no contraindications (eg, unprotected airway). A partial reversal with digoxin-Fab based on an available digoxin concentration or with empirical treatment should be enough for clinical improvement.

Empirical treatment: 2 to 4 vials every 15 to 30 minutes as needed.

Based on digoxin level drawn at least 6 hours after last dose.

Number of vials = (digoxin level in nmol/L × 0.00781) × weight in kg
Number of vials = (digoxin level in ng/L × weight in kg)/100

However, in case of cardiac arrest, a complete reversal should be targeted (10 vials).[38]

In *chronic toxicity*, one vial of digoxin-Fab at a time should be sufficient for reversal.[25]

There is general agreement that digoxin-Fab is indicated for patients with life-threatening tachy-bradydysrhythmias. Additional indications include hemodynamic instability with concentrations (eg, digoxin higher than 2.6 nmol/L or 2 μ g/L) that support digoxin as a contributing cause or hyperkalemia (higher than 5–6 mmol/L) in acute poisoning.[24]

If a digoxin level is assessed, it is recommended to wait up to 6 hours after the last dose to allow the drug to disperse into clinically representative concentrations.[12] There is a 10-fold to 20-fold rise in the total measured digoxin concentration (which includes the Fab-digoxin complex) following the administration of digoxin-Fab for over 32 hours, suggesting prolonged and continuous redistribution of digoxin from the tissue to the plasma.[24] Therefore, dosing based on digoxin levels after the administration of digoxin-Fab is irrelevant.

Supportive measures such as atropine or epinephrine for the treatment of brady-cardia can be considered while waiting for digoxin-Fab; however, cardiac pacing was associated with life-threatening dysrhythmias in an observational study,[39] which was not replicated in a group of patients with chronic digoxin toxicity paced transvenously.[40] If a patient presented with tachydysrhythmias, the use of Class Ib weak sodium channel blockers (phenytoin, lidocaine) was reported, although these were rarely used.[41] Furthermore, the administration of calcium for the treatment of hyperkalemia is still controversial. It is not useful in treating acute overdose and can instead be potentially dangerous. When intracellular hypercalcemia is already present, the administration of calcium can result in dysrhythmias, cardiac dysfunction secondary to hypercontractility, and cardiac arrest.[42] Although an animal study[42] and a retrospective study[43] did not reveal these side effects, experts have recommended avoiding this treatment.[44]

Sodium Channel Blockers

Sodium channel blockade results from several types of poisoning (eg, tricyclic antidepressants, diphenhydramine, carbamazepine, chloroquine, hydroxychloroquine, quinine, cocaine, venlafaxine) on top of Class I antidysrhythmic poisonings.[16] Therefore, the overall management of the patient will depend on which other mechanisms of toxicity are involved. In early presentation of acute overdose, the administration of activated charcoal should be considered if there are no contraindications (eg, unprotected airway). In cases of QRS widening with signs of sodium channel blockade (prominent R wave in aVR and deep S wave in lead 1) or dysrhythmias with QRS widening, the administration of a bolus of 1 to 2 mEq/kg of sodium bicarbonate should be considered and repeated as needed.[27] In addition, hypertonic saline can be an alternative if the patient is already hypokalemic, alkalemic, or has another contraindication to the administration of sodium bicarbonate. Bicarbonate infusion can be considered in patients poisoned with an agent known to respond to a change in pH. Lipid emulsion can be considered in refractory life-threatening toxicity. The usual dose is a 1.5-mL/kg bolus, followed by an infusion of 0.25 mL/kg per minute, but clinicians should be careful not to give more than 10 mL/kg per day because more side effects have been documented with higher doses (eg, laboratory analytical interferences, hypersensitivity, fat overload syndrome, extracorporeal machine circuit obstruction).[20] A safer alternative may be to give boluses of 1.5 mL/kg at a time to keep a better count of what has been administered. Ultimately, extracorporeal life support can serve as a rescue therapy.

DISCUSSION
State of Research and Controversies

The current evidence available for the management of cardiotoxic drug poisoning is of low to very low quality. Therefore, current expert consensus and guidelines are likely to change over time as more evidence becomes available. The use of rescue therapies, such as lipid emulsion or extracorporeal life support, is a subject of controversies. Many will claim that they would be more successful if used earlier, but better evidence is available for other therapies. Moreover, decontamination practices are highly variable. An expert consensus is currently ongoing for the use of activated charcoal, but the underlying evidence has been scant for most agents.

Future Directions

Controlled trials should be considered for treatments more often used, such as activated charcoal, calcium, high-dose regular insulin, and sodium bicarbonate.

Once such evidence is better documented, scientists should evaluate which knowledge translation tools are the best to guide clinicians, eventually improving patient care.

SUMMARY

While managing unstable patients poisoned with cardiotoxic drugs, clinicians should follow a structured approach, including excellent support measures. In addition, they should consider decontamination in early presentation and, as initial therapies, the ones for which there exist more evidence and fewer side effects. Management algorithms are proposed for CCB and BB poisonings. For unstable patients poisoned with cardiac glycosides, the administration of digoxin-Fab is key, and this antidote should be readily available. Finally, despite the sparse evidence supporting the use of a sodium bicarbonate bolus, few side effects have been documented when using it to reverse the toxicity of sodium channel blockers. Consequently, its administration should be part of the treatment of these poisonings.

CLINICS CARE POINTS

- Decontamination should be considered during early presentation of cardiovascular drug toxicity, although the evidence does not allow one to make a clear recommendation.
- First-line therapies for CCB poisoning include the administration of calcium, epinephrine/norepinephrine, and high-dose regular insulin.
- First-line therapies for BB poisoning include the administration of epinephrine/norepinephrine and high-dose regular insulin. In addition, sodium bicarbonate boluses may be administered for BBs with sodium blockade effect.
- In CCB and BB poisonings, if a patient is not responding to an increase in high-dose regular insulin (up to 10 U/kg per hour), lipid emulsion (except for hydrosoluble BBs) and extracorporeal life support can be considered.
- In acute cardiac glycoside overdoses, the administration of activated charcoal should be considered if there are no contraindications, and digoxin-Fab should be administered if indications are met. A partial reversal based on an available digoxin concentration or with empirical treatment should be enough for clinical improvement. However, in the case of cardiac arrest, a complete reversal should be targeted.
- In chronic cardiac glycoside toxicity, involvement of a pharmacist is key, correction of hypokalemia and hypomagnesemia is important, and digoxin-Fab should be administered if indications are met. One vial at a time should be enough for clinical improvement.
- The administration of sodium bicarbonate is the first-line therapy for sodium channel blocker toxicity.

DISCLOSURE

Dr M. St-Onge has no conflict of interest.

REFERENCES

1. Gummin DD, Mowry JB, Spyker DA, et al. 2016 Annual report of the American Association of Poison Control Centers' National Poison Data System (NPDS): 34th annual report. Clin Toxicol 2017;55(10):1072–254.

2. Brassard E, Archambault P, Lacombe G, et al. To call or not to call: behavioral determinants influencing the decision of intensivist to consult poison centers for calcium channel blocker poisoning. Clin Toxicol 2020;58(9):913–21.

3. Centre antipoison du Québec – CIUSSS de la Capitale nationale. Available at: https://www.ciusss-capitalenationale.gouv.qc.ca/centre-antipoison-du-quebec/professionnels-de-la-sante/aide-memoire-guidant-les-5-premieres-minutes-de-la-reanimation. Accessed January 25, 2021.

4. Vaughan Williams EM. Classification of antidysrhythmic drugs. Pharmacol Ther 1975;1(1):115–38.

5. Srinivasan A. Drugs affecting the cardiac action potential. Available at: https://en.wikipedia.org/wiki/Antiarrhythmic_agent#/media/File:Cardiac_action_potential.png. Accessed January 25, 2021.

6. Knollmann BC, Roden DM. Chapter 30: antiarrhythmic drugs. In: Brunton LL, Hilal-Dandan R, Knollmann BC, editors. Goodman & Gilman's the pharmacological basis of therapeutics. 13th edition. McGraw-Hill Education; 2018.

7. Ebihara T, Morita M, Kawada M, et al. Efficacy of isoproterenol for treating amlodipine overdose resulting in bradycardia. Acute Med Surg 2017;4(3):353–7.

8. Hang D. Chapter 60: calcium channel blockers. In: Nelson LS, Howland MA, Lewin NA, et al, editors. Goldfrank's toxicologic emergencies. 11th edition. McGraw-Hill Education; 2019. p. 945–52.

9. Levine M, Boyer EW, Pozner CN, et al. Assessment of hyperglycemia after calcium channel blocker overdoses involving diltiazem or verapamil. Crit Care Med 2007;35(9):2071–5.

10. Brubacher JR. Chapter 59: β-adrenergic antagonists. In: Nelson LS, Howland MA, Lewin NA, et al, editors. Goldfrank's toxicologic emergencies. 11th edition. McGraw-Hill Education; 2019. p. 926–40.

11. Rathore SS, Curtis JP, Wang Y, et al. Association of serum digoxin concentration and outcomes in patients with heart failure. JAMA 2003;289:871–8.

12. Hack JB. Chapter 62: Cardioactive steroids. In: Nelson LS, Howland MA, Lewin NA, et al, editors. Goldfrank's toxicologic emergencies. 11th edition. McGraw-Hill Education; 2019. p. 969–76.

13. Bismuth C, Gaultier M, Conso F, et al. Hyperkalemia in acute digitalis poisoning: prognostic significance and therapeutic implications. Clin Toxicol 1973;6:153–62.

14. Chan BS, Isbister GK, Page CB, et al. Clinical outcomes from early use of digoxin-specific antibodies versus observation in chronic digoxin poisoning (ATMO-4). Clin Toxicol 2019;57(7):638–43.

15. ECG & echo learning. Available at: https://ecgwaves.com/wp-content/uploads/2016/09/bidirectional_VT.jpg. Accessed January 25, 2021.

16. Yates C, Manini AF. Utility of the electrocardiogram in drug overdose and poisoning: theoretical considerations and clinical implications. Curr Cardiol Rev 2012;8:137–51.

17. St-Onge M, Dubé PA, Gossein S, et al. Treatment for calcium channel blocker poisoning: a systematic review. Clin Toxicol 2014;52(9):926–44.

18. Holger JS, Stellpflug SJ, Cole JB, et al. High-dose insulin: a consecutive case series in toxin-induced cardiogenic shock. Clin Toxicol 2011;49(7):653–8.

19. Holger JS, Dries DJ, Barringer KW, et al. Cardiovascular and metabolic effects of high-dose insulin in a porcine septic shock model. Acad Emerg Med 2010;17(4):429–35.

20. Gosselin S, Hoegberg LCG, Hoffman RS, et al. Evidence-based recommendations on the use of intravenous lipid emulsion therapy in poisoning. Clin Toxicol 2016;54(10):899–923.

21. Rotella JA, Greene SL, Koutsogiannis Z, et al. Treatment for beta-blocker poisoning: a systematic review. Clin Toxicol 2020;58(10):943–83.
22. Peterson CD, Leeder JS, Sterner S. Glucagon therapy for beta-blocker overdose. Drug Intell Clin Pharm 1984;18(5):394–8.
23. Hartel G, Manninen V, Reissell P. Treatment of digoxin intoxication. Lancet 1973; 2(7821):158.
24. Chan BSH, Buckley NA. Digoxin-specific antibody fragment in the treatment of digoxin toxicity. Clin Toxicol 2014;52:824–36.
25. Chan BS, Isbister GK, Page CB, et al. Clinical outcomes from early use of digoxin-specific antibodies versus observation in chronic digoxin poisoning (ATOM-4). Clin Toxicol 2019;57(7):638–43.
26. Chan BS, Isbister GK, O'Leary M, et al. Efficacy and effectiveness of anti-digoxin antibodies in chronic digoxin poisonings from the DORA study (ATOM-1). Clin Toxicol 2016;54(6):488–94.
27. Bruccoleri RE, Burns MM. A literature review of the use of sodium bicarbonate for the treatment of QRS widening. J Med Toxicol 2016;12(1):121–9.
28. Seger DL, Hantsch C, Zavoral T, et al. Variability of recommendations for serum alkalinization in tricyclic antidepressant overdose: a survey of US Poison Center medical directors. Clin Toxicol 2003;41(4):331–8.
29. McCabe JL, Menegazzi JJ, Cobaugh DJ, et al. Recovery from severe cyclic antidepressant overdose with hypertonic saline/dextran in a swine model. Acad Emerg Med J 1994;1(2):111–5.
30. Scalabrini A, Simonetti MP, Velasco IT, et al. Hypertonic NaCl antagonizes cardiac arrhythmia induced by bupivacaine. Braz Med Biol Res 1989;22(2):249–52.
31. Auzinger GM, Scheinkestel CD. Successful extracorporeal life support in a case of severe flecainide intoxication. Crit Care Med 2001;29(4):887–90.
32. Reynolds JC, Judge BS. Successful treatment of flecainide-induced cardiac arrest with extracorporeal membrane oxygenation in the ED. Am J Emerg Med 2015;33(10):1542.e1–2.
33. Sivalingam SK, Gadiraju VT, Hariharan MV, et al. Flecainide toxicity-treatment with intravenous fat emulsion and extra-corporeal life-support. Acute Cardiol Care 2013;15(4):90–2.
34. St-Onge M, Anseeuw K, Cantrell FL, et al. Expert consensus recommendations for the management of calcium channel blocker poisoning in adults. Crit Care Med 2017;45(3):e306–15.
35. Warrick BJ, Tataru AP, Smolinske S. A systematic analysis of methylene blue for drug-induced shock. Clin Toxicol 2016;54(7):547–55.
36. Centre antipoison du Québec – CIUSSS de la Capitale nationale. Available at: https://www.ciusss-capitalenationale.gouv.qc.ca/sites/default/files/images/guideantidore CAPQ/algorithme_bb_ang_02_2020.pdf?lang=en. Accessed January 25, 2021.
37. Patocka J, Nepovimova E, Wu W, et al. Digoxin: pharmacology and toxicology – a review. Environ Toxicol Pharmacol 2020;79:103400.
38. Centre antipoison du Québec – CIUSSS de la Capitale nationale. Available at: https://www.ciusss-capitalenationale.gouv.qc.ca/digoxin-specific-antibodies?lang=en. Accessed January 25, 2021.
39. Taboulet P, Baud FJ, Bismuth C, et al. Acute digitalis intoxication – is pacing still appropriate? Clin Toxicol 1993;31(2):261–73.
40. Chen JY, Liu PY, Chen JH, et al. Safety of transvenous temporary cardiac pacing in patient with accidental digoxin overdose and symptomatic bradycardia. Cardiology 2004;102(30):152–5.

41. Rumack BH, Wolfe RR, Gilfrich H. Phenytoin (diphenylhydantoin) treatment of massive digoxin overdose. Br Heart J 1974;36:405–8.
42. Hack JB, Woody JH, Lewis DE, et al. The effect of calcium chloride in treating hyperkalemia due to acute digoxin toxicity in a porcine model. Clin Toxicol 2004; 42(4):337–42.
43. Levine M, Nikkanen H, Pallin DJ. The effects of intravenous calcium in patients with digoxin toxicity. J Emerg Med 2011;40(1):41–6.
44. Gupta A, Su M, Greller H, et al. Digoxin and calcium: the verdict is still out. J Emerg Med 2010;39(1):102.

Toxicology of Medications for Diabetes Mellitus

Kevin Baumgartner, MD*, Jason Devgun, MD

KEYWORDS

- Toxicology ● Overdose ● Poisoning ● Insulin ● Metformin ● Sulfonylurea
- SGLT2 inhibitor ● Diabetes mellitus

KEY POINTS

- Insulin overdose may produce severe and prolonged hypoglycemia.
- Sulfonylurea poisoning should be treated with octreotide, sparing intravenous dextrose where possible.
- Acute metformin *overdose* may lead to life-threatening acidosis with elevated lactate concentrations, which may require hemodialysis.
- Glucagon-like peptide 1 agonists and dipeptidyl peptidase 4 inhibitors appear to be benign in overdose in diabetic patients but may produce profound hypoglycemia in *nondiabetic* patients.
- Euglycemic diabetic ketoacidosis may develop in critically ill patients taking sodium-glucose co-transporter 2 inhibitors.

INTRODUCTION

Diabetes mellitus (DM) is one of the most common chronic diseases; the worldwide prevalence of DM in adults may be as high as 7.7% (439 million adults) by 2030.[1] As such, medications for the treatment of DM are commonly prescribed, with more than 18 million adults in the United States filling a prescription for antidiabetic drugs in 2012.[2]

Toxicity from medications for DM may occur for many reasons. Some patients deliberately overdose on medications. In other cases, therapeutic misadventures and medication administration errors cause unintentional poisoning; this circumstance is especially common with insulin.[3] Finally, some patients may become poisoned due to changes in renal function, which render a previously therapeutic medication dose toxic; this is a particular risk with the sulfonylurea class.

Many patients who are poisoned by medications for DM may be appropriately cared for at home, discharged from the emergency department, or admitted to a general

The authors have no conflicts of interest to disclose.
Department of Emergency Medicine, Division of Medical Toxicology, Washington University School of Medicine, 660 South Euclid Avenue, Campus Box 8072, St Louis, MO 63110, USA
* Corresponding author.
E-mail address: baumgartner.k@wustl.edu

medical floor. However, some may require admission to the intensive care unit (ICU), typically due to a need for aggressive dextrose supplementation and frequent blood glucose monitoring, but occasionally due to severe systemic illness, as in metformin-associated lactic acidosis (MALA).

This article reviews the mechanism of action and pharmacology of commonly prescribed classes of medications for DM and discusses the clinical presentation and treatment of poisoning by these medications, with particular attention to care in the ICU.

DISCUSSION
Insulins

Insulin use is quite common: approximately 7.4 million Americans use one or more formulations of insulin to manage type 1 and type 2 DM.[4] All pharmacologic insulins replicate the function of endogenously produced insulin, which triggers the uptake of glucose into cells, suppresses ketosis, and promotes the storage of energy in fatty acids, among many other actions. Clinicians may now choose from a large array of insulin analogues with different pharmacokinetic profiles, which are classified by their duration of action (**Table 1**).[5]

Insulin poisoning may be intentional, as in suicide or homicide attempts, or unintentional, as in administration errors or accumulation due to renal insufficiency. Unintentional overdoses typically produce milder clinical effects and may frequently be managed at home.[6] The primary toxicity of insulin poisoning is hypoglycemia, which may be life-threatening if not promptly recognized and treated. Hypokalemia has also been reported and is usually mild. A systematic review of predominantly intentional insulin overdoses reported a median serum potassium of 3.2 mmol/L. However, in some cases, hypokalemia may be severe and associated with dysrhythmias.[7] Hypomagnesemia and hypophosphatemia also may occur.[8]

The primary challenge in management of insulin poisoning is predicting the duration of hypoglycemia, which varies considerably depending on the formulation and amount of insulin administered. Larger overdoses tend to produce longer periods of hypoglycemia.[9] Poisoning by the long-acting insulins typically produces more prolonged hypoglycemia than poisoning by the short-acting insulins.

The duration of hypoglycemia in overdose can be much longer than the duration of action of the agent in clinical use. For example, an overdose of 300 units of insulin lispro produced hypoglycemia that persisted for more than 11 hours,[10] an overdose of

Table 1 Insulins		
Duration of Action	**Generic Name**	**Common Trade Name(s)**
Short	Lispro	Humalog
	Aspart	Novolog
	Glulisine	Apidra
	Regular	Humulin, Novolin
Moderate	Neutral protamine Hagedorn (NPH)	Humulin N, Novolin N
Long	Detemir	Levemir
	Glargine	Lantus, Basaglar, Toujeo
	Degludec	Tresiba

2700 units of insulin glargine produced recurrent hypoglycemic episodes as late as 96 hours postexposure,[11] and a patient who self-administered 2500 units of neutral protamine Hagedorn insulin required intravenous (IV) dextrose for 6 days.[12] Patient characteristics are also important; nondiabetic patients who overdose on insulin are more likely to have recurrent hypoglycemia than patients with DM.[13]

The mainstay of treatment for insulin poisoning is IV dextrose, typically administered as a bolus followed by an infusion.[7] Selection of the dose of dextrose to administer is typically guided by the severity of hypoglycemia and the patient's clinical status; for example, a patient who is awake and alert with mild hypoglycemia may not require any bolus, whereas a patient with severe hypoglycemia or neurologic compromise due to hypoglycemia will typically be treated with a bolus of 50% dextrose. The dextrose infusion rate should be titrated to maintain euglycemia, and frequent blood glucose testing is essential. Patients requiring large amounts of dextrose may require highly concentrated dextrose infusions to avoid volume overload. If a patient's hypoglycemia is not correcting with standard infusions of 5% or 10% dextrose, it may be necessary to administer 20% dextrose, which requires a central line. ICU admission due to the intensity of nursing care is usually required; in one systematic review of insulin overdoses, 38% of patients spent part of their hospitalization in the ICU.[7] Careful monitoring of electrolytes and fluid status is also required.

In rare cases, adjunctive therapies have been used to treat insulin poisoning. Glucagon may be used in the prehospital setting. Octreotide, a somatostatin analogue, has been used in some cases with equivocal results.[14,15] Octreotide may suppress endogenous insulin secretion provoked by dextrose administration in patients with type 2 diabetes. Hydrocortisone and other steroids have been used to induce insulin resistance in severe cases.[16] Finally, there are older case reports of surgical incision of the subcutaneous tissue at the site of insulin injection, which theoretically removes a "depot" of unabsorbed insulin.[17,18] This therapy is of questionable efficacy and is not typically performed today.

Sulfonylureas

Sulfonylureas promote secretion of insulin from beta islet cells by promoting closure of the K_{ATP} potassium channel, which induces depolarization of the cell and allows calcium influx. Calcium influx then leads to exocytosis of insulin.[19] Because sulfonylureas directly induce insulin release regardless of the blood glucose level, they can produce dangerous hypoglycemia in therapeutic use and in overdose. Sulfonylurea prescribing has declined in the past decades, likely due to the development of alternative agents not associated with hypoglycemia.[20]

Sulfonylurea poisoning may occur due to deliberate overdose, therapeutic error, pediatric exploratory ingestion, or accumulation due to impaired renal elimination. Most cases are unintentional,[21] but cases of intentional poisoning typically have more serious outcomes, likely due to the higher doses involved.[22]

The time to onset of hypoglycemia in sulfonylurea poisoning can vary considerably, making decisions regarding required medical observation time complex. In particular, pediatric exposures can cause significant delayed onset of hypoglycemia (in some cases, more than 8 hours postexposure), especially if food or dextrose is given.[23] Onset of hypoglycemia in adult poisoning is typically more rapid.[19] Hypoglycemia may be prolonged or recurrent, especially in poisonings by sulfonylureas with long half-lives. This is especially true in patients with impaired renal function.[24,25]

Although the administration of IV dextrose would seem to be the most appropriate treatment for sulfonylurea-induced hypoglycemia, it should actually be *avoided* as much as possible. Administration of parenteral dextrose to patients with sulfonylurea poisoning *promotes* insulin release even when blood glucose levels are normal, and may contribute to severe rebound hypoglycemia.[19] In addition, *prophylactic* IV dextrose administration may be associated with delayed onset of clinical hypoglycemia[23] and should be avoided.

Administration of parenteral dextrose boluses is sometimes unavoidable, as in patients with significant changes in mental status, seizures, or neurologic deficits. After the initial symptomatic hypoglycemia is corrected, or if patients are initially mildly hypoglycemic or euglycemic, oral consumption of complex carbohydrates should be encouraged.[19] Food taken orally (especially in the form of complex carbohydrates, proteins, or fat) produces slower and more sustained increases in blood glucose than parenteral dextrose, and does not usually cause the aggressive "spike" in insulin secretion that can accompany IV dextrose administration. If additional IV dextrose is required, it should be provided by *infusion* to avoid the abrupt increases in blood glucose that can provoke rebound insulin secretion.

The antidote of choice for sulfonylurea poisoning is octreotide. Octreotide is a somatostatin analogue that suppresses insulin release from beta islet cells by preventing calcium influx. Because calcium influx is downstream from K_{ATP} channel closure in the cascade of events that leads to insulin release, octreotide interrupts the stimulus for insulin secretion promoted by sulfonylureas.

The use of octreotide is well supported by evidence. A review of published case reports of octreotide therapy for sulfonylurea poisoning showed that octreotide treatment decreased the average number of hypoglycemic episodes from 3.3 before treatment to 0.4 after treatment.[26] A retrospective single-center case review demonstrated a decrease in hypoglycemic episodes (3.2 to 0.2 on average) and dextrose requirements (72.5 g dextrose to 5 g on average).[27] A prospective, double-blind, placebo-controlled trial of octreotide plus standard therapy (dextrose and oral carbohydrates) versus standard therapy alone showed that patients treated with octreotide had higher glucose levels and fewer episodes of recurrent hypoglycemia.[28]

The optimal octreotide dosing regimen is not known. Octreotide may be given by IV infusion or by subcutaneous (SQ) injection; there is no evidence that either route is superior. A reasonable dosing regimen for adults would be 50 µg SQ every 6 hours.[29] In children, 1 to 1.5 µg/kg IV or SQ every 6 hours may be reasonable.[29] The optimal duration of treatment is also unclear. Either continuous infusion or repeat dosing is necessary in most cases, as octreotide has a very short half-life compared with the duration of action of the sulfonylureas, especially in overdose. Some investigators suggest planning for a total of 3 to 4 doses.[29] In any case, it is important to monitor blood glucose for a prolonged period (up to 24 hours) following discontinuation of octreotide to ensure that hypoglycemia does not recur due to persistent sulfonylurea effect.

The use of glucagon is not routinely recommended in sulfonylurea poisoning, as it induces insulin release and is effective only in patients with adequate glycogen stores.[19] Intramuscular glucagon may have a role in prehospital treatment of severe symptomatic hypoglycemia when IV access is not available. Hemodialysis is typically not indicated in sulfonylurea poisoning, as sulfonylureas are highly protein bound and treatment with octreotide and supportive therapy is usually adequate.

Biguanides

Metformin is the most commonly prescribed medication for DM and the only biguanide used in the United States. Metformin has a complex mechanism of action that includes inhibition of hepatic gluconeogenesis, improvement of insulin sensitivity in peripheral tissues, alteration of lipid metabolism, and enhanced glucose utilization in the gastrointestinal (GI) tract.[30,31] In therapeutic use, metformin may cause GI upset, vitamin B12 deficiency, and rarely hemolytic anemia.[32] Metformin does *not* appear to cause excessive lactate production or metabolic acidosis when used therapeutically in patients with intact renal function.[33] Metformin undergoes minimal hepatic metabolism and is predominantly excreted unchanged in the urine.[32]

The most feared complication of metformin poisoning is MALA. We use the term "MALA" here because it is well-known and widely accepted, but it is important to note that it is more precise to describe metformin toxicity as producing an elevated anion gap metabolic acidosis and an elevated lactate concentration.[32] MALA may occur in acute metformin overdose, when impairment in renal function leads to accumulation of metformin taken at therapeutic doses, or when patients taking metformin therapeutically develop an intercurrent illness.

At toxic levels, metformin is a metabolic poison that disrupts gluconeogenesis and aerobic respiration. Metformin directly inhibits complex I in the electron transport chain, impairing the transfer of electrons from second messengers such as NADH and $FADH_2$ into the electron transport chain.[34] This reaction causes an increase in the concentration of reduced second messengers that cannot unload their electrons, altering the overall redox state of the cell. This altered redox state impairs metabolism of pyruvate to acetyl-CoA and favors the production of lactate from pyruvate.

In addition, the inhibition of the electron transport chain disrupts oxidative phosphorylation, preventing the production of adenosine triphosphate (ATP) via aerobic respiration. This forces the cell to rely on less efficient glycolysis for ATP production. The disrupted oxidative phosphorylation system cannot appropriately recycle and use protons produced by normal cellular metabolism. These protons then leak out of the mitochondria and contribute to the development of metabolic acidosis.[32]

The clinical presentation of MALA is vague and can present a diagnostic challenge, especially in the absence of a known large overdose. Patients may present with nausea, vomiting, fatigue, altered mental status, or frank shock.[32] Hypoglycemia is unusual in metformin poisoning.[35,36]

In MALA related to *acute metformin overdose*, blood pH and serum lactate appear to have significant prognostic value. A systematic review found that no patient with acute metformin overdose died whose nadir blood pH was greater than 6.9 or whose peak serum lactate concentration was less than 25 mmol/L.[37] Patients with MALA in the setting of acute overdose have survived without significant neurologic sequelae after presenting with a blood pH as low as 6.38.[38] Hepatic activity as measured by prothrombin activity also may be a useful prognostic factor; in one retrospective case series, prothrombin activity less than 50% was independently associated with death,[39] although this study included metformin-poisoned patients without acute overdose.

It is more difficult to predict prognosis in patients who develop MALA in the absence of an acute overdose. A retrospective case series of 49 such patients (most with acute impairment of renal function) found no prognostic value of the serum lactate or the plasma metformin concentration.[40] Some suggest that in the absence of an acute metformin overdose, patients die because of underlying medical conditions (such as septic shock or renal failure), *not* due to the toxic effects of metformin, despite high lactate concentrations.[41]

The cornerstone of treatment in MALA is supportive care, including volume resuscitation, management of electrolyte and acid-base disturbances, and hemodynamic support. In severe cases, extracorporeal treatment may be required. Hemodialysis is effective in correcting acidosis, clearing lactate, and removing metformin from the body.[42] The Extracorporeal Treatment in Poisoning Workgroup recommends extracorporeal treatment in severe metformin poisoning (**Box 1**).[42] Intermittent

> **Box 1**
> **Indications for hemodialysis in metformin-associated lactic acidosis[42]**
>
> Lactate concentration greater than 20 mmol/L
>
> pH less than or equal to 7.0
>
> Shock
>
> Failure of standard supportive measures
>
> Decreased level of consciousness

hemodialysis is the preferred extracorporeal treatment, but continuous renal replacement therapy may be a reasonable alternative if the patient cannot tolerate hemodialysis.[42]

The use of sodium bicarbonate for blood alkalinization in MALA is controversial. Sodium bicarbonate use in patients with severe metabolic acidosis is not uncommon clinically and may be a plausible bridge therapy to maintain pH in a near-physiologic range while the underlying cause of acidosis is being treated. There are minimal data regarding the use of sodium bicarbonate in MALA. One retrospective review of patients treated with metformin, buformin, or phenformin who developed metabolic acidosis and elevated lactate showed that treatment with sodium bicarbonate did not improve survival.[43]

Other therapies for MALA remain somewhat speculative. Some investigators suggest administration of glucose and insulin; there is no direct evidence for this therapy in MALA, but it appeared to improve survival in severe *phenformin* toxicity.[44] Methylene blue has been used in several cases of severe metformin toxicity as an adjunctive treatment with good results.[45,46] The mechanism of action of methylene blue is unclear, but it may serve as an alternative electron carrier that can receive electrons from NADH and deliver them to the electron transport chain, thus bypassing the metformin-poisoned complex I.[47] Methylene blue also may counteract metformin-induced vasoplegia by scavenging nitric oxide.[32] It may be reasonable to consider methylene blue therapy in severe MALA refractory to standard supportive therapy while extracorporeal treatment is being arranged.

Glucagon-like Peptide-1 Receptor Agonists

Glucagon-like peptide 1 receptor agonists (GLP-1 RAs) are a class of noninsulin injectable medications for type 2 DM originally derived from a hormone found in Gila monster venom. Agents currently available in the United States are listed in **Table 2**. They bind to the GLP-1 receptor and exert a number of beneficial effects, including suppression of glucagon secretion, enhanced synthesis and secretion of insulin, delayed gastric emptying, and reduction of food intake.[48] Because insulin secretion provoked by GLP-1 RAs is glucose-dependent, hypoglycemia is not typically a concern.[49] Adverse effects of therapeutic use include GI upset, drug-induced liver injury, and a possible link to pancreatitis and endocrine malignancies, although this association is not definite and has been questioned.[50]

GLP-1 RA overdose does not appear to cause serious toxicity. Large overdoses, both intentional and unintentional, are associated with GI upset, but *not* with significant hypoglycemia or pancreatitis.[51-57] Even quite massive overdoses (up to 70-fold)[53] and repeated overdoses over a long period (daily 10-fold overdose for 7 months)[52] produced GI upset but no significant hypoglycemia. There are 2 cases in which GLP-1 RA poisoning produced borderline hypoglycemia (65 mg/dL and

Table 2
GLP-1 RAs, DPP-4 inhibitors, and SGLT2 inhibitors available in the United States

GLP-1 RAs		DPP-4 Inhibitors		SGLT2 Inhibitors	
Agent	Trade Name(s)	Agent	Trade Name(s)	Agent	Trade Name(s)
Dulaglutide	Trulicity	Alogliptin	Nesina	Canagliflozin	Invokana
Exenatide	Bydureon Byetta	Linagliptin	Tradjenta	Dapagliflozin	Farxiga
Liraglutide	Saxenda Victoza	Saxagliptin	Onglyza	Empagliflozin	Jardiance
Lixisenatide	Adlyxin	Sitagliptin	Januvia	Ertugliflozin	Steglatro
Semaglutide	Ozempic Rybelsus				

Abbreviations: DPP-4, dipeptidyl peptidase 4; GLP-1 RA, glucagon-like peptide 1 receptor agonist; SGLT2, sodium-glucose co-transporter 2.

69 mg/dL). In one case no treatment was required,[58] and in the other the hypoglycemia corrected with a 1-time dose of 10% dextrose and did not recur.[59]

There is 1 published case of severe hypoglycemia following an intentional overdose of liraglutide in a *nondiabetic* patient; this patient's blood glucose on presentation was 23 mg/dL, and he required dextrose-containing fluids for 48 hours.[56] It is possible that nondiabetic patients are at risk of hypoglycemia following GLP-1 RA poisoning as compared with diabetic patients because of differential expression of GLP-1 receptors.[60] It is reasonable to monitor blood sugar closely and expect hypoglycemia in *nondiabetic* patients with GLP-1 RA poisoning.

Interestingly, it appears that GLP-1 RA poisoning may significantly delay absorption of orally ingested medication. A 58-year-old woman who injected 600 μg exenatide and ingested large amounts of sedating medications experienced no alteration of mental status until 14 hours postingestion.[59] The markedly delayed symptom onset suggests that exenatide may have impaired absorption of the orally ingested medications, likely due to the inhibitory effects of GLP-1 on gastric emptying.

Dipeptidyl Peptidase-4 Inhibitors

Dipeptidyl peptidase 4 (DPP-4) is an enzyme that breaks down GLP-1 and other incretins. DPP-4 inhibitors suppress DPP-4 activity and thus indirectly increase GLP-1 and incretin signaling, leading to the same downstream effects as the GLP-1 RAs. Unlike GLP-1 RAs, DPP-4 inhibitors are orally bioavailable. Agents currently available in the United States are listed in **Table 2**. Like the GLP-1 RAs, they may cause GI upset, but are generally well-tolerated with few serious adverse effects of therapeutic use.[61]

Clinical experience with DPP-4 inhibitor poisoning is quite limited, but existing data suggest that this class is benign in overdose. A review of isolated DPP-4 inhibitor ingestions from the National Poison Database System (NPDS) identified 650 cases, of which only 9 (2%) had moderate clinical effects and only 1 (0.002%) had major clinical effects. The case with major clinical effects involved a *nondiabetic* patient, who developed recurrent hypoglycemia requiring prolonged infusion of dextrose-containing fluids.[62] A review of data from a state poison center during the same period identified 62 cases, of whom none had moderate or major clinical effects, and none experienced hypoglycemia.[63] A separate review of a different state poison center database found no cases of hypoglycemia in isolated DPP-4 inhibitor overdose.[64]

Case reports of DPP-4 inhibitor poisoning are scarce. One diabetic patient ingested 1700 mg sitagliptin (17 times greater than the approved maximum dose) and developed no clinical symptoms and no hypoglycemia.[65] A 17 year old *nondiabetic* patient ingested 8 to 9 tablets of sitagliptin 50 mg/metformin 500 mg and developed hypoglycemia and seizures, requiring prolonged treatment with IV dextrose.[66] As with the GLP-1 RAs, it seems reasonable to expect hypoglycemia in *nondiabetic* patients following DPP-4 inhibitor poisoning.

Sodium-Glucose Co-transporter 2 Inhibitors

Sodium-glucose co-transporter 2 (SGLT2) inhibitors disrupt reabsorption of glucose in the proximal convoluted tubule of the nephron, leading to excretion of excess glucose in the urine, thereby lowering blood glucose levels. The increase in glucose excretion appears to be proportional to the blood glucose level and is insulin-independent, suggesting that SGLT2 inhibitors are unlikely to induce hypoglycemia.[67] Agents currently available in the United States are listed in **Table 2**.

SGLT2 inhibitors have several important adverse effects in therapeutic use. Perhaps the most dangerous is euglycemic diabetic ketoacidosis (eDKA). The enhanced glucose excretion promoted by SGLT2 inhibitors may mask hyperglycemia in DKA, making the diagnosis of DKA more challenging. SGLT2 inhibitors may also trigger the onset of DKA. The mechanism by which this occurs is not clear, but may involve suppression of insulin release (due to decreases in blood glucose) and potentially direct stimulation of glucagon release.[68] Patients taking SGLT2 inhibitors appear to be most at risk of eDKA when exposed to additional precipitating factors (**Box 2**).[69] It may be reasonable to stop SGLT2 inhibitors in patients hospitalized with severe acute illness to prevent eDKA.[69] Clinicians should maintain a high level of suspicion for eDKA in patients taking SGLT2 inhibitors and should not be falsely reassured by normal or near-normal blood glucoses. Assessment of blood or urine ketones, venous pH, and anion gap is critical, even if glucose is normal or near-normal, and the presence of ketonemia or ketonuria with an anion gap acidosis should prompt initiation of treatment. Treatment is similar to treatment of standard DKA, with the caveat that dextrose-containing fluids should be started immediately.[70]

SGLT2 inhibitors have also been linked to increased rates of genitourinary infections, including genital candidiasis, bacterial urinary tract infections, and life-threatening Fournier's gangrene.[71,72] It is possible that the glycosuria induced by SGLT2 inhibitors creates a genitourinary milieu that favors the growth of fungi and bacteria. The strength of the association between SGLT2 inhibitor use and increased rates of urinary tract infections and Fournier gangrene has been questioned, and serious infectious complications are rare overall.[73]

Box 2
Factors that may precipitate euglycemic diabetic ketoacidosis in patients taking sodium-glucose co-transporter 2 inhibitors

Inappropriate reduction or omission of insulin

Acute infectious illness

Other acute illness (myocardial infarction, stroke)

Bariatric surgery

Other major surgical procedures

Dietary restriction (especially low-carbohydrate)

Physical exertion

Excessive alcohol intake

There is minimal published evidence regarding acute SGLT2 inhibitor poisoning. A retrospective review of poison center data from 6 states identified 88 cases of isolated SGLT2 inhibitor exposure. Eighty patients (91%) had no symptoms, and no patients developed hypoglycemia.[74] A separate review of national NPDS data during a similar time period identified 627 isolated SGLT2 inhibitor exposures. No patient had clinically important hypoglycemia, and the most common clinical effect was eDKA in therapeutic use, as described previously.[75] A single case report of SGLT2 inhibitor overdose has been published in English. A 32-year-old *nondiabetic* patient ingested 1500 mg ipragliflozin and never developed hypoglycemia.[76] An additional case report published in German describes a 74-year-old woman who attempted suicide by ingestion of empagliflozin and did not develop hypoglycemia.[77]

SUMMARY

Medications used to treat DM are heterogeneous, with widely differing safety profiles in therapeutic use and in overdose. A thorough understanding of the mechanisms of action and toxicology of these agents is essential to critical care practice.

CLINICS CARE POINTS

- Anticipate *severe, prolonged hypoglycemia* after large intentional insulin overdoses. Monitor glucose and potassium closely. Consider octreotide and/or glucocorticoids in severe or refractory cases.

- Sulfonylurea poisoning should be treated with octreotide, sparing IV dextrose where possible.

- Acute metformin *overdose* may lead to potentially life-threatening acidosis and elevated lactate requiring hemodialysis. Patients taking metformin *therapeutically* who develop an acute illness may develop elevated lactate concentrations and acidosis.

- GLP-1 receptor agonists and DPP-4 inhibitors appear to be benign in overdose in diabetic patients but may cause profound hypoglycemia in *nondiabetic* patients.

- SGLT2 inhibitors may predispose patients to euglycemic DKA, especially in the context of an acute physiologic stressor such as critical illness or surgery. Euglycemic DKA should be suspected in patients taking SGLT2 inhibitors who develop an anion gap metabolic acidosis.

REFERENCES

1. Shaw JE, Sicree RA, Zimmet PZ. Global estimates of the prevalence of diabetes for 2010 and 2030. Diabetes Res Clin Pract 2010;87(1):4–14.
2. Hampp C, Borders-Hemphill V, Moeny DG, et al. Use of antidiabetic drugs in the U.S., 2003-2012. Diabetes Care 2014;37(5):1367–74.
3. Hodges NL, Spiller HA, Casavant MJ, et al. Non-health care facility medication errors resulting in serious medical outcomes. Clin Toxicol (Phila) 2018;56(1):43–50.
4. Cefalu WT, Dawes DE, Gavlak G, et al. Insulin access and affordability working group: conclusions and recommendations. Diabetes Care 2018;41(6):1299–311.
5. Mathieu C, Gillard P, Benhalima K. Insulin analogues in type 1 diabetes mellitus: getting better all the time. Nat Rev Endocrinol 2017;13(7):385–99.
6. Beuhler MC, Spiller HA, Aleguas A. Demographics and outcome of unintentional insulin overdoses managed by three poison centers. Clin Toxicol (Phila) 2013;51(8):789–93.

7. Johansen NJ, Christensen MB. A systematic review on insulin overdose cases: clinical course, complications and treatment options. Basic Clin Pharmacol Toxicol 2018;122(6):650–9.
8. Matsumura M, Nakashima A, Tofuku Y. Electrolyte disorders following massive insulin overdose in a patient with type 2 diabetes. Intern Med 2000;39(1):55–7.
9. Ohyama T, Saisho Y, Muraki A, et al. Prediction of recovery time from hypoglycemia in patients with insulin overdose. Endocr J 2011;58(7):607–11.
10. Brvar M, Mozina M, Bunc M. Prolonged hypoglycaemia after insulin lispro overdose. Eur J Emerg Med 2005;12(5):234–5.
11. Lu M, Inboriboon PC. Lantus insulin overdose: a case report. J Emerg Med 2011; 41(4):374–7.
12. Samuels MH, Eckel RH. Massive insulin overdose: detailed studies of free insulin levels and glucose requirements. J Toxicol Clin Toxicol 1989;27(3):157–68.
13. Stapczynski JS, Haskell RJ. Duration of hypoglycemia and need for intravenous glucose following intentional overdoses of insulin. Ann Emerg Med 1984;13(7): 505–11.
14. Groth CM, Banzon ER. Octreotide for the treatment of hypoglycemia after insulin glargine overdose. J Emerg Med 2013;45(2):194–8.
15. Dewaal CM, McGillis E, Mink M, et al. Octreotide for the treatment of intentional insulin aspart overdose in a non-diabetic patient. CJEM 2018;20(4):643–7.
16. Tariq K, Tariq S, Denney Queen AM. Role of steroids in refractory hypoglycemia due to an overdose of 10,000 units of insulin glargine: a case report and literature review. AACE Clin Case Rep 2018;4(1):e70–4.
17. McIntyre AS, Woolf VJ, Burnham WR. Local excision of subcutaneous fat in the management of insulin overdose. Br J Surg 1986;73(7):538.
18. Levine DF, Bulstrode C. Managing suicidal insulin overdose. Br Med J Clin Res Ed 1982;285(6346):974–5.
19. Klein-Schwartz W, Stassinos GL, Isbister GK. Treatment of sulfonylurea and insulin overdose. Br J Clin Pharmacol 2016;81(3):496–504.
20. Kitten AK, Kamath M, Ryan L, et al. National ambulatory care non-insulin antidiabetic medication prescribing trends in the United States from 2009 to 2015. PLoS One 2019;14(8):e0221174.
21. Mowry JB, Spyker DA, Cantilena LR, et al. 2013 annual report of the American Association of Poison Control Centers' National Poison Data System (NPDS): 31st annual report. Clin Toxicol (Phila) 2014;52(10):1032–283.
22. Forrester MB. Adult glyburide ingestions reported to Texas poison control centers, 1998–2005. Hum Exp Toxicol 2007;26(7):563–71.
23. Lung DD, Olson KR. Hypoglycemia in pediatric sulfonylurea poisoning: an 8-year poison center retrospective study. Pediatrics 2011;127(6):e1558–64.
24. Mifsud S, Schembri EL, Fava S. A case of severe relapsing sulphonylurea-induced hypoglycaemia. BMJ Case Rep 2019;12(12):e231368.
25. Krepinsky J, Ingram AJ, Clase CM. Prolonged sulfonylurea-induced hypoglycemia in diabetic patients with end-stage renal disease. Am J Kidney Dis 2000; 35(3):500–5.
26. Dougherty PP, Klein-Schwartz W. Octreotide's role in the management of sulfonylurea-induced hypoglycemia. J Med Toxicol 2010;6(2):199–206.
27. McLaughlin SA, Crandall CS, McKinney PE. Octreotide: an antidote for sulfonylurea-induced hypoglycemia. Ann Emerg Med 2000;36(2):133–8.
28. Fasano CJ, O'Malley G, Dominici P, et al. Comparison of octreotide and standard therapy versus standard therapy alone for the treatment of sulfonylurea-induced hypoglycemia. Ann Emerg Med 2008;51(4):400–6.

29. Glatstein M, Scolnik D, Bentur Y. Octreotide for the treatment of sulfonylurea poisoning. Clin Toxicol (Phila) 2012;50(9):795–804.
30. Rena G, Hardie DG, Pearson ER. The mechanisms of action of metformin. Diabetologia 2017;60(9):1577–85.
31. Pernicova I, Korbonits M. Metformin–mode of action and clinical implications for diabetes and cancer. Nat Rev Endocrinol 2014;10(3):143–56.
32. Wang GS, Hoyte C. Review of biguanide (metformin) toxicity. J Intensive Care Med 2019;34(11–12):863–76.
33. Salpeter SR, Greyber E, Pasternak GA, et al. Risk of fatal and nonfatal lactic acidosis with metformin use in type 2 diabetes mellitus. Cochrane Database Syst Rev 2010;(4):CD002967.
34. El-Mir MY, Nogueira V, Fontaine E, et al. Dimethylbiguanide inhibits cell respiration via an indirect effect targeted on the respiratory chain complex I. J Biol Chem 2000;275(1):223–8.
35. Forrester MB. Adult metformin ingestions reported to Texas poison control centers, 2000-2006. Hum Exp Toxicol 2008;27(7):575–83.
36. Spiller HA, Weber JA, Winter ML, et al. Multicenter case series of pediatric metformin ingestion. Ann Pharmacother 2000;34(12):1385–8.
37. Dell'Aglio DM, Perino LJ, Kazzi Z, et al. Acute metformin overdose: examining serum pH, lactate level, and metformin concentrations in survivors versus nonsurvivors: a systematic review of the literature. Ann Emerg Med 2009;54(6):818–23.
38. Ahmad S, Beckett M. Recovery from pH 6.38: lactic acidosis complicated by hypothermia. Emerg Med J 2002;19(2):169–71.
39. Seidowsky A, Nseir S, Houdret N, et al. Metformin-associated lactic acidosis: a prognostic and therapeutic study. Crit Care Med 2009;37(7):2191–6.
40. Lalau JD, Race JM. Lactic acidosis in metformin-treated patients. Prognostic value of arterial lactate levels and plasma metformin concentrations. Drug Saf 1999;20(4):377–84.
41. Blumenberg A, Benabbas R, Sinert R, et al. Do patients die with or from metformin-associated lactic acidosis (MALA)? Systematic review and meta-analysis of pH and lactate as predictors of mortality in MALA. J Med Toxicol 2020;16(2):222–9.
42. Calello DP, Liu KD, Wiegand TJ, et al. Extracorporeal treatment for metformin poisoning: systematic review and recommendations from the extracorporeal treatments in poisoning workgroup. Crit Care Med 2015;43(8):1716–30.
43. Luft D, Schmülling RM, Eggstein M. Lactic acidosis in biguanide-treated diabetics: a review of 330 cases. Diabetologia 1978;14(2):75–87.
44. Misbin RI. Phenformin-associated lactic acidosis: pathogenesis and treatment. Ann Intern Med 1977;87(5):591–5.
45. Graham RE, Cartner M, Winearls J. A severe case of vasoplegic shock following metformin overdose successfully treated with methylene blue as a last line therapy. BMJ Case Rep 2015;2015. bcr2015210229.
46. Warrick BJ, Tataru AP, Smolinske S. A systematic analysis of methylene blue for drug-induced shock. Clin Toxicol (Phila) 2016;54(7):547–55.
47. Wen Y, Li W, Poteet EC, et al. Alternative mitochondrial electron transfer as a novel strategy for neuroprotection. J Biol Chem 2011;286(18):16504–15.
48. Drucker DJ. Mechanisms of action and therapeutic application of glucagon-like peptide-1. Cell Metab 2018;27(4):740–56.
49. Aroda VR, Ratner R. The safety and tolerability of GLP-1 receptor agonists in the treatment of type 2 diabetes: a review. Diabetes Metab Res Rev 2011;27(6):528–42.

50. Drab SR. Glucagon-like peptide-1 receptor agonists for type 2 diabetes: a clinical update of safety and efficacy. Curr Diabetes Rev 2016;12(4):403–13.
51. Madsen LR, Christiansen JJ. A 45-fold liraglutide overdose did not cause hypoglycaemia. Ugeskr Laeger 2015;177(5):V11140595 [in Danish].
52. Bode SFN, Egg M, Wallesch C, et al. 10-fold liraglutide overdose over 7 months resulted only in minor side-effects. J Clin Pharmacol 2013;53(7):785–6.
53. Nakanishi R, Hirose T, Tamura Y, et al. Attempted suicide with liraglutide overdose did not induce hypoglycemia. Diabetes Res Clin Pract 2013;99(1):e3–4.
54. Nafisah SB, Almatrafi D, Al-Mulhim K. Liraglutide overdose: a case report and an updated review. Turk J Emerg Med 2020;20(1):46–9.
55. Krishnan L, Dhatariya K, Gerontitis D. No clinical harm from a massive exenatide overdose: a short report. Clin Toxicol (Phila) 2013;51(1):61.
56. Solverson KJ, Lee H, Doig CJ. Intentional overdose of liraglutide in a non-diabetic patient causing severe hypoglycemia. CJEM 2018;20(S2):S61–3.
57. Bowler M, Nethercott DR. Two lessons from the empiric management of a combined overdose of liraglutide and amitriptyline. Case Rep 2014;2(3):28–30.
58. Elmehdawi RR, Elbarsha AM. An accidental liraglutide overdose: case report. Libyan J Med 2014;9(1):23055.
59. Payen C, Thouret JM, Vial T, et al. Mild hypoglycaemia and delayed effects of co-ingestions following acute exenatide (Bayetta) poisoning. Presented at the 2012 International Congress of the European Association of Poisons Centres and Clinical Toxicologists, 25 May–1 June 2012, London, UK.
60. Cho YM, Fujita Y, Kieffer TJ. Glucagon-like peptide-1: glucose homeostasis and beyond. Annu Rev Physiol 2014;76:535–59.
61. Williams-Herman D, Engel SS, Round E, et al. Safety and tolerability of sitagliptin in clinical studies: a pooled analysis of data from 10,246 patients with type 2 diabetes. BMC Endocr Disord 2010;10:7.
62. Russell JL, Casavant MJ, Spiller HA, et al. Clinical effects of exposure to DPP-4 inhibitors as reported to the national poison data system. J Med Toxicol 2014;10(2):152–5.
63. Darracq MA, Toy JM, Chen T, et al. A retrospective review of isolated gliptin-exposure cases reported to a state poison control system. Clin Toxicol (Phila) 2014;52(3):226–30.
64. Whitney IJ, Borys DJ, Morgan DL. Incidence of hypoglycemia in sitagliptin overdose. Presented at the 2009 North American Congress of Clinical Toxicology Annual Meeting, September 21–26, 209, San Antonio, Texas, USA.
65. Furukawa S, Kumagi T, Miyake T, et al. Suicide attempt by an overdose of sitagliptin, an oral hypoglycemic agent: a case report and a review of the literature. Endocr J 2012;59(4):329–33.
66. Bahulikar A, Kulkarni V, Phalgune D. A case of janumet poisoning. J Clin Diagn Res 2017;11(11):OD01–2.
67. List JF, Whaley JM. Glucose dynamics and mechanistic implications of SGLT2 inhibitors in animals and humans. Kidney Int Suppl 2011;120:S20–7.
68. Ogawa W, Sakaguchi K. Euglycemic diabetic ketoacidosis induced by SGLT2 inhibitors: possible mechanism and contributing factors. J Diabetes Investig 2016;7(2):135–8.
69. Goldenberg RM, Berard LD, Cheng AYY, et al. SGLT2 inhibitor-associated diabetic ketoacidosis: clinical review and recommendations for prevention and diagnosis. Clin Ther 2016;38(12):2654–64.e1.
70. Goldenberg RM, Gilbert JD, Hramiak IM, et al. Sodium-glucose co-transporter inhibitors, their role in type 1 diabetes treatment and a risk mitigation strategy for

preventing diabetic ketoacidosis: the STOP DKA protocol. Diabetes Obes Metab 2019;21(10):2192–202.

71. Liu J, Li L, Li S, et al. Effects of SGLT2 inhibitors on UTIs and genital infections in type 2 diabetes mellitus: a systematic review and meta-analysis. Sci Rep 2017; 7(1):2824.

72. Bersoff-Matcha SJ, Chamberlain C, Cao C, et al. Fournier gangrene associated with sodium-glucose cotransporter-2 inhibitors: a review of spontaneous postmarketing cases. Ann Intern Med 2019;170(11):764–9.

73. Scheen AJ. An update on the safety of SGLT2 inhibitors. Expert Opin Drug Saf 2019;18(4):295–311.

74. Schaeffer SE, DesLauriers C, Spiller HA, et al. Retrospective review of SGLT2 inhibitor exposures reported to 13 poison centers. Clin Toxicol (Phila) 2018;56(3): 204–8.

75. Smith K, Gomez L, Smith L, et al. How sweet it is: sodium glucose co-transporter 2 inhibitor ingestions reported to U.S. poison centers. Presented at the 2017 North American Congress of Clinical Toxicology, October 11–15, 2017, Vancouver, British Columbia, Canada.

76. Nakamura M, Nakade J, Toyama T, et al. Severe intoxication caused by sodium-glucose cotransporter 2 inhibitor overdose: a case report. BMC Pharmacol Toxicol 2020;21(1):5.

77. Schneider A, Lengenfelder B. Suizidversuch mit dem SGLT-2-inhibitor Empagliflozin rettet Patientin das Leben. Diabetologia 2018;14(2):99–100.

Antithrombotic and Antiplatelet Drug Toxicity

David B. Liss, MD*, Michael E. Mullins, MD

KEYWORDS

- Anticoagulants • Antiplatelets • Reversal agents • Hemorrhage • Toxicity

KEY POINTS

- Anticoagulants and antiplatelet agents target various points in the coagulation cascade.
- The primary toxicity associated with these agents is hemorrhage.
- In hemorrhage, bleeding control and resuscitation are the primary actions.
- Reversal agents exist for most of the anticoagulants with variable efficacy.
- Antiplatelet agents do not have readily available reversal agents.

INTRODUCTION

Significant progress has been made in the development of medications to prevent thrombosis and platelet aggregation. These drugs target specific components of the coagulation cascade or platelet activation and aggregation process (**Fig. 1**). Morbidity related to these medications is primarily due to hemorrhage. This review covers the pharmacology of each drug class, typical use of the medications, pharmacodynamic monitoring, and available reversal agents.

ANTICOAGULANTS
Vitamin K Antagonists

The vitamin K antagonists are derivatives of dicoumarol. Although the terminology is pervasive, these drugs do not directly antagonize vitamin K, but achieve anticoagulation by inhibiting the enzymes that recycle oxidized vitamin K.

Warfarin

Warfarin, an antagonist of vitamin K reduction, is derived from the coumarins and is the only drug within this class still in use in the United States.[1] The active form of vitamin K aids in the gamma-carboxylation of factors II, VII, IX, and X, as well as proteins C and S.[2] Warfarin depletes factor VII (half-life 3–6 hours) and protein C (half-life

Department of Emergency Medicine, Division of Medical Toxicology, Washington University in St. Louis, 660 South Euclid Avenue, CB 8072, St Louis, MO 63110, USA
* Corresponding author.
E-mail address: lissd@wustl.edu

Crit Care Clin 37 (2021) 591–604
https://doi.org/10.1016/j.ccc.2021.03.012
0749-0704/21/© 2021 Elsevier Inc. All rights reserved.

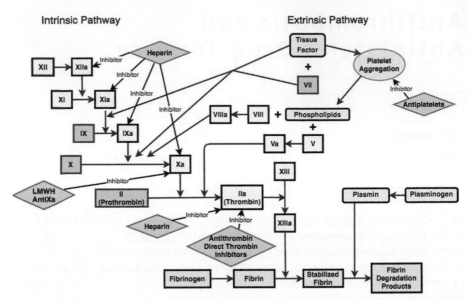

Fig. 1. Simplified coagulation cascade with platelet aggregation. Factors affected by warfarin in pink.

6–8 hours) and subsequently factors IX and X (half-lives of 18–30 hours) (see **Fig. 1**).[3] Prothrombin (factor II) has the longest half-life of vitamin-K–dependent factors of 60 to 100 hours.[1,3] Because of the differing rates of clotting factor and protein depletion, therapeutic antithrombosis does not occur immediately and some patients remain at increased risk for thrombosis during the initial treatment period due to the reduction of anticoagulant proteins C and S.

Warfarin sodium is rapidly and completely absorbed via the oral route. It exhibits a wide range of apparent half-lives of elimination, 15 to 58 hours, with a mean of 42 hours.[4,5] Time to anticoagulation varies widely between individuals partly because of variation in pharmacokinetics including genetic variation in CYP450 metabolism as well as co-administered drug and diet effects on absorption and metabolism.[6] Extensive CYP450 metabolism of warfarin presents the potential for numerous drug-drug, herb-drug, and food-drug interactions. Most interactions involve inhibition of CYP450 isoenzymes, which may increase the anticoagulant effects of warfarin.[7,8] However, induction of CYP450 isoenzymes as well as P-glycoprotein may reduce the effectiveness of a given dose of warfarin.

Warfarin sodium has US Food and Drug Administration (FDA) approval for use in the treatment and prophylaxis of venous thromboembolism, thromboembolic complications from atrial fibrillation and/or cardiac valve replacement, and for anticoagulation for patients with prosthetic heart valves.[9,10] It also has been used for reducing the risk of death, recurrent myocardial infarction, and thromboembolic events, including stroke, after myocardial infarction.[5]

The anticoagulant effects of warfarin can be measured with the prothrombin time/international normalized ratio (PT/INR) assay.[7,8] In either overdose of warfarin or bleeding complications due to therapeutic over-anticoagulation by warfarin, the INR is the recommended test for evaluation.[11,12]

The primary toxicity related to patients taking warfarin is hemorrhage. Spontaneous hemorrhage risk increases with INR elevation, renal dysfunction, age, presence of

VKORC1 and *CYP2C9* mutations, duration of warfarin use, and concurrent aspirin use.[13,14] Warfarin overdose also occurs and places patients at risk of hemorrhage.[12] However, in a case series of 23 patients with warfarin poisoning, only 3 had bleeding events, one described as "major," with all patients recovering.[12]

Warfarin can paradoxically produce life-threatening skin necrosis. Although the exact mechanism is not proven, this outcome is more common in either congenital or acquired deficiencies of proteins C or S or antithrombin deficiency.[15] These proteins function as anticoagulants and the resultant loss of anticoagulation produces microvascular thrombosis and eventually skin necrosis.[15,16] Systemic atheroemboli and cholesterol microemboli are also produced with warfarin therapy. Numerous varying symptoms can result depending on the eventual location of emboli.[17] One syndrome related to these emboli is the "purple or blue toe syndrome" in which patients develop painful purple/blue discoloration of the toes and feet after 3 to 8 weeks of therapy with warfarin.[17–20] Development should prompt discontinuation of warfarin and replacement with another agent.

As the primary life-threatening adverse reaction to warfarin, moderate to severe hemorrhage requires consideration of reversal. Varying algorithms and recommendations exist regarding warfarin reversal.[21–25] As with all bleeding, the highest priority is to address the site of bleeding with manual compression or surgical intervention. Our approach is summarized in **Table 1**.[22,26,27] Four factor prothrombin complex concentrates (4F-PCC) are a lyophilized mixture of factors II, VII, IX, and X, as well as proteins C and S. It is preferred over alternative measures; 3-factor PCC lacks a significant quantity of factor VII, fresh frozen plasma requires blood typing and significant volume administration to reverse anticoagulation, and recombinant factor VIIa (rFVIIa) does not replace 3 of the missing factors and increases risks of clotting.[27,28]

Warfarin overdose is a rare poisoning, but management is similar to warfarin reversal. A review of all cases over a 25-year period at 2 academic medical centers revealed 23 cases, with a median reported dose of 100 mg (interquartile range [IQR] 75–216 mg).[12] All patients developed coagulopathy, defined as INR greater than 1.4, 3 developed hemorrhage, but all recovered. Seventeen of these 23 patients were treated with vitamin K, either oral or intravenous, with a median dose of 15 mg (IQR 10–50 mg). In warfarin overdose, our recommendation is 5 to 10 mg oral vitamin K_1 daily until the INR is less than 2.

Superwarfarins

Analogues to warfarin with significantly increased duration of effect were developed as rodenticides. Intentional and accidental human poisoning with these agents also

Table 1
Approach to warfarin reversal

Asymptomatic INR Elevation	Mild Hemorrhage	Moderate Hemorrhage	Severe or Life-Threatening Hemorrhage
Hold warfarin until INR <2	Hold warfarin until INR <2	Vitamin K_1 5–10 mg IV	Vitamin K_1 5–10 mg IV
		Blood product resuscitation including fresh frozen plasma	Blood product resuscitation including fresh frozen plasma
			4F-PCC

Abbreviations: 4F-PCC, 4 factor prothrombin complex concentrates; INR, international normalized ratio; IV, intravenous.

occurs.[29,30] The most commonly encountered clinically are brodifacoum and broma-diolone. Large intentional ingestions produce profound and prolonged anticoagulation, at times lasting months in duration.[30] A rise in INR may be delayed 1 to 2 days similarly to that seen in warfarin. Patients from an outbreak associated with brodifacoum adulterated synthetic cannabinoids in March 2018 were treated with oral vitamin K_1. However a shortage of this medication complicated the management.[29] Varying treatment regimens have been described with dosing ranging from oral vitamin K_1 50 to 150 mg/d typically given in divided doses every 6 to 8 hours. Serious or life-threatening hemorrhage should be treated similarly to that associated with warfarin therapy.

Heparins

Named for compounds isolated from canine liver, this group of anticoagulants consists of varying preparations of naturally derived heparins.[31] Members of this class in current usage include unfractionated heparin (UFH) and the low molecular weight heparins (LMWHs). Multiple available forms of LMWH exist but only enoxaparin, dalteparin, and tinzaparin are FDA approved in the United States.[32] These drugs vary in their molecular weights and in their ratio of anti-Xa/anti-IIa activity.[33]

The primary mechanism of action of this class is activation of antithrombin, which then inhibits either thrombin (factor IIa) or factor Xa (see **Fig. 1**).[34] UFH is made up of a heterogeneous group of glycosaminoglycans, ranging from 3000 to 30,000 Da in molecular weight.[35] LMWH is produced by depolymerizing UFH, which yields a mixture with an average molecular weight of 5000 Da.[34] The active site of the heparin molecule is a specific pentasaccharide sequence that causes a conformational change in antithrombin, increasing its activity on thrombin and factor Xa.[33]

LMWH has a more predictable efficacy due to longer half-life, better bioavailability, and less dose-dependent clearance.[34] UFH is highly protein bound and has faster renal clearance than LMWH, although the half-life of UFH is difficult to predict and increases with dose.[35] The anticoagulant effects of UFH also vary between individuals due to its high protein binding, which inhibits its effect on antithrombin. Both UFH and LMWH are used in the prevention and treatment of venous thromboembolism as well as coronary artery disease.[33–35]

As UFH inhibits both factors IIa and Xa, the activated partial thromboplastin time (aPTT), which measures activity in the intrinsic and common pathways, is an excellent measure of anticoagulation effect from this drug (see **Fig. 1**).[36] Some controversy exists over the need to monitor therapy with LMWH; however, some recommendations include the special populations of pregnant patients, small children, patients at extremes of body mass, and those with renal insufficiency.[35,37,38] Although UFH has a dose-response effect on the aPTT, as the molecular weight of the heparin decreases, so does its effect on the aPTT. LMWH is better monitored by the anti-factor Xa activity level.[34,39]

The primary toxicity associated with the heparins is hemorrhage and thrombosis. Cancer and renal insufficiency increase the risk of bleeding. In animal models, UFH causes an increased risk of bleeding; however, in human trials, there does not appear to be a reduction in bleeding risk with LMWH.[34,39] Additional toxicity related to the heparins includes heparin-induced thrombocytopenia (HIT), non–immune-mediated heparin-associated thrombocytopenia (HAT, formerly HIT 1), purple toe syndrome, and heparin-induced osteoporosis.[34,40,41]

Thrombosis with heparin therapy is paradoxically related to HIT. This condition results from immunoglobulin G antibodies that recognize an epitope of platelet factor 4 (PF4) combined with either heparin or LMWH.[42] The Fc portion of these antibodies crosslink platelets and monocytes leading to thrombocytopenia, thrombin generation, and clotting.[43] Typically HIT begins 5 to 10 days after initiation of heparin therapy and results in thrombosis or thromboembolism in up to 50% of cases.[44] HIT is identified by a drop in platelets and detection of the antibody to PF4-heparin. This antibody has high sensitivity but low specificity for HIT and must be confirmed by a platelet activation assay, such as a serotonin-release assay.[45] Diagnosis of HIT requires immediate cessation of UFH or LMWH and initiation of direct thrombin inhibitor treatment.[41,45,46] Warfarin should be avoided, as it may exacerbate thrombosis through protein C depletion.

Because of its large number of negatively charged amino acids, heparin can be neutralized by the arginine-rich protamine sulfate. Derived from fish semen, this protein binds UFH, effectively reversing anticoagulation. The dosing ratio is 1 mg intravenous protamine per 100 units of heparin with the caveat that heparin infusions have a short half-life and only the heparin received in the prior 2.5 hours should be used in dose calculation.[47] LMWH can also be bound by protamine; however, human evidence of efficacy is lacking. A suggested dose for LMWH given within the preceding 8 hours is 1 mg per 100 anti-Xa units (1 mg of enoxaparin is approximately 100 anti-Xa units), up to a maximum of 50 mg. A second dose of 0.5 mg per 100 anti-Xa units can be administered for continued bleeding.[47] Protamine causes hypotension and bradycardia and should be administered slowly. In addition, there is concern that fish allergy, prior exposure to protamine, history of vasectomy, or exposure to neutral protamine Hagedorn insulin may predispose the patient to anaphylaxis.[47,48]

Direct Thrombin Inhibitors

Direct thrombin inhibitors (DTIs) inhibit factor IIa and prevent conversion of fibrinogen to fibrin (see **Fig. 1**). The class includes the bivalent DTIs (lepirudin, desirudin, and bivalirudin) and the univalent DTIs (argatroban and dabigatran).

Dabigatran acts at the last step of the coagulation cascade and does not alter coagulation factor concentrations. For this reason, commonly available measures of coagulation, such as INR and aPTT, are insensitive indicators of dabigatran effect. The aPTT may be elevated in acute or chronic overdose, however, a normal aPTT neither confirms nor excludes therapeutic use of dabigatran.[49] Point-of-care INR tests may yield falsely elevated results in the presence of dabigatran.[50] Tests that more directly measure effect of dabigatran include ecarin clotting time (ECT), ecarin chromogenic assay, HEMOCLOT thrombin inhibitor, and thrombin generation assay, but these tests are not widely available.

Several case reports of acute or acute-on-chronic overdoses of dabigatran show a consistent pattern.[51–56] Dabigatran concentrations, when available, were 8 to 20 times higher than the concentration seen in therapeutic use. Thrombin time (TT) and aPTT were markedly long for up to approximately 2 days. Two patients received antidotal treatment with idarucizumab, although their outcomes were similar to those who received oral activated charcoal.[53,54]

Two poison control center studies illustrate a low risk of bleeding complications.[57,58] Major and fatal outcomes concentrated among adults older than 65 years with bleeding as an adverse drug reaction. Renal insufficiency was a contributing factor in approximately one-quarter of these cases. Adults and adolescents with acute, intentional overdoses seldom had any bleeding despite abnormal clotting studies for up to 2 days.

The pharmacokinetics of dabigatran are generally favorable for removal by hemodialysis (HD).[59] Case reports and case series illustrate successful removal of dabigatran by HD in patients with acute hemorrhage while taking therapeutic doses of dabigatran.[60,61]

Treatment with blood clotting factors is generally ineffective in reversing dabigatran. Dabigatran acts primarily on thrombin at the end of the common pathway in the coagulation cascade. The factors in 4F-PCC all act earlier in the coagulation cascade before the site of action of dabigatran (see **Fig. 1**). A randomized controlled trial of 4F-PCC in human volunteers showed no effect on aPTT, TT, or ECT when given after dabigatran.[62]

Idarucizumab is a specific monoclonal antibody fragment that binds dabigatran.[63] The usual dose is 5 g for life-threatening bleeding or need for emergency surgery while taking dabigatran. Although indicated for dabigatran exposure with life-threatening bleeding, 2 case reports describe its use in large overdoses of dabigatran with markedly abnormal coagulation studies but no clinical bleeding.[53,54] Idarucizumab 5 g rapidly reduced the dabigatran concentration to zero and normalized the PT, aPTT, and TT in both cases. Other reports with 3 patients describe cases of incomplete reversal of dabigatran with 5 g of idarucizumab.[64,65] Such cases may require additional idarucizumab or factor VIII inhibitor bypass activity or HD.

Factor Xa Inhibitors

This class includes apixaban, rivaroxaban, and edoxaban. All are reversible inhibitors of free and clot-bound factor Xa (see **Fig. 1**). This prevents factor Xa from forming prothrombinase and in turn prevents conversion of prothrombin to thrombin.[7,22]

As with the DTIs, INR and aPTT are insensitive measures of anti-Xa effect but may be abnormal in acute or chronic overdose. Some hospitals have anti-Xa activity testing calibrated for therapeutic heparin monitoring (as an alternative to aPTT). This is a semiquantitative test for the anti-Xa inhibitor drugs. An elevated anti-Xa activity alone is not a sufficient indication for antidotal treatment.

Andexanet alfa is a "decoy" receptor for factor Xa.[66,67] It rapidly and effectively binds rivaroxaban and apixaban. It effectively reduces the free drug concentration and restores the clotting activity to normal for the duration of the infusion.

If andexanet is not available, the 4F-PCC will provide additional factor X to overcome the effect of anti-Xa agents. In a double-blind, crossover randomized controlled trial, 4F-PCC given after rivaroxaban 20 mg twice a day normalized the PT and endogenous thrombin potential in volunteers.[62]

Andexanet alfa also binds UFH, and patients who need therapeutic anticoagulation with UFH may have heparin resistance. Two patients who received andexanet before undergoing cardiac surgery required much larger doses of UFH and had difficulty achieving the target activated clotting time.[66,67]

Table 2 provides information on other factor Xa and thrombin inhibitors that are not reviewed in detail.

ANTIPLATELETS
Aspirin

Aspirin, or acetylsalicylic acid, is a weak organic acid that irreversibly acetylates 2 prostaglandin synthases commonly known as cyclooxygenase 1 and 2 (COX-1 and COX-2).[73] These enzymes catalyze the conversion of arachidonic acid to prostaglandin H_2 (PGH$_2$). Platelets require PGH$_2$ to produce thromboxane A_2 (TXA$_2$), which causes platelet aggregation and vasoconstriction (see **Fig. 1**). Aspirin is rapidly absorbed with a relatively short half-life of 15 to 20 minutes, however platelet inhibition is irreversible.[74] Given the irreversible effect on platelet COX-1, aspirin has antiplatelet

Table 2
Additional factor Xa and thrombin inhibitors

Drug/Class	Mechanism	Monitoring	Reversal
Fondaparinux	Pentasaccharide heparin analogue, inhibits factor Xa	Anti-factor Xa activity	None, rFVIIa has been suggested
Bivalirudin	Hirudin analogue, direct thrombin inhibitor	ACT or aPTT	None, short half-life, stop infusion
Argatroban	Arginine derivative, direct thrombin inhibitor	ACT or aPTT	None, short half-life, stop infusion

Abbreviations: ACT, activated clotting time; aPTT, activated partial thromboplastin time; rFVIIa, recombinant factor VIIa.
Data from Refs.[47,68–72]

effects long after the concentration is undetectable. Platelet function assays that measure pharmacodynamic effects of aspirin on platelets can be used to detect platelet inhibition.[75]

The risk of major intracranial or extracranial hemorrhage associated with aspirin is less than 1% per year.[74] Platelet transfusion does not appear to improve outcomes in human studies with life-threatening intracranial or extracranial hemorrhage in the setting of aspirin use.[76–78] Platelet function assays can precede the administration of platelets if there is a question of whether aspirin was taken recently. In one prospective study, platelet transfusion before neurosurgical intervention in the setting of a positive platelet function assay showed improved outcomes.[79] Desmopressin has a low side-effect profile combined with some evidence of efficacy, and a single dose is recommended in the setting of intracranial hemorrhage with recent aspirin use.[76] Blood product resuscitation and hemorrhage source control are paramount.

In the setting of poisoning, a salicylate concentration is necessary to guide treatment.[80] Salicylate poisoning exerts a direct stimulatory effect on the medulla, causing increased respiration and a resulting respiratory alkalosis. At high concentrations, aspirin also uncouples oxidative phosphorylation and the citric acid cycle, producing a metabolic acidosis.[80,81] The presentation varies depending on acute or chronic toxicity with severe toxicity causing pulmonary edema, cerebral edema, seizures, or coma.[80]

Treatment for aspirin poisoning begins with crystalloid fluid resuscitation. Once stabilized, if the mental status permits, activated charcoal should be administered if there is

Table 3
Additional antiplatelet agents

Drug/Class	Mechanism	Monitoring	Reversal
Dipyridamole	Inhibits phosphodiesterase, increases cAMP	None	None, hypotension can be treated with caffeine or aminophylline
GIIb/IIIa inhibitors (abciximab, eptifibatide, tirofiban)	Inhibit GIIb/IIIa on platelets, prevents aggregation	Platelet count	Platelets, eptifibatide and tirofiban have short half-lives, stop infusion

Abbreviation: cAMP, cyclic adenosine monophosphate.
Data from Refs.[74,88–91]

suspicion of continued aspirin absorption (rising serial concentrations). Although these patients may appear to be in respiratory distress, intubation should be performed only with both clinical and laboratory evidence of hypoventilation.[82] A sodium bicarbonate infusion may enhance elimination by alkalinizing the urine with caution not to increase the arterial pH above 7.5.[80] Hypokalemia is common and should be corrected, as the urine will not properly alkalinize. Hemodialysis is recommended if the salicylate concentration is >100 mg/dL or greater than 90 mg/dL with renal impairment, altered mental status, or new hypoxemia requiring oxygen therapy.[83] Hemodialysis is also recommended after failure of standard therapy if the concentration is >90 mg/dL or greater than 80 mg/dL with renal impairment, or if the blood pH is <7.20.[83]

Table 4
Summary of anticoagulants and antiplatelet agents

Drug Class (Agents)	Mechanism	Monitoring	Reversal Agent
Vitamin K antagonists (warfarin)	Inhibit vitamin K reductase preventing formation of factors II, VII, IX, and X	INR	Vitamin K, FFP, 4F-PCC
Heparins (unfractionated heparin, low molecular weight heparin)	Inhibit factor IIa (heparin) and/or factor Xa (UFH, LMWH)	aPTT, ACT	Protamine sulfate (UFH)
Oral direct thrombin inhibitors (dabigatran)	Direct thrombin inhibitor	ECT, ECA, HTI, TGA, TT	Idarucizumab, possibly hemodialysis
Xa inhibitors (apixaban, rivaroxaban, edoxaban)	Inhibit free and clot-bound Xa	Anti-factor Xa activity	Andexanet alfa, 4F-PCC
Aspirin	COX-1 and COX-2 inhibition, prostaglandin inhibition	Aspirin level for overdose; platelet function assay	Desmopressin, platelet transfusion not recommended unless intracranial surgery
Dipyridamole	Inhibits phosphodiesterase, increases cAMP	None	None for hemorrhage. Possibly aminophylline or caffeine for overdose
ADP antagonists (ticlopidine, prasugrel, clopidogrel, ticagrelor, cangrelor)	ADP receptor antagonists, prevent platelet aggregation	Platelet function assay	No specific antidote

Abbreviations: 4F-PCC, 4 factor prothrombin complex concentrates; ACT, activated clotting time; ADP, adenosine diphosphate; aPTT, activated partial thromboplastin time; cAMP, cyclic adenosine monophosphate; COX, cyclooxygenase; ECA, ecarin chromogenic assay; ECT, ecarin clotting time; FFP, fresh frozen plasma; HTI, HEMOCLOT thrombin inhibitor; INR, international normalized ratio; TGA, thrombin generation assay; TT, thrombin time.

Adenosine Diphosphate Antagonists

The thienopyridine class, ticlopidine, prasugrel, and clopidogrel, are adenosine diphosphate (ADP) receptor antagonists. They irreversibly inhibit the P2Y$_{12}$ receptor on platelets, which prevents their aggregation (see **Fig. 1**). They are all prodrugs that require metabolism to exert their effects. Clopidogrel requires activation by CYP2C19, and a significant portion of the population has been found to have loss-of-function polymorphisms, prompting some recommendations for genetic testing before clopidogrel therapy, as in-stent thrombosis has occurred in these patients.[74,84] Ticagrelor and cangrelor are reversible ADP antagonists that do not require metabolic activation.[85]

Monitoring of antiplatelet effect may occur with dynamic platelet function testing, such as the VerifyNow P2Y12 assay or light transmittance aggregometry, to detect high on-treatment platelet activity during routine clinical care.[74,86] These tests are not efficacious in the setting of life-threatening hemorrhage to guide management.[87]

No reversal agents exist for these medications. Platelet transfusion is suggested; however, clinical trials in the setting of intracranial hemorrhage did not improve outcomes.[78]

Table 3 provides additional information on other antiplatelet agents.

SUMMARY

With the exception of aspirin, the primary toxicity of these agents is related to uncontrollable life-threatening hemorrhage or thrombosis. By knowing the mechanism of action of each class, the correct reversal agent may be used (**Table 4**). However, rapid hemorrhage source control and appropriate resuscitation remain the principal objectives.

CLINICS CARE POINTS

- Life-threatening bleeding should be managed with manual compression, surgical hemorrhage control, and blood product resuscitation, including plasma and platelets.

- Severe warfarin-associated bleeding should be treated with 4F-PCC in addition to blood product resuscitation and IV vitamin K.

- Protamine can reverse UFH, however its effects on LMWH are less certain.

- HIT is a life-threatening immune-mediated disease that requires surveillance to detect and prompt treatment with an alternative anticoagulant.

- Dabigatran can be reversed with idarucizumab and removed by hemodialysis.

- Rivaroxaban and apixaban can be reversed with either andexanet alfa or 4F-PCC.

- Aspirin toxicity requires aggressive fluid resuscitation, urine alkalinization, and possibly hemodialysis.

DISCLOSURE

The authors have no commercial benefits, financial support, or financial conflicts of interest to disclose.

REFERENCES

1. Deykin D. Warfarin therapy. 1. N Engl J Med 1970;283(13):691–4.

2. Wessler S, Gitel SN. Warfarin. N Engl J Med 1984;311(10):645–52.

3. Bos MHA, van't Veer C, Reitsma PH. Molecular biology and biochemistry of the coagulation factors and pathways of hemostasis. In: Kaushansky K, Lichtman MA, Prchal JT, et al, editors. Williams hematology. 9th edition. New York: McGraw-Hill Education; 2015. p. 1–3.

4. O'Reilly RA, Aggeler PM, Leong LS. Studies on the coumarin anticoagulant drugs: the pharmacodynamics of warfarin in man. J Clin Invest 1963;42(10): 1542–51.

5. Bristol-Myers Squibb Company. Coumadin® (Warfarin sodium) [package insert]. U.S. Food and Drug Administration website. 2011. Available at: www.accessdata. fda.gov/drugsatfda_docs/label/2011/009218s107lbl.pdf. Accessed October 30, 2020.

6. Cropp JS, Bussey HI. A review of enzyme induction of warfarin metabolism with recommendations for patient management. Pharmacotherapy 1997;17(5): 917–28.

7. Fawzy AM, Lip GYH. Pharmacokinetics and pharmacodynamics of oral anticoagulants used in atrial fibrillation. Expert Opin Drug Metab Toxicol 2019;15(5): 381–98.

8. Hirsh J, Dalen JE, Anderson DR, et al. Oral anticoagulants: mechanism of action, clinical effectiveness, and optimal therapeutic range. Chest 1998;114(5, Supplement):445S–69S.

9. Whitlock RP, Sun JC, Fremes SE, et al. Antithrombotic and thrombolytic therapy for valvular disease: antithrombotic therapy and prevention of thrombosis, 9th ed: American College of Chest Physicians Evidence-Based Clinical Practice Guidelines. Chest 2012;141(2 Suppl):e576S–600S.

10. Nishimura RA, Otto CM, Bonow RO, et al. 2017 AHA/ACC Focused update of the 2014 AHA/ACC guideline for the management of patients with valvular heart disease: a report of the American College of Cardiology/American heart association Task Force on clinical practice guidelines. Circulation 2017;135(25):e1159–95.

11. Holbrook A, Schulman S, Witt DM, et al. Evidence-based management of anticoagulant therapy: antithrombotic therapy and prevention of thrombosis, 9th ed: American College of Chest Physicians Evidence-Based Clinical Practice Guidelines. Chest 2012;141(2):e152S–84S.

12. Levine M, Pizon AF, Padilla-Jones A, et al. Warfarin overdose: a 25-year experience. J Med Toxicol 2014;10(2):156–64.

13. Garcia DA, Regan S, Crowther M, et al. The risk of hemorrhage among patients with warfarin-associated coagulopathy. J Am Coll Cardiol 2006;47(4):804–8.

14. Limdi MA, Crowley MR, Beasley TM, et al. Influence of kidney function on risk of hemorrhage among patients taking warfarin: a cohort study. Am J Kidney Dis 2013;61(2):354–7.

15. Fred HL. Skin necrosis induced by coumarin congeners. Tex Heart Inst J 2017; 44(4):233–6.

16. Chan YC, Valenti D, Mansfield AO, et al. Warfarin induced skin necrosis. Br J Surg 2000;87(3):266–72.

17. Hyman BT, Landas SK, Ashman RF, et al. Warfarin-related purple toes syndrome and cholesterol microembolization. Am J Med 1987;82(6):1233–7.

18. Feder W, Auerbach R. "Purple toes": an uncommon sequela of oral coumarin drug therapy. Ann Intern Med 1961;55:911–7.

19. Lebsack CS, Weibert RT. "Purple toes" syndrome. Postgrad Med 1982; 71(5):81–4.

20. Akle CA, Joiner CL. Purple toe syndrome. J R Soc Med 1981;74(3):219.

21. Witt DM, Clark NP, Kaatz S, et al. Guidance for the practical management of warfarin therapy in the treatment of venous thromboembolism. J Thromb Thrombolysis 2016;41(1):187–205.

22. Lip GYH, Banerjee A, Boriani G, et al. Antithrombotic therapy for atrial fibrillation: CHEST guideline and expert panel report. Chest 2018;154(5):1121–201.

23. Hemphill JC, Greenberg SM, Anderson CS, et al. Guidelines for the management of spontaneous intracerebral hemorrhage. Stroke 2015;46(7):2032–60.

24. Milling TJ, Pollack CV. A review of guidelines on anticoagulation reversal across different clinical scenarios – is there a general consensus? Am J Emerg Med 2020;38(9):1890–903.

25. Spahn DR, Bouillon B, Cerny V, et al. Management of bleeding and coagulopathy following major trauma: an updated European guideline. Crit Care 2013; 17(2):R76.

26. Sarode R, Milling TJ, Refaai MA, et al. Efficacy and safety of a 4-factor prothrombin complex concentrate in patients on vitamin K antagonists presenting with major bleeding: a randomized, plasma-controlled, phase IIIb study. Circulation 2013;128(11):1234–43.

27. Tran HA, Chunilal SD, Harper PL, et al. An update of consensus guidelines for warfarin reversal. Med J Aust 2013;198(4):198–9.

28. Quinlan DJ, Eikelboom JW, Weitz JI. Four-factor prothrombin complex concentrate for urgent reversal of vitamin K antagonists in patients with major bleeding. Circulation 2013;128(11):1179–81.

29. Chong Y-K, Mak TW-L. Superwarfarin (long-acting anticoagulant rodenticides) poisoning: from pathophysiology to laboratory-guided clinical management. Clin Biochem Rev 2019;40(4):175–85.

30. Moritz E. Notes from the Field: outbreak of severe illness linked to the vitamin K antagonist brodifacoum and use of synthetic cannabinoids — Illinois, March–April 2018. MMWR Morb Mortal Wkly Rep 2018;67:607–8.

31. Wardrop D, Keeling D. The story of the discovery of heparin and warfarin. Br J Haematol 2008;141(6):757–63.

32. U.S. Food and Drug Administration. Generic enoxaparin questions and Answers. Available at: https://www.fda.gov/drugs/postmarket-drug-safety-information-patients-and-providers/generic-enoxaparin-questions-and-answers. Accessed November 25, 2020.

33. Gray E, Mulloy B, Barrowcliffe TW. Heparin and low-molecular-weight heparin. Thromb Haemost 2008;99(5):807–18.

34. Weitz JI. Low-molecular-weight heparins. N Engl J Med 1997;337(10):688–99.

35. Hirsh J. Heparin. N Engl J Med 1991;324(22):1565–74.

36. Gallus AS, Hirsh J. Antithrombotic drugs: Part I. Drugs 1976;12(1):41–68.

37. Harenberg J. Is laboratory monitoring of low-molecular-weight heparin therapy necessary? Yes. J Thromb Haemost 2004;2(4):547–50.

38. Cadroy Y, Pourrat J, Baladre MF, et al. Delayed elimination of enoxaparin in patients with chronic renal insufficiency. Thromb Res 1991;63(3):385–90.

39. Harenberg J, Heene DL. Pharmacology and special clinical applications of low-molecular-weight heparins. Am J Hematol 1988;29(4):233–40.

40. Hirsh J. Laboratory monitoring of low-molecular-weight heparin therapy. J Thromb Haemost 2004;2(6):1003.

41. Greinacher A. Heparin-induced thrombocytopenia. N Engl J Med 2015;373(3): 252–61.

42. Brandt S, Krauel K, Gottschalk KE, et al. Characterisation of the conformational changes in platelet factor 4 induced by polyanions: towards in vitro prediction of antigenicity. Thromb Haemost 2014;112(1):53–64.

43. Kelton JG, Sheridan D, Santos A, et al. Heparin-induced thrombocytopenia: laboratory studies. Blood 1988;72(3):925–30.

44. Warkentin TE, Kelton JG. A 14-year study of heparin-induced thrombocytopenia. Am J Med 1996;101(5):502–7.

45. East JM, Cserti-Gazdewich CM, Granton JT. Heparin-induced thrombocytopenia in the critically ill patient. Chest 2018;154(3):678–90.

46. Linkins L-A, Dans AL, Moores LK, et al. Treatment and prevention of heparin-induced thrombocytopenia: antithrombotic therapy and prevention of thrombosis, 9th ed: American College of chest physicians evidence-based clinical practice guidelines. Chest 2012;141(2 Suppl):e495S–530S.

47. Garcia DA, Baglin TP, Weitz JI, et al. Parenteral anticoagulants: antithrombotic therapy and prevention of thrombosis, 9th ed: American College of chest physicians evidence-based clinical practice guidelines. Chest 2012;141(2 Suppl): e24S–43S.

48. Levy JH, Schwieger IM, Zaidan JR, et al. Evaluation of patients at risk for protamine reactions. J Thorac Cardiovasc Surg 1989;98(2):200–4.

49. Douxfils J, Ageno W, Samama C-M, et al. Laboratory testing in patients treated with direct oral anticoagulants: a practical guide for clinicians. J Thromb Haemost 2018;16(2):209–19.

50. DeRemer CE, Gujral JS, Thornton JW, et al. Dabigatran falsely elevates point of care international normalized ratio results. Am J Med 2011;124(9):e5–6.

51. Woo JS, Kapadia N, Phanco SE, et al. Positive outcome after intentional overdose of dabigatran. J Med Toxicol 2013;9(2):192–5.

52. Vlad I, Armstrong J, Ridgley J, et al. Dabigatran deliberate overdose: two cases and suggestions for laboratory monitoring. Clin Toxicol Phila Pa 2016;54(3): 286–9.

53. Shapiro S, Bhatnagar N, Khan A, et al. Idarucizumab for dabigatran overdose in a child. Br J Haematol 2018;180(3):457–9.

54. Peetermans M, Pollack C, Reilly P, et al. Idarucizumab for dabigatran overdose. Clin Toxicol Phila Pa 2016;54(8):644–6.

55. Gorodetsky RM, Sankoh F, Pereira J, et al. Conservative management of dabigatran overdose: case report and review of literature. Asia Pac J Med Toxicol 2016; 5(1):25–7.

56. Hajšmanová Z, Šigutová P, Lavičková A. Repeated administration of idarucizumab to a patient with dabigatran overdose. Hamostaseologie 2018;38(1):39–42.

57. Stevenson JW, Minns AB, Smollin C, et al. An observational case series of dabigatran and rivaroxaban exposures reported to a poison control system. Am J Emerg Med 2014;32(9):1077–84.

58. Conway SE, Schaeffer SE, Harrison DL. Evaluation of dabigatran exposures reported to poison control centers. Ann Pharmacother 2014;48(3):354–60.

59. Liesenfeld K-H, Staab A, Härtter S, et al. Pharmacometric characterization of dabigatran hemodialysis. Clin Pharmacokinet 2013;52(6):453–62.

60. Chen BC, Sheth NR, Dadzie KA, et al. Hemodialysis for the treatment of pulmonary hemorrhage from dabigatran overdose. Am J Kidney Dis 2013;62(3):591–4.

61. Singh T, Maw TT, Henry BL, et al. Extracorporeal therapy for dabigatran removal in the treatment of acute bleeding: a single center experience. Clin J Am Soc Nephrol 2013;8(9):1533–9.

62. Eerenberg ES, Kamphuisen PW, Sijpkens MK, et al. Reversal of rivaroxaban and dabigatran by prothrombin complex concentrate: a randomized, placebo-controlled, crossover study in healthy subjects. Circulation 2011;124(14):1573–9.

63. Pollack CV, Reilly PA, Eikelboom J, et al. Idarucizumab for dabigatran reversal. N Engl J Med 2015;373(6):511–20.

64. Simon A, Domanovits H, Ay C, et al. The recommended dose of idarucizumab may not always be sufficient for sustained reversal of dabigatran. J Thromb Haemost 2017;15(7):1317–21.

65. Steele AP, Lee JA, Dager WE. Incomplete dabigatran reversal with idarucizumab. Clin Toxicol 2018;56(3):216–8.

66. Eche IM, Elsamadisi P, Wex N, et al. Intraoperative unfractionated heparin unresponsiveness during endovascular repair of a ruptured abdominal aortic aneurysm following administration of andexanet alfa for the reversal of rivaroxaban. Pharmacotherapy 2019;39(8):861–5.

67. Watson CJ, Zettervall SL, Hall MM, et al. Difficult intraoperative heparinization following andexanet alfa administration. Clin Pract Cases Emerg Med 2019; 3(4):390–4.

68. Babin JL, Traylor KL, Witt DM. Laboratory monitoring of low-molecular-weight heparin and fondaparinux. Semin Thromb Hemost 2017;43(3):261–9.

69. Piran S, Schulman S. Treatment of bleeding complications in patients on anticoagulant therapy. Blood 2019;133(5):425–35.

70. Bijsterveld NR, Moons AH, Boekholdt SM, et al. Ability of recombinant factor VIIa to reverse the anticoagulant effect of the pentasaccharide fondaparinux in healthy volunteers. Circulation 2002;106(20):2550–4.

71. Lee CJ, Ansell JE. Direct thrombin inhibitors. Br J Clin Pharmacol 2011;72(4): 581–92.

72. Swan SK, Hursting MJ. The pharmacokinetics and pharmacodynamics of argatroban: effects of age, gender, and hepatic or renal dysfunction. Pharmacotherapy 2000;20(3):318–29.

73. Burch JW, Stanford N, Majerus PW. Inhibition of platelet prostaglandin synthetase by oral aspirin. J Clin Invest 1978;61(2):314–9.

74. Eikelboom JW, Hirsh J, Spencer FA, et al. Antiplatelet drugs: antithrombotic therapy and prevention of thrombosis, 9th ed: American College of Chest Physicians evidence-based clinical practice guidelines. Chest 2012;141(2 Suppl): e89S–119S.

75. Le Quellec S, Bordet J-C, Negrier C, et al. Comparison of current platelet functional tests for the assessment of aspirin and clopidogrel response. A review of the literature. Thromb Haemost 2016;116(4):638–50.

76. Frontera JA, Lewin JJ, Rabinstein AA, et al. Guideline for reversal of antithrombotics in intracranial hemorrhage: a statement for healthcare professionals from the Neurocritical care Society and Society of Critical Care Medicine. Neurocrit Care 2016;24(1):6–46.

77. Nagalla S, Sarode R. Role of platelet transfusion in the reversal of anti-platelet therapy. Transfus Med Rev 2019;33(2):92–7.

78. Baharoglu MI, Cordonnier C, Al-Shahi Salman R, et al. Platelet transfusion versus standard care after acute stroke due to spontaneous cerebral haemorrhage associated with antiplatelet therapy (PATCH): a randomised, open-label, phase 3 trial. Lancet 2016;387(10038):2605–13.

79. Li X, Sun Z, Zhao W, et al. Effect of acetylsalicylic acid usage and platelet transfusion on postoperative hemorrhage and activities of daily living in patients with

acute intracerebral hemorrhage: clinical article. J Neurosurg 2013;118(1): 94–103.

80. Palmer BF, Clegg DJ. Salicylate toxicity. N Engl J Med 2020;382(26):2544–55.

81. Smith MJH, Dawkins PD. Salicylate and enzymes. J Pharm Pharmacol 1971; 23(10):729–44.

82. Greenberg MI, Hendrickson RG, Hofman M. Deleterious effects of endotracheal intubation in salicylate poisoning. Ann Emerg Med 2003;41(4):583–4.

83. Juurlink DN, Gosselin S, Kielstein JT, et al. Extracorporeal treatment for salicylate poisoning: systematic review and recommendations from the EXTRIP Workgroup. Ann Emerg Med 2015;66(2):165–81.

84. Mega JL, Simon T, Collet J-P, et al. Reduced-function CYP2C19 genotype and risk of adverse clinical outcomes among patients treated with clopidogrel predominantly for PCI: a meta-analysis. JAMA 2010;304(16):1821–30.

85. Ferri N, Corsini A, Bellosta S. Pharmacology of the new P2Y12 receptor inhibitors: insights on pharmacokinetic and pharmacodynamic properties. Drugs 2013; 73(15):1681–709.

86. Jeong Y-H, Bliden KP, Antonino MJ, et al. Usefulness of the VerifyNow P2Y12 assay to evaluate the antiplatelet effects of ticagrelor and clopidogrel therapies. Am Heart J 2012;164(1):35–42.

87. Maas MB, Naidech AM, Kim M, et al. Medication history versus point-of-care platelet activity testing in patients with intracerebral hemorrhage. J Stroke Cerebrovasc Dis 2018;27(5):1167–73.

88. Fitzgerald GA. Dipyridamole. N Engl J Med 1987;316(20):1247–57.

89. Chen ZC, Kwan CM, Chen JH. Profound shock resulting from a large dose of dipyridamole. Int J Cardiol 1994;46(1):75–8.

90. Stangl PA, Lewis S. Review of currently available GP IIb/IIIa inhibitors and their role in peripheral vascular interventions. Semin Interv Radiol 2010;27(4):412–21.

91. Kalra K, Franzese CJ, Gesheff MG, et al. Pharmacology of antiplatelet agents. Curr Atheroscler Rep 2013;15(12):371.

Toxicity of Immunotherapeutic Agents

Cristina Gutierrez, MD[a],*, Colleen McEvoy, MD[b], Daniel Reynolds, MD[c],
Joseph L. Nates, MD, MBA[a]

KEYWORDS

- Immunotherapy • Toxicities • Intensive care unit • Chimeric antigen receptor T-cells
- Immune checkpoint inhibitors • Monoclonal antibodies

KEY POINTS

- As the cancer population increases and immunotherapy becomes widely utilized, severe toxicities from these treatments will become more prevalent.
- The most common immunotherapies that cause toxicities leading to critical illness are chimeric antigen receptor T cells, monoclonal antibodies, and immune checkpoint inhibitors.
- Toxicities from immunotherapy can be immune mediated (an inflammatory response that causes organ failure) or antigen mediated (recognition of the tumoral antigen leads to undesired effects).
- The wide spectrum of toxicities is unique and can mimic other causes of organ failure in the cancer population, concomitantly treating and ruling out other common causes of organ failure is necessary.
- A multidisciplinary team of intensivists, oncologists, and other specialists is essential to assist with diagnosis and rapid management of these toxicities.

INTRODUCTION

Cytotoxic chemotherapy has been the mainstream of cancer therapy, but in the past 3 decades immunotherapy increasingly has been used to treat a variety of malignancies.[1] This change has shown promising results while at the same time having better patient tolerance. Despite this, toxicities from immunotherapy sometimes can be severe enough to

[a] Department of Critical Care, Division of Anesthesiology and Critical Care, The University of Texas MD Anderson Cancer Center, 1515 Holcombe Boulevard. Houston, TX 77030, USA; [b] Stem Cell Transplant and Oncology Intensive Care Unit, Division of Pulmonary and Critical Care Medicine, Washington University School of Medicine, 4523 Clayton Ave, St Louis, MO 63110, USA; [c] Division of Pulmonary and Critical Care Medicine, Washington University School of Medicine, 4523 Clayton Ave, St Louis, MO 63110, USA
* Corresponding author. Department of Critical Care and Respiratory Care, Division of Anesthesiology, Critical Care & Pain Medicine, The University of Texas MD Anderson Cancer Center, 1515 Holcombe Boulevard, Unit #112, Houston, TX 77030.
E-mail address: cgutierrez4@mdanderson.org

Crit Care Clin 37 (2021) 605–624
https://doi.org/10.1016/j.ccc.2021.03.004
0749-0704/21/© 2021 Elsevier Inc. All rights reserved.

require intensive care unit (ICU) admission. The spectrum of these toxicities is unique and can mimic other causes of organ failure in the cancer population; when not recognized early, they can have significant morbidity and mortality.[1] As the cancer population increases and as immunotherapy becomes widely utilized, awareness by the ICU team of these toxicities and their presentations is imperative.

Overall, immunotherapy engages the host's immune system to inhibit proliferation and dissemination of cancer cells in addition to producing long-lasting tolerance against recurrence of the malignancy. Immunotherapy is a broad category, but those with severe toxicities include (1) chimeric antigen receptor (CAR) T-cell therapy; (2) monoclonal antibodies (mAbs); and (3) immune checkpoint inhibitors (ICIs). Toxicities from these therapies can be divided into (1) immune mediated (ICIs and CAR T-cell therapy), in which an inflammatory response causes organ failure, and (2) antigen mediated (on-target off-tumor by cell therapies and mAbs), when the recognition of the tumoral antigen can have unwanted effects and lead to organ failure.

This review focuses on the most common therapies and their toxicities that lead to critical illness. A multidisciplinary team is essential to assist with diagnosis and management of these patients. As these therapies become more common in nonspecialized centers, a therapy-type and organ-system approach is necessary to reduce morbidity and mortality when severe toxicities occur (**Fig. 1**).

CHIMERIC ANTIGEN RECEPTOR T CELLS

CARs are artificially engineered receptors inserted into immune cells, such as T cells, natural killer (NK) cells, and myeloid cells, modified to express a single-chain antibody.[2] The CAR recognizes specific antigens on tumor cells, resulting in T-cell activation and selective destruction of the malignant cells. Autologous CAR T-cell therapy begins with collection of a patient's T-cells via leukapheresis, and they then are

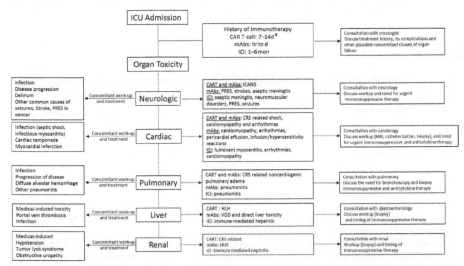

Fig. 1. Approach to the ICU cancer patient with possible immunotherapy related toxicity. [a] Some can present as late as 30 days. CART, CAR T-cells; CRS, cytokine release syndrome; HUS, hemolytic uremic syndrome; HLH, hemophagocytic lymphohistiocytosis; mAbs, monoclonal antibodies; MRI, magnetic resonance imaging; nICI, immune checkpoint inhibitor; PRES, posterior reversible encephaloapthy syndrome; VOD, veno-occlussive disease.

genetically engineered to express a CAR via a viral vector. The patient receives a conditioning regimen, typically fludarabine and/or cyclophosphamide, followed by infusion of the CAR T cells. CD19 CAR T cells, the most investigated cells, recognize the CD19 antigen expressed on B-cell–related malignancies. Three CD19 products (tisagenlecleucel, axicabtagene ciloleucel, and Brexucabtagene autoleucel) now are approved for treatment of refractory B-cell malignancies.[3–6] Additional CAR T-cell therapies are being considered for regulatory approval or in clinical trials.

The profound immune activation that results from CAR T-cell activation, beneficial for tumor destruction and response, can at the same time drive the most common and unique toxicities seen with this therapy: cytokine release syndrome (CRS) and immune effector cell–associated neurotoxicity syndrome (ICANS). CRS and ICANS, along with sepsis, are the most common and life-threatening complications observed in patients.

Cytokine Release Syndrome

CRS results from an uncontrolled and profound systemic inflammation. In the setting of CAR T-cell therapy, CRS is a clinical syndrome related to CAR T-cell expansion and marked elevations of serum inflammatory markers, which occur after antigen recognition, activation, and proliferation of T cells. This inflammatory milieu further causes secondary activation of other inflammatory cells, such as T cells, B cells, NK cells, and macrophages. Elevations in C-reactive protein (CRP), ferritin, interferon (IFN)-γ, tumor necrosis factor (TNF)-α, interleukin (IL)-6, and IL-10 are observed as the syndrome progresses.[7–9] CRP often is used as a biomarker, because higher levels correspond to increased severity of CRS.[8] The prevalence of CRS depends on the malignancy being treated and the CAR cell construct and can occur in 60% to 93% of patients.[3–6,10] Risk factors for severe CRS are listed in **Box 1**.[11]

The hallmark clinical features of CRS include fever, hypotension, and hypoxemia, which the new American Society for Transplantation and Cellular Therapy (ASTCT) consensus grading is based on (**Table 1**).[12] The severity of CRS can be graded

---

Box 1
Risk factors associated with specific toxicities from immunotherapy

Type of Therapy	Toxicity	Risk Factors
CAR T-cell therapy	CRS	High dose of infused CAR T cells High disease burden CAR products with CD28 costimulatory domain
	ICANS	Concomitant grade 3 and grade 4 CRS High disease burden CAR products with CD28 costimulatory domain
ICIs	Pneumonitis	NSCLC COPD or pulmonary fibrosis Advanced age Use of EGFR TKIs Radiation therapy
	Myocarditis	Diabetes Sleep apnea High BMI

Abbreviations: BMI, body mass index; COPD, chronic obstructive pulmonary disease; CRS, cytokine release syndrome; EGFR, epidermal growth factor receptor; NSCLC, non–small cell lung carcinoma; TKI, tyrosine kinase inhibitors.

Table 1
American Society for Transplantation and Cellular Therapy guidelines for cytokine release syndrome grading

Cytokine Release Syndrome Parameter	Grade 1	Grade 2	Grade 3	Grade 4
Fever	Temperature ≥38.0°C	Temperature ≥38.0° C	Temperature ≥38.0° C	Temperature ≥38.0°C
Hypotension	None	Not requiring vasopressors	Requiring a vasopressor with or without vasopressin	Requiring multiple vasopressors (excluding vasopressin)
Hypoxia	None	Requiring low-flow nasal cannula or blow-by	Requiring high-flow nasal cannula, facemask, nonrebreather, or Venturi mask	Requiring positive pressure (CPAP, BiPAP, IMV)

Abbreviations: BiPAP, bilevel positive airway pressure; CPAP, continuous positive airway pressure; IMV, invasive mechanical ventilation.
From Lee DW, Santomasso BD, Locke FL, et al. ASTCT Consensus Grading for Cytokine Release Syndrome and Neurologic Toxicity Associated with Immune Effector Cells. Biol Blood Marrow Transplant. 2019;25(4):625-638. http://doi.org/10.1016/j.bbmt.2018.12.758.

from mild symptoms (grade 1), including fever and tachycardia, and can progress to severe symptoms manifesting with respiratory failure, shock, and multiple organ failure (grades 3–5). Symptoms typically occur within 5 days to 7 days but can be seen up to 10 days to 14 days after infusion.[11] Hypercytokinemia causes vasodilation and capillary leak syndrome, which can lead to shock, noncardiogenic pulmonary edema, and organ failure.

Cardiovascular toxicities concomitantly observed with CRS include dysrhythmias, heart blocks, and acute cardiomyopathy, which develop in 5% to 10% of patients with greater than grade 2 CRS.[13,14] Acute hepatic and renal failure and severe coagulopathy also occur with increasing severity of CRS.[11] Macrophage activation syndrome/hemophagocytic lymphohistiocytosis (HLH) has been described and can be considered in the presence of greater than or equal to grade 3 CRS with multiple organ failure in the presence of an elevated serum ferritin greater than 10,000 ng/mL.[4,11,15]

The treatment of CRS aims to suppress the inflammatory response, without completely inhibiting CAR T-cell proliferation. Tocilizumab, a monoclonal anti–IL-6 receptor antibody, should be used as first-line treatment of any grade of CRS.[2,11,16] Corticosteroids are mainstay of treatment of grades 2 to 4 toxicities and should be used cautiously to avoid inhibition of CAR T-cell proliferation.[2,11,16] Research on additional therapies, such as anakinra, have shown an effective reduction of inflammation while reducing the need of high dose corticosteroids.[17] Best practices for management of CRS include development of institutional guidelines and close observation of symptoms to guide appropriate escalation or de-escalation of treatment.[16]

Immune Effector Cell–Associated Neurotoxicity Syndrome

Neurotoxicity after CAR T-cell therapy, referred to as ICANS, can occur in up to 70% to 80% of patients, with 13% to 40% presenting with greater than or equal to grade 3 toxicity.[3–6] ICANS may present within the first 7 days after an infusion of cells, typically in conjunction with CRS; a second phase of ICANS can be seen within days to weeks after resolution of CRS.[7,11] Although ICANS usually is reversible, a lack of recognition and prompt treatment may lead to death.[11]

The pathophysiology of ICANS remains poorly defined. Although ICANS often occurs with CRS, it can occur in its absence, which suggests a degree of independence from the mechanism of CRS. Conversely, severe ICANS is associated with higher levels of systemic inflammation and with severe CRS.[18,19] Disruption of the blood-brain barrier plays an important role, because patients with severe neurotoxicity have elevated proinflammatory cytokine levels, such as IL-6, IFN-γ, granulocyte-macrophage colony-stimulating factor, and CAR T cells, in cerebrospinal fluid (CSF).[7,19]

Risk factors for severe ICANS are listed in **Box 1**.[11] The clinical presentation initially can be mild symptoms, manifesting with confusion, lack of attention, aphasia, and dysgraphia.[2,12] As the clinical syndrome progresses, patients can develop worsening level of consciousness, motor deficits, and convulsive and nonconvulsive seizures that can progress to status epilepticus.[2,12] Cerebral edema is a rare, idiosyncratic manifestation that has a rapid onset and is potentially fatal.[11] The ASTCT consensus developed a grading system for severity of ICANS, including a 10-point screening tool **(Table 2)**.[12]

The management of neurotoxicity greater than or equal to grade 2 mainly is corticosteroids and supportive care.[11] As the severity of symptoms progress, more interventions and intensive care often are required.[16] A recent survey showed that although all patients with grade 3 toxicities are admitted to the ICU, up to 70% of centers admit patients with grade 1 to grade 2 toxicities for close monitoring.[20] In grade 2 or higher

Table 2
American Society for Transplantation and Cellular Therapy guidelines for immune effector cell–associated neurotoxicity syndrome grading

Neurotoxicity Domain	Grade 1	Grade 2	Grade 3	Grade 4
ICE score	7–9	3–6	0–2	0 (unarousable and unable to perform)
Depressed level of consciousness	Awakens spontaneously	Awakens to voice	Awakens only to tactile stimulus	Unarousable or requires vigorous or repetitive tactile stimuli to arouse; stupor or coma
Seizure	N/A	N/A	Any clinical seizure focal or generalized that resolves rapidly or nonconvulsive seizures on EEG that resolve with intervention	Life-threatening prolonged seizure (>5 min); or repetitive clinical or electrical seizures without return to baseline in between
Motor findings	N/A	N/A	N/A	Deep focal motor weakness, such as hemiparesis or paraparesis
Elevated ICP/cerebral edema	N/A	N/A	Focal/local edema on neuroimaging	Diffuse cerebral edema on neuroimaging: decerebrate or decorticate posturing; or CN VI palsy; or papilledema; or Cushing's triad

Abbreviations: CN, cranial nerve; ICE, immune effector cell–associated encephalopathy; ICP, intracranial pressure.
From Lee DW, Santomasso BD, Locke FL, et al. ASTCT Consensus Grading for Cytokine Release Syndrome and Neurologic Toxicity Associated with Immune Effector Cells. Biol Blood Marrow Transplant. 2019;25(4):625-638. http://doi.org/10.1016/j.bbmt.2018.12.758.

toxicity, CSF sampling and imaging of the central nervous system is recommended to exclude other pathologies, especially when patients are not improving.[11,16] Seizures, seen in grade 3 ICANS, are a known complication with nonconvulsive status epilepticus occurring in 10% of patients.[4] Electroencephalogram (EEG) monitoring and antiepileptics are required, with many institutions using prophylactic antiepileptics.[20] Tocilizumab is recommended only in patients with concurrent CRS; however, its use is not recommended in the absence of CRS.[7,11,18]

Other Complications

Infectious complications after CAR T-cell therapy are a major source of morbidity and mortality. Infections may occur independent of CRS, concurrent with CRS, or as a complication of treatment of CRS and ICANS. Infections occur in 23% to 60% of patients who receive CAR T cells and occur typically within the first month after treatment; up to 30% of patients who develop CRS have an infection.[21–23] The most common infections are bacterial, but fungal and viral pathogens are also common.[21,22] Tumor lysis syndrome has been described after pretreatment with lymphodepleting chemotherapy but also after CAR proliferation.[11] Other hematological complications include cytopenias and hypogammaglobulinemia.[11] B-cell aplasia leading to hypogammaglobulinemia, lasting up to 2 years, increases the risk of infectious complications and may require therapy with intravenous immunoglobulin (IVIG).[11]

MONOCLONAL ANTIBODIES

More than 14 mAbs (excluding ICIs) have been approved for cancer therapy.[24] Due to the large range of antigens they target, each mAb has a unique mechanism of action and range of toxicities (**Table 3**). mAbs are proteins designed to bind tumoral antigens and prompt cell death.[24,25] The most common toxicities associated with mAbs are infusion and hypersensitivity reactions. Other toxicities are related to secondary effects of the receptors and antigens.

Hypersensitivity and Other Infusion Reactions

Many mAbs now are of chimeric and human origin, but immunization still can occur after infusion of many of these agents.[26,27] Alterations in amino acids, their positions, and antibody structure can lead to immune-mediated responses independent of the origin of the mAb.[28] Reactions to mAbs have different mechanisms, which can overlap, making it difficult to differentiate one form of reaction from another. Overall, immune-mediated reactions to mAbs can be divided into (1) type I (IgE) hypersensitivity reactions, (2) non-IgE and complement-mediated reactions; and (3) delayed-type IV reactions.[27] Awareness, early recognition, and creation of treatment protocols can improve patient safety and outcomes.

Hypersensitivity or type I reactions

IgE-mediated hypersensitivity reactions present immediately after infusion.[26,29] Severe cases present with angioedema, bronchospasm, and dyspnea (in some cases leading to respiratory failure), hypotension, and anaphylactic shock.[28–30] Some of the agents associated with severe hypersensitivity include cetuximab, rituximab, tositumomab, ibritumomab, trastuzumab, and pertuzumab.[27] Although the use of skin tests has not been standardized, they can be beneficial in some patients to predict further infusion reactions. Unfortunately, these tests not always are positive, such as in the case of rituximab; therefore, caution should be used in interpretation.[27] Treatment of hypersensitivity reactions due to mAbs does not differ from that of other

Table 3
Toxicities of monoclonal antibodies

Monoclonal Antibody	Target	Toxicity	Characteristics	Treatment
Rituximab Ofatumumab Obinutuzumab Ibritumomab Tositumomab	CD20	Infusion reactions		Premedication (acetaminophen, antihistamines, and corticosteroids)
		Hypersensitivity reactions	Skin test not adequate for rituximab	Discontinuation or desensitization Corticosteroids Antihistamines Epinephrine
		Delayed infusion reactions	Rituximab (Stevens-Johnson syndrome)	Discontinuation, corticosteroids and management as a burn patient if necessary
		CRS	Same as CAR T cell with rituximab, ofatumumab	Corticosteroids and organ support
		Cardiotoxicity	Rituximab-dysrhythmias	Supportive treatment of arrhythmias
		Pulmonary toxicity	Rituximab-ILD, pneumonitis, COP	Corticosteroids
Inotuzumab Moxetumomab	CD22	Infusion reaction	Occurs shortly after infusion despite premedication	Premedication with acetaminophen, antihistamines, and corticosteroids
		Cardiotoxicity	QTc prolongation with inotuzumab	Avoid other medications that could worsen QTc
		Capillary leak syndrome	Moxetumomab	Supportive care with vasopressors to avoid further organ damage
		Liver toxicity and VOD	Inotuzumab	Defibrotide, supportive care for liver failure
		HUS	Moxetumomab (resolved)	
Daratumumab Brentuximab	CD30	Infusion reactions	Anaphylaxis like	Premedication (acetaminophen, antihistamines and corticosteroids) Epinephrine

Drug	Target	Toxicity	Description	Management
Blinatumomab	CD19/CD3	CRS/neurotoxicity	Similar to CAR T-cell toxicity	Corticosteroids Dose escalation
Bevacizumab	VEGF	Neurotoxicity	Ischemic and hemorrhagic stroke PRES	Supportive care
		Other vascular-associated complications	Bleeding Perforation Arterial and venous thrombosis	Supportive care
Trastuzumab Pertuzumab	HER-2	Infusion reactions	In as many as 40% of patients	Premedication (acetaminophen, antihistamines, and corticosteroids)
		Hypersensitivity reactions	Trastuzumab-respiratory symptoms Pertuzumab-anaphylactic shock	Discontinuation or desensitization Corticosteroids Antihistamines Epinephrine
		Cardiac toxicity	Cardiomyopathy	Cardiac optimization of heart failure, inotropic support if needed
		Capillary leak syndrome		Supportive care with vasopressors to avoid further organ damage
Gemtuzumab	CD33	VOD		Defibrotide, supportive care for liver failure
Tagraxofusp	CD123	Capillary leak syndrome		Supportive care with vasopressors to avoid further organ damage
Alemtuzumab	CD52	Cardiotoxicity Pulmonary toxicity	Arrhythmias Alveolar hemorrhage	Supportive treatment of arrhythmias Corticosteroids

(continued on next page)

Table 3
(continued)

Monoclonal Antibody	Target	Toxicity	Characteristics	Treatment
Cetuximab	EGFR	Delayed infusion reactions	Stevens-Johnson syndrome	Discontinuation, corticosteroids and management as a burn patient if necessary
				Corticosteroids
				Antihistamines
				Epinephrine
		Hypersensitivity reactions	Rare	Discontinuation or desensitization
		Cardiotoxicity	Cardiomyopathy, MI, pericarditis, dysrhythmias, myocarditis	Supportive cardiac management according to toxicity and clinical presentation
		Neurotoxicity	Aseptic meningitis	Corticosteroids
		Pulmonary toxicity	Interstitial lung disease, noncardiogenic pulmonary edema	Corticosteroids

Abbreviations: COP, cryptogenic organizing pneumonia; CRS, cytokine release syndrome; EGFR, epidermal growth factor; HER, human epidermal growth factor receptor; HUS, hemolytic uremic syndrome; ILD, interstitial lung disease; MI, myocardial infarction; VEGF, vascular endothelial growth factor; VOD, veno-occlussive disease.

allergic reactions. Corticosteroids, antihistamines, respiratory support, and hemodynamic support with epinephrine are recommended.[30]

Infusion reactions
Overall, infusion reactions are the most common adverse events (AEs) associated with mAbs, with incidences as high as 50% to 80%.[27,31] In general, these reactions occur within hours of infusion and are mild, well tolerated, and self-limited. Although the pathophysiology of these reactions might overlap and clinically look similar to hypersensitivity reactions, these are thought to be mediated by IgG and complement.[29] Tumor burden and the antibody's concentration at the target play a role in these reactions; therefore, spacing and decreasing the dose of mAbs have improved their safety profile.[25,26,29,31] The most common presentations of infusion reactions are fever, tachycardia, myalgia, and chills.[27,28] Severe cases, usually rare, can progress to hypotension, shock, dyspnea, and respiratory failure.[28] Treatment of these reactions is similar to hypersensitivity reactions, and premedication with antihistamines, acetaminophen, and corticosteroids can reduce their incidence. Hemodynamic and respiratory support might be required in patients with severe presentations.

Delayed-type IV reactions
Although rare, delayed-type IV reactions have been described with rituximab and cetuximab.[1] These reactions are T-cell mediated and appear within days to weeks after infusion. Commonly, they present as mild cutaneous manifestations but can evolve to Stevens-Johnson syndrome and toxic epidermal necrolysis (TEN).[27] Treatment should include discontinuation of the causative agent, corticosteroids, airway protection for patients with significant mucosal involvement, and transfer to a burn center for specialized care.

Cytokine Release Syndrome
CRS occurs when recognition of the antigen by the mAb leads to cell apoptosis and secondary release of proinflammatory cytokines.[29] CRS from mAbs can be difficult to differentiate from infusion reactions because it also presents hours after infusion but usually is not observed after repeat doses of the mAb.[29] Antibodies reported to cause CRS include alemtuzumab, rituximab, ofatumumab (CD20), and blinatumomab (CD3 [T cells] and CD19 [B cells]).[25,28,32] The clinical presentation and management are similar to that described for CAR T-cell–induced CRS.

Cardiotoxicity
Cardiotoxicity is observed with use of mAbs, such as trastuzumab, pertuzumab (both HER-2/neu), cetuximab (epidermal growth factor receptor [EGFR]), and alemtuzumab (CD52).[26,33] Cardiotoxicity from trastuzumab and pertuzumab is due to binding to HER-2, which is found in cardiomyocytes and plays a pivotal role in cell survival.[26,33] In the case of cetuximab, EGFR is thought to be involved in myocardial cell physiology.[33] Other cardiac toxicities described with EGFR mAbs include dysrhythmias, myocardial infarction, pericarditis, myocarditis, and cardiomyopathies.[28,33] These complications can be observed within hours to days after the infusion; therefore, close monitoring and awareness of these complications are imperative. Risk factors include a prior cardiac history, treatment with anthracyclines, older age, and radiation to the chest.[26,27] Dysrhythmias are observed with rituximab and alemtuzumab and QTc prolongation with inotuzumab.[27,32]

Neurotoxicity

Severe neurologic manifestations are uncommon with mAbs but are observed with bevacizumab, cetuximab, and blinatumomab. Posterior reversible encephalopathy syndrome (PRES) is described in patients receiving bevacizumab and is thought to be secondary to endothelial dysfunction caused by vascular endothelial growth factor (VEGF) binding.[28] The clinical presentation is typical with uncontrolled hypertension, headache, visual loss, seizures, and, in severe cases, coma. Treatment, besides discontinuation of the mAb, is mainly supportive, including blood pressure control and treatment of seizures. Bevacizumab also is known to be associated with ischemic and hemorrhagic strokes.[1] Neurotoxicity with blinatumomab presents in as many as 30% of patients, and its presentation is similar to the neurotoxicity observed with CAR T-cell therapy.[32] Treatment consists of corticosteroids, and supportive care for the management of delirium and seizures.

Less Common Toxicities

Capillary leak syndrome presenting as shock, hypoalbuminemia, and generalized edema has been described with trastuzumab, moxetumomab (CD22), and tagraxofusp (CD123).[25] Treatment of this syndrome mainly is supportive, with vasopressors and judicious intravenous fluids to avoid further third spacing and organ failure.

Liver toxicity and veno-occlusive disease (VOD) with inotuzumab (anti-CD22) and gemtuzumab (anti-CD33) are reported in patients post–stem cell transplant.[25,31,32] Management is challenging and includes prevention of further hepatotoxicity, close monitoring, and defibrotide.

Pulmonary toxicity manifesting as diffuse alveolar hemorrhage, interstitial pneumonitis, and cryptogenic organizing pneumonia is described with cetuximab, rituximab, alemtuzumab, and trastuzumab.[27,30] In general, these toxicities are rare (<1% in most cases) but as many 8% of patients receiving rituximab can develop interstitial lung disease.[30] Treatment includes discontinuation of the mAb and corticosteroids; responses to treatment are variable.

Reactivation of infections, such as tuberculosis, hepatitis, and John Cunningham virus, are observed with rituximab and brentuximab.[27,28,30] Neutropenia, although not common, has been described with brentuximab, elotuzumab, pertuzumab, and trastuzumab.[27,31] Suspicion and early treatment of opportunistic and viral infections are essential.

Arterial and venous thromboembolic events, gastrointestinal bleeding, and bowel perforation have been reported with bevacizumab, due to its effects on angiogenesis.[26,27] Reversible hemolytic uremic syndrome was reported in patients receiving moxetumomab for hairy cell leukemia.[31]

IMMUNE CHECKPOINT INHIBITORS

ICIs now are used to treat 17 types of cancer.[34] The percentage of patients receiving ICIs increased to 43.6% in 2018, and, as such, the number of patients presenting with severe toxicities will increase.[35] The mechanism of action of these antibodies involves blocking inhibitory receptors on T-cell lymphocytes: (1) cytotoxic T-lymphocyte–associated protein-4 (CTLA-4) (ipilimumab and tremelimumab); (2) the programmed cell death protein (PD-1) receptor (nivolumab and pembrolizumab); and (3) program death-ligand (PDL-1) (atezolizumab, durvalumab, and avelumab) (**Table 4**). Targeting these receptors disrupts inhibitory signals that follow T-cell activation and consequently trigger an antitumor response by the immune system. Unfortunately, this

Table 4
Immune-related toxicities from immune checkpoint inhibitors. Adverse effects of immune checkpoint inhibitors

System	Toxicity	Rates
All	Due to PD1/PD-L1	Grades 1–2: 60%–85%; grades 3–4: 10%–27%
All	Due to combined PD1/PD-L1 + CTLA-4	Grades 1–2: 95%; grades 3–4: 55%
Dermatologic	Rash, pruritus, vitiligo, alopecia areata, stomatitis, xerosis cutis, photosensitivity, Stevens-Johnson syndrome, TEN, DRESS, acute febrile neutrophilic dermatosis (Sweet syndrome)	15%–40%
Ophthalmologic	Peripheral ulcerative keratitis, retinitis, Sjögren syndrome, uveitis, orbital inflammation, such as dacryoadenitis, Vogt-Koyanagi-Harada syndrome	<1%
Neurologic	Peripheral neuropathy, posterior reversible encephalopathy, Guillain-Barré syndrome, paraneoplastic syndromes leading to neurologic symptoms, encephalitis, meningitis, encephalopathy presenting with confusion/fever/seizures, myasthenia gravis, transverse myelitis, bulbar myopathy	1%–12%
Respiratory	Multiple respiratory symptoms, pneumonitis, and a range of different radiographic pathologies associated with acute lung injury and acute respiratory distress syndrome	5%–19%
Cardiovascular	Arrhythmias or conduction defects, acute coronary syndrome, takotsubo-like cardiomyopathy, myocarditis, pericarditis, heart failure	<2%
Gastrointestinal	Bloody diarrhea, abdominal pain, intestinal perforation, enterocolitis, colitis, immune-related hepatitis	<20%–45%
Renal	Acute tubular interstitial nephritis (the most frequent of all presentations), glomerulonephritis (pauci-immune, membranous), immunoglobulin A nephropathy, amyloid A	<1%–5.1%
Hematological	Anemia, neutropenia, lymphopenia, aplastic anemia, autoimmune hemolytic anemia, immune thrombocytopenic purpura	
Endocrine	Hypothyroidism and hyperthyroidism, thyrotoxicosis secondary to thyroiditis or Graves disease, hypophysitis with hypopituitarism, central adrenal insufficiency and hypogonadotropic hypogonadism, diabetes mellitus type 1	1%–13%

(continued on next page)

Table 4
(continued)

System	Toxicity	Rates
Rheumatological	Arthralgia, myalgia, vasculitides (giant cell arteritis), myalgia, polymyalgia rheumatica, systemic lupus erythematosus, polymyositis,	<15%
Musculoskeletal	Necrotizing myositis, rhabdomyolysis	<1%

Abbreviations: DRESS, drug rash with eosinophilia and systemic symptoms; TEN, toxic epidermal necrolysis.

secondary activation of the immune system can lead to serious immune-related AEs (irAEs) that can affect any organ (see **Table 4**).

Factors associated with ICI therapy that can affect the incidence and severity of toxicity include dosing, the use of monotherapy or combined therapy (higher incidence with the latter), and its target (some toxicities being more common with anti–CTLA-4 than with anti–PD-1/PDL-1).[36,37] A recent systematic review and meta-analysis of 106 studies with 20,128 patients reported an overall presence of at least 1 AE in 66% of patients and 14% of patients developed greater than or equal to grade 3 AEs.[38] The most common causes of death were respiratory; among 75 deaths, 52% were caused by respiratory AEs. The second group was associated with cardiac events (11%), followed by infectious (9%), hematologic (7%), hepatic disorders (4%), and cerebrovascular (3%).[39] The time of onset of irAEs after ICI treatment varies, but commonly they present after 3 months but can range between weeks to a year post-treatment.[37]

Multiple guidelines exist to guide treatment of irAEs. Overall, the treatment of all severe irAEs is discontinuation of the ICI and corticosteroids. The dose and duration of corticosteroids vary according to the grade and type of toxicity.[37,40,41] As many as 10% of patients with severe irAEs fail corticosteroids and require other immunosuppressive therapies.[42] Some of the treatments used include IVIG, cyclophosphamide, and anticytokine therapy (IL-6, IL-1, and TNF-α blockade), among others.[37,40–42] Although it is recommended to have a step-by-step approach, some toxicities, such as myocarditis and myasthenia gravis, might require a more urgent approach with early, high-dose, and multiagent immunosuppression. Use of tissue biopsy findings and serum biomarkers to tailor therapy is under evaluation.[42] Due to the spectrum of presentations of irAEs and their wide differential diagnosis, a multidisciplinary team, including oncologists, intensivists, and other specialists, to guide work-up and treatment is important.

Neurotoxicity

The incidence of neurologic toxicity in patients receiving monotherapy is 4% to 6% and increases to 12% when combining both anti–CTLA-4 and anti–PD-1/PDL-1 therapy.[37,43] Although severe toxicities ($\geq$grade 3) are rare (<1%), the presentations are serious with syndromes, such as Guillain-Barré, myasthenia gravis, granulomatous inflammation of the central nervous system, transverse myelitis, multifocal central nervous system demyelination, PRES, enteric neuropathy, encephalitis, aseptic meningitis, facial nerve palsy, Tolosa-Hunt syndrome, and bulbar myopathy.[44,45]

Laboratory tests and imaging should be utilized to promptly rule out other common neurologic complications in cancer patients. Specific treatment of neuromuscular syndromes includes plasmapheresis, IVIG, pyridostigmine, and proteasome inhibitors (bortezomib) to inhibit cytotoxic T cells.[37,40,41,45] Avoiding medications that can trigger cholinergic crisis is recommended (eg, ciprofloxacin and β-blockers). Multidisciplinary team involvement is recommended because many cases are refractory and require long-term immunosuppression. The prognosis is guarded and mortality associated with these AEs has been reported, especially when associated with myocarditis.[45]

Pulmonary Toxicity

The incidence of pulmonary toxicity has been reported to be less than 5% in patients treated with ICIs, but recent publications suggest a higher incidence (19%).[40,46] Risk factors for pneumonitis are listed in **Box 1**. Pneumonitis usually presents within 4 months or as late as 1 year following therapy.[47] Symptoms usually begin with dyspnea and can progress to hypoxemic respiratory failure requiring ventilator support. Typical radiographic features include ground-glass opacities but can be complicated with other patterns, such as reticular fibrotic pattern, diffuse peripheral reticular infiltrates, and patchy nonsegmental airspace consolidations.[47,48] The roles of bronchoscopy and biopsy for diagnosis are yet to be determined, but they can be useful to rule out other causes of respiratory failure.[46] In these patients, a variety of agents also may lead to pulmonary toxicity and coexisting infections, making it difficult to determine the actual cause of respiratory failure. Treatment guidelines recommend long periods of corticosteroids with a 6-week taper.[37,40,41] In severe and refractory cases, infliximab, IVIG, and cyclophosphamide can be considered.[37,40,41]

Cardiotoxicity

ICI-related cardiotoxicity manifests as electrophysiologic defects with dysrhythmias, conduction defects, acute coronary syndrome, pericardial effusion, takotsubo-like cardiomyopathy, and myocarditis.[49–51] Although the incidence of ICI-associated cardiotoxicity is low (<2%), its prognosis is very poor, with mortality between 33% and 46%.[49,51] Risk factors associated with myocarditis are listed in **Box 1**. Common cardiac diagnostic tools, such as biomarkers and electrocardiogram, are useful but seem to work better in combination. Echocardiography can be useful, but as many as 50% of patients who have a normal echocardiogram still can develop a fulminant event.[49] A cardiology consult is recommended to discuss work-up, such as cardiac computed tomography, magnetic resonance imaging, and cardiac catheterization with biopsy.

Management is dependent on severity grade and clinical presentation. Grade 3 cardiac irAEs (symptoms with mild activity) demand aggressive therapies. Standard cardiac therapies (eg, pericardiocentesis, antiarrhythmic medications, and cardioversion) should be delivered concomitantly with immunosuppression. High-dose corticosteroids with prednisone or methylprednisolone (1 g/d) are recommended.[37,41,50] If steroids fail, escalation to mycophenolate mofetil, infliximab, antithymocyte globulin, and IVIG is recommended.[37,41,50]

Other Toxicities

Gastrointestinal toxicity manifests mainly with diarrhea (which can lead to severe electrolyte derangements), colitis, and liver failure.[52]

Renal toxicity is rare, and a recent study reported 16 cases among 6412 patients who received ICIs.[53] The cases ranged from acute tubular interstitial nephritis (the most frequent of all presentations), to glomerulonephritis (pauci-immune or membranous), to immunoglobulin A nephropathy, and to amyloid A.[53] These findings suggested multiple complex mechanisms, requiring further investigation. The investigators suggested to performing kidney biopsy in toxicities grade 2 or above.[53]

Other significant toxicities include endocrine toxicities with hypothyroidism as the most frequent (all-grade incidence 6%), panhypopituitarism with adrenal crisis, and diabetes.[38] Hematologic toxicities can occur and cytopenias, such as anemia (including autoimmune hemolytic anemia), lymphopenia, and neutropenia, are frequent.[38]

SUMMARY

Although immunotherapy provides lifesaving therapeutic options in a significant proportion of cancer patients, a wide range of associated toxicities is recognized. Severe toxicities can lead to discontinuation of the therapy with the detrimental consequences of disease progression and, in the most severe cases, even to death. As more patients receive these therapies, severe toxicities from these treatments will be more prevalent, and awareness by the ICU team of their presentations is imperative. Early suspicion and recognition are crucial to improve patients' outcomes.

CLINICS CARE POINTS

- Differential diagnosis in the critically ill cancer patient requires a system-based approach in which immunotherapy as a cause of organ failure needs to be ruled out.
- Having a timeline of when each therapy was received can help rule out these treatments as the culprit of the ongoing clinical presentation.
- Treating rapidly and concomitantly other common causes of multiorgan failure in cancer patients, especially sepsis, is extremely important in this patient population.

DISCLOSURE

C. Gutierrez served in the advisory board for Legend Biotech and Janssen in August 2020 and January 2021.

REFERENCES

1. Gutierrez C, McEvoy C, Munshi L, et al. Critical care management of toxicities associated with targeted agents and immunotherapies for cancer. Crit Care Med 2020;48(1):10–21.
2. Neelapu SS, Tummala S, Kebriaei P, et al. Chimeric antigen receptor T-cell therapy - assessment and management of toxicities. Nat Rev Clin Oncol 2017;15(1):47–62.
3. Maude SL, Laetsch TW, Buechner J, et al. Tisagenlecleucel in children and young adults with B-cell lymphoblastic leukemia. N Engl J Med 2018;378(5):439–48.
4. Neelapu SS, Locke FL, Bartlett NL, et al. Axicabtagene ciloleucel CAR T-cell therapy in refractory large B-cell lymphoma. N Engl J Med 2017;377(26):2531–44.
5. Schuster SJ, Bishop MR, Tam CS, et al. Tisagenlecleucel in adult relapsed or refractory diffuse large B-cell lymphoma. N Engl J Med 2019;380(1):45–56.
6. Wang M, Munoz J, Goy A, et al. KTE-X19 CAR T-cell therapy in relapsed or refractory mantle-cell lymphoma. N Engl J Med 2020;382(14):1331–42.
7. Gust J, Hay KA, Hanafi LA, et al. Endothelial activation and blood-brain barrier disruption in neurotoxicity after adoptive immunotherapy with CD19 CAR-T cells. Cancer Discov 2017;7(12):1404–19.
8. Lee DW, Gardner R, Porter DL, et al. Current concepts in the diagnosis and management of cytokine release syndrome. Blood 2014;124(2):188–95.
9. Maude SL, Barrett D, Teachey DT, et al. Managing cytokine release syndrome associated with novel T cell-engaging therapies. Cancer J 2014;20(2):119–22.
10. Raje N, Berdeja J, Lin Y, et al. Anti-BCMA CAR T-cell therapy bb2121 in relapsed or refractory multiple myeloma. N Engl J Med 2019;380(18):1726–37.
11. Maus MV, Alexander S, Bishop MR, et al. Society for Immunotherapy of Cancer (SITC) clinical practice guideline on immune effector cell-related adverse events. J Immunother Cancer 2020;8(2):e001511.
12. Lee DW, Santomasso BD, Locke FL, et al. ASTCT consensus grading for cytokine release syndrome and neurologic toxicity associated with immune effector cells. Biol Blood Marrow Transplant 2019;25(4):625–38.
13. Ganatra S, Redd R, Hayek SS, et al. Chimeric Antigen Receptor T-cell therapy-associated cardiomyopathy in patients with refractory or relapsed non-hodgkin lymphoma. Circulation 2020;142(17):1687–90.
14. Alvi RM, Frigault MJ, Fradley MG, et al. Cardiovascular events among adults treated with chimeric antigen receptor T-cells (CAR-T). J Am Coll Cardiol 2019;74(25):3099–108.

15. Shah NN, Highfill SL, Shalabi H, et al. CD4/CD8 T-Cell selection affects chimeric antigen receptor (CAR) T-cell potency and toxicity: Updated results from a phase I anti-CD22 CAR T-cell trial. J Clin Oncol 2020;38(17):1938–50.

16. Gutierrez C, McEvoy C, Mead E, et al. Management of the critically ill adult chimeric antigen receptor-T cell therapy patient: a critical care Perspective. Crit Care Med 2018;46(9):1402–10.

17. Strati P, Ahmed S, Kebriaei P, et al. Clinical efficacy of anakinra to mitigate CAR T-cell therapy-associated toxicity in large B-cell lymphoma. Blood Adv 2020; 4(13):3123–7.

18. Rubin DB, Al Jarrah A, Li K, et al. Clinical predictors of neurotoxicity after chimeric antigen receptor T-cell therapy. JAMA Neurol 2020;77(12):1–7.

19. Santomasso BD, Park JH, Salloum D, et al. Clinical and Biological correlates of neurotoxicity associated with CAR T-cell therapy in patients with B-cell acute lymphoblastic leukemia. Cancer Discov 2018;8(8):958–71.

20. Gutierrez C, Brown ART, Herr MM, et al. The chimeric antigen receptor-intensive care unit (CAR-ICU) initiative: Surveying intensive care unit practices in the management of CAR T-cell associated toxicities. J Crit Care 2020;58:58–64.

21. Hill JA, Li D, Hay KA, et al. Infectious complications of CD19-targeted chimeric antigen receptor-modified T-cell immunotherapy. Blood 2018;131(1):121–30.

22. Haidar G, Garner W, Hill JA. Infections after anti-CD19 chimeric antigen receptor T-cell therapy for hematologic malignancies: timeline, prevention, and uncertainties. Curr Opin Infect Dis 2020;33(6):449–57.

23. Wudhikarn K, Palomba ML, Pennisi M, et al. Infection during the first year in patients treated with CD19 CAR T cells for diffuse large B cell lymphoma. Blood Cancer J 2020;10(8):79.

24. Glassman PM, Balthasar JP. Mechanistic considerations for the use of monoclonal antibodies for cancer therapy. Cancer Biol Med 2014;11(1):20–33.

25. Jabbour E, O'Brien S, Ravandi F, et al. Monoclonal antibodies in acute lymphoblastic leukemia. Blood 2015;125(26):4010–6.

26. Tabrizi MA, Roskos LK. Preclinical and clinical safety of monoclonal antibodies. Drug Discov Today 2007;12(13–14):540–7.

27. Baldo BA. Adverse events to monoclonal antibodies used for cancer therapy: Focus on hypersensitivity responses. Oncoimmunology 2013;2(10):e26333.

28. Hansel TT, Kropshofer H, Singer T, et al. The safety and side effects of monoclonal antibodies. Nat Rev Drug Discov 2010;9(4):325–38.

29. Picard M, Galvao VR. Current knowledge and management of hypersensitivity reactions to monoclonal antibodies. J Allergy Clin Immunol Pract 2017;5(3):600–9.

30. Meisel K, Rizvi S. Complications of monoclonal antibody therapy. Med Health R 2011;94(11):317–9.

31. Simon F, Garcia Borrega J, Brockelmann PJ. Toxicities of novel therapies for hematologic malignancies. Expert Rev Hematol 2020;13(3):241–57.

32. Jain T, Litzow MR. Management of toxicities associated with novel immunotherapy agents in acute lymphoblastic leukemia. Ther Adv Hematol 2020;11. 2040620719899897.

33. Chaudhary P, Gajra A. Cardiovascular effects of EGFR (epidermal growth factor receptor) monoclonal antibodies. Cardiovasc Hematol Agents Med Chem 2010; 8(3):156–63.

34. Johnson DB, Reynolds KL, Sullivan RJ, et al. Immune checkpoint inhibitor toxicities: systems-based approaches to improve patient care and research. Lancet Oncol 2020;21(8):e398–404.

35. Haslam A, Prasad V. Estimation of the percentage of US patients with cancer who are Eligible for and Respond to checkpoint inhibitor immunotherapy drugs. JAMA Netw Open 2019;2(5):e192535.

36. Postow MA, Sidlow R, Hellmann MD. Immune-related adverse events associated with immune checkpoint blockade. N Engl J Med 2018;378(2):158–68.

37. Haanen J, Carbonnel F, Robert C, et al. Management of toxicities from immuno-therapy: ESMO Clinical Practice Guidelines for diagnosis, treatment and follow-up. Ann Oncol 2017;28(suppl_4):iv119–42.

38. Wang Y, Zhou S, Yang F, et al. Treatment-Related Adverse Events of PD-1 and PD-L1 inhibitors in clinical trials: a systematic review and meta-analysis. JAMA Oncol 2019;5(7):1008–19.

39. Wang DY, Salem JE, Cohen JV, et al. Fatal toxic effects associated with immune checkpoint inhibitors: a systematic review and meta-analysis. JAMA Oncol 2018; 4(12):1721–8.

40. Puzanov I, Diab A, Abdallah K, et al. Managing toxicities associated with immune checkpoint inhibitors: consensus recommendations from the society for immuno-therapy of cancer (SITC) toxicity management working group. J Immunother Can-cer 2017;5(1):95.

41. Brahmer JR, Lacchetti C, Schneider BJ, et al. Management of immune-related adverse events in patients treated with immune checkpoint inhibitor therapy: american society of clinical oncology clinical practice guideline. J Clin Oncol 2018;36(17):1714–68.

42. Martins F, Sykiotis GP, Maillard M, et al. New therapeutic perspectives to manage refractory immune checkpoint-related toxicities. Lancet Oncol 2019;20(1): e54–64.

43. Spiers L, Coupe N, Payne M. Toxicities associated with checkpoint inhibitors-an overview. Rheumatology (Oxford) 2019;58(Suppl 7):vii7–16.

44. Zimmer L, Goldinger SM, Hofmann L, et al. Neurological, respiratory, musculo-skeletal, cardiac and ocular side-effects of anti-PD-1 therapy. Eur J Cancer 2016;60:210–25.

45. Dubey D, David WS, Reynolds KL, et al. Severe neurological toxicity of immune checkpoint inhibitors: growing spectrum. Ann Neurol 2020;87(5):659–69.

46. Sears CR, Peikert T, Possick JD, et al. Knowledge gaps and research priorities in immune checkpoint inhibitor-related pneumonitis. an official american thoracic society research statement. Am J Respir Crit Care Med 2019;200(6):e31–43.

47. Naidoo J, Wang X, Woo KM, et al. Pneumonitis in patients treated with anti-programmed death-1/programmed death ligand 1 therapy. J Clin Oncol 2017; 35(7):709–17.

48. Nishino M, Giobbie-Hurder A, Hatabu H, et al. Incidence of programmed cell death 1 inhibitor-related pneumonitis in patients with advanced cancer: a system-atic review and meta-analysis. JAMA Oncol 2016;2(12):1607–16.

49. Mahmood SS, Fradley MG, Cohen JV, et al. Myocarditis in patients treated with immune checkpoint inhibitors. J Am Coll Cardiol 2018;71(16):1755–64.

50. Chen DY, Huang WK, Chien-Chia Wu V, et al. Cardiovascular toxicity of immune checkpoint inhibitors in cancer patients: a review when cardiology meets im-muno-oncology. J Formos Med Assoc 2020;119(10):1461–75.

51. Ball S, Ghosh RK, Wongsaengsak S, et al. Cardiovascular toxicities of immune checkpoint inhibitors: JACC review topic of the week. J Am Coll Cardiol 2019; 74(13):1714–27.

52. Grover S, Rahma OE, Hashemi N, et al. Gastrointestinal and hepatic toxicities of checkpoint inhibitors: algorithms for management. Am Soc Clin Oncol Educ Book 2018;38:13–9.

53. Mamlouk O, Selamet U, Machado S, et al. Nephrotoxicity of immune checkpoint inhibitors beyond tubulointerstitial nephritis: single-center experience. J Immunother Cancer 2019;7(1):2.

Iatrogenic Toxicities in the Intensive Care Unit

Lama H. Nazer, PharmD, BCPS, FCCM[a],*, Anne Rain T. Brown, PharmD, BCCCP, FCCM[b],
Wedad Awad, PharmD[a]

KEYWORDS

- Iatrogenic disease • Drug-related side effects and adverse reactions
- Adverse drug reactions • Critical illness • Intensive care units

KEY POINTS

- Drug therapy is associated with various types of iatrogenic toxicities in critically ill patients.
- The underlying comorbidities, along with the patient's critical illness, increase the risk of developing drug-induced toxicities, but also complicates the ability to diagnose and identify the contributing factor(s).
- Management of drug-induced toxicities typically involves the discontinuation of therapy and if needed, supportive therapy to treat the underlying manifestations.

INTRODUCTION

Drug-induced iatrogenic toxicities are common in critically ill patients and have been associated with increased morbidity and mortality. Critically ill patients are at increased risk of iatrogenic toxicities due to the underlying critical illness, comorbidities, complexity of care, and increased number of administered medications. Early recognition and management of iatrogenic toxicities is essential.[1,2]

This review discusses several types of iatrogenic toxicities associated with medications used in the intensive care unit (ICU). We describe the mechanism of such toxicities, clinical presentation and diagnosis, as well as management. Although intravenous fluids and parenteral nutrition are considered drug therapy, this review does not address iatrogenic toxicities associated with such therapies.

DISCUSSION
Acid Base Disorders

Acid base disorders (ABDs) are among the most common complications encountered in critically ill patients.[3] Although ABDs may be a sign of severe underlying

[a] King Hussein Cancer Center, Queen Rania Al-Abdallah Street, PO Box 1269, Amman 11941, Jordan; [b] University of Texas MD Anderson Cancer Center, 1515 Holcombe Boulevard, Houston, TX 77030, USA
* Corresponding author. Department of Pharmacy, King Hussein Cancer Center, Queen Rania Al-Abdallah Street, PO Box 1269, Amman 11941, Jordan.
E-mail address: lnazer@khcc.jo

Crit Care Clin 37 (2021) 625–641
https://doi.org/10.1016/j.ccc.2021.03.008
0749-0704/21/© 2021 Elsevier Inc. All rights reserved.

pathophysiology, in the case of iatrogenic ABDs life-threatening imbalances are a result of treatment modalities applied to critically ill patients. Drug-induced ABDs can be divided into categories based on accumulation of acid or base through either an exogenous source or decreased elimination, acid or base loss, or respiratory disorders resulting from drug-induced depression or hyperventilation.[4] **Table 1** depicts the most common medications associated with ABDs and the mechanisms for the toxicities.

Drug-related metabolic acidosis can be attributed to increased H+ load, inability to excrete H+, or HCO3− loss. Metabolic acidosis associated with increased H+ load may be caused by several medications that result in increased acid production through direct accumulation of lactic acid or ketones, attributed to mitochondrial toxicity. Typically, lactate is converted into pyruvate, relying on mitochondria and intact oxidative metabolism. Medications thought to induce metabolic acidosis through interference with this process include biguanides, nucleoside reverse transcriptase inhibitors, linezolid, isoniazid, propofol, valproic acid, and statins.[4–7]

Several medications affect the body's ability to clear acid despite an adequate glomerular filtration rate, resulting in conditions broadly characterized as renal tubular acidosis (RTA). Classic type 1 RTA is commonly associated with amphotericin, which may cause dose-related impairment of urinary H+ excretion in the distal tubule.[8,9] Acetazolamide is the most notable culprit associated with type 2 RTA resulting in ineffective bicarbonate resorption in the proximal tubule and inadequate proximal acidification through its inhibition of carbonic anhydrase, albeit this side effect is typically a desired effect when used to combat diuretic induced alkaloses.[10] Several medications noted in **Table 1** are implicated in the development of a type 4 RTA where distal renal sodium absorption along with impaired K+ and H+ excretion results in hyperkalemia, hyperchloremia, and normal anion gap metabolic acidosis.[11,12]

Drug-related metabolic alkalosis can be attributed to the loss of anions or the retention of cations. Most commonly, bicarbonate clearance is disturbed by a decrease in

Table 1
Drug-induced acid base toxicities

Acid Base Disorder	Medication	Mechanism of Toxicity
Metabolic acidosis[3–5]		
Elevated anion gap metabolic acidosis	Linezolid, metformin, propofol, valproic acid	Mitochondrial toxicity, type B lactic acidosis
	Medications containing propylene glycol	Propylene glycol metabolized to lactic acid
Normal anion gap metabolic acidosis	Carbonic anhydrase inhibitors	Decrease bicarbonate reabsorption in the proximal tubule
	Angiotensin-converting enzyme inhibitors, cyclosporine, heparin, potassium-sparing diuretics, tacrolimus, trimethoprim, pentamidine	Hyperchloremic metabolic acidosis, inhibition of Na + reabsorption, type 4 renal tubular acidosis
	Amphotericin B	Type 1 renal tubular acidosis
Metabolic alkalosis[4]		
Metabolic alkalosis	Loop and thiazide diuretics	Distal H+ and Cl⁻ excretion and associated HCO_3^- reabsorption
	Penicillins	Increased aldosterone synthesis and K+ secretion

effective arterial blood volume, but metabolic alkalosis may also be the result of high aldosterone and high distal sodium delivery. Most commonly seen with high doses of loop and thiazide diuretics, distal renal acid loss without equivalent bicarbonate diuresis results in a metabolic contraction alkalosis. Associated chloride loss may also further influence bicarbonate reabsorption.[13]

Respiratory acidosis resulting from iatrogenic conditions are typically derived from sedating toxins that are addressed in the Cristina Gutierrez and colleagues' article "Toxicity of Immunotherapeutic Agents," elsewhere in this issue. Respiratory alkalosis may be the most frequently encountered acid base disorder and hyperventilation is the most common iatrogenic cause.[14] Medication-induced respiratory alkalosis is most frequently the result of salicylate intoxication.

Clinical presentation and diagnosis

Signs and symptoms of the associated ABD are typically related to compensatory responses, either respiratory or metabolic depending on the primary ABD.[5] For example, a patient with drug-induced metabolic acidosis may first present with hyperventilation (if breathing spontaneously). In the absence of cardiopulmonary findings, the clinician should consider systemic acidosis. Additional information on clinical manifestations due to propofol and propylene glycol toxicity is provided in sections below.

Analysis of ABDs should be performed in a systematic manner. A thorough clinical evaluation and medical history is paramount, particularly to determine if any medications may be the cause for the ABD.[15] One must then determine the primary ABD and the secondary response, followed by calculation of the anion gap, and in certain cases, evaluation of the osmolar gap (see the James A. Chenoweth and colleagues' article, "Carbon Monoxide Poisoning," elsewhere in this issue).[5] Interpretation of the ABD must also be evaluated in the context of the clinical situation and diagnosis.

Management

In most cases, removal of the offending agent along with supportive care is sufficient to manage the condition. When the disorder is readily reversible, facilitating respiratory compensation also can be used. Correction of any electrolyte disturbances associated with ABD should be made, such as hyperkalemia which may accompany metabolic acidosis, or hypokalemia, which may accompany metabolic alkalosis.

In acute severe metabolic acidosis with a pH less than 7.15, intravenous sodium bicarbonate may be considered. Clinicians should monitor for adverse effects associated with sodium bicarbonate excess including hypernatremia, hyperosmolality, hypokalemia, hypocalcemia, and hypophosphatemia.[16]

In the case of diuretic-induced metabolic alkalosis, volume status should be assessed, and if correction of extracellular volume losses is possible, saline-based fluids should be administered. However, if the patient has increased extracellular volume with bicarbonate excess, acetazolamide may be administered.[17]

Electrolyte Disorders

Electrolyte disturbances are common in critically ill patients. Such disturbances are attributed mainly to the patients' critical illness and underlying comorbidities, as well as iatrogenic complications such as those associated with various medications.[18] The commonly encountered drug-induced electrolyte disorders in the ICU involve sodium, potassium, calcium, phosphate, and magnesium. **Table 2** outlines the various electrolyte disorders associated with medications commonly used in critically ill patients and the mechanisms involved with such disturbances. In general, electrolyte

Table 2
Drug-induced electrolyte toxicities

Electrolyte Disorder	Medications	Mechanism of Toxicity
Sodium disorders[19-22]		
Hyponatremia	Mannitol	Fluid expansion/increased osmolality
	Diuretics (mostly thiazides)	Impairs renal dilution capacity
	Angiotensin-converting enzyme (ACE) inhibitors, amiodarone, barbiturates, carbamazepine, desmopressin, morphine, nonsteroidal anti-inflammatory drugs	Impairs secretion and/or effect of antidiuretic hormone
	Trimethoprim/sulfamethoxazole	Renal salt-wasting
Hypernatremia	Hypertonic intravenous fluids (eg, hypertonic saline, hypertonic sodium bicarbonate)	Increase sodium administration
	Antibiotics with high sodium content (eg, ampicillin, nafcillin, penicillin G sodium, piperacillin/tazobactam)	
	Loop diuretics	Water loss
	Aminoglycosides, amphotericin B, diuretics, dopamine, foscarnet	Acquired nephrogenic diabetes insipidus
	Phenytoin	Central diabetes insipidus
	Osmotic cathartic agents (eg, lactulose, sorbitol)	Gastrointestinal water loss
Potassium disorders[19,23]		
Hypokalemia	Beta-2 receptor agonists, dobutamine, epinephrine, insulin methylxanthines	Stimulate Na+/K+ ATPase pump (potassium shift to intracellular space)
	Aminoglycosides, amphotericin B, corticosteroids, diuretics (mainly loop and thiazide), penicillins	Increase urinary excretion of potassium
	Osmotic diuretics	Increase osmolality of the glomerular filtrate
Hyperkalemia	Potassium-containing medications (eg, potassium supplements, penicillin G potassium, enteral and parenteral feeding formulations)	Increase potassium administration
	Stored blood products	
	Amino acids, beta-blockers (mostly nonselective), digoxin, mannitol, succinylcholine, verapamil	Inhibit Na+/K+ ATPase pump (potassium shift to extracellular space)
	ACE inhibitors, angiotensin receptor blockers, direct renin inhibitors, unfractionated heparin, low-molecular weight heparin	Reduce aldosterone secretion resulting in reduced renal potassium excretion
	Aldosterone antagonists, trimethoprim/sulfamethoxazole, pentamidine	Tubular resistance to aldosterone
	Nonsteroidal anti-inflammatory drugs	Prostaglandin-mediated decrease in renin release

Calcium disorders[19,24-26]

Hypocalcemia	H2-blockers	Decrease gastrointestinal absorption of calcium
	Bisphosphonates, calcitonin	Decrease bone resorption
	Citrate in blood products, ethylenediaminetetraacetic acid (EDTA)-containing medications (propofol and contrast dye), foscarnet, phosphate-containing laxatives and enemas	Calcium chelation
	Medications associated with hypomagnesemia: aminoglycosides, amphotericin B, loop diuretics	Decrease parathyroid hormone secretion/action (secondary to hypomagnesemia or hypermagnesemia)
	Medications associated with hypermagnesemia: magnesium-containing laxatives and antacids	
	Carbamazepine, isoniazid, phenytoin, phenobarbital, rifampin, theophylline	Vitamin D deficiency/resistance
	Loop diuretics	Increase urinary excretion of calcium
	Corticosteroids	Decrease gastrointestinal absorption of calcium, decrease bone resorption, increase urinary excretion of calcium
	Proton pump inhibitors	Decrease gastrointestinal absorption of calcium, decrease bone resorption, decrease parathyroid hormone secretion/action secondary to hypomagnesemia
	Gadolinium-based contrast agents	Interfere with laboratory assessment (pseudohypocalcemia)
Hypercalcemia	Vitamin A, Vitamin D	Increase gastrointestinal absorption of calcium
	Vitamin D	Increase bone resorption
	Thiazide diuretics	Decrease urinary excretion of calcium

Phosphate disorders[19,25,27]

Hypophosphatemia	Antacids (aluminum, magnesium, and calcium-containing), sucralfate	Decrease gastrointestinal absorption of phosphate
	Albuterol, catecholamines (epinephrine, dopamine), erythropoietin, granulocyte colony-stimulating factors, insulin, sodium bicarbonate	Transcellular shift of phosphate to the intracellular space
	Acyclovir, aminoglycosides, diuretics (acetazolamide being the most potent), rifampicin, valproic acid	Increase urinary excretion of phosphate
	Corticosteroids	Decrease gastrointestinal absorption of phosphate, increase urinary excretion of phosphate
	Mannitol	Interferes with laboratory assessment (pseudohypophosphatemia)

(continued on next page)

Table 2
(continued)

Electrolyte Disorder	Medications	Mechanism of Toxicity
Hyperpho-sphatemia	Phosphate-containing enemas and laxatives Liposomal amphotericin B (high doses)	Increase phosphate administration Interferes with laboratory assessment (pseudohyperphosphatemia)
Magnesium disorders[19,28]		
Hypoma-gnesemia	Proton pump inhibitors Salbutamol/albuterol, theophylline, insulin Aminoglycosides, amphotericin B, cyclosporine, colony-stimulating factors, digoxin. diuretics (loop diuretics being the most potent), foscarnet, pentamidine	Decrease gastrointestinal absorption of magnesium Transcellular shift of magnesium to the intracellular space Increased urinary excretion of magnesium
Hyperma-gnesemia	Magnesium-containing medications (laxatives, enemas, antacids)	Increase magnesium administration

disorders are due to an increase or decrease in the total body electrolyte concentration or due to electrolyte shift between the intracellular and extracellular space.

Clinical presentation and diagnosis

Patients typically present with signs and symptoms that are consistent with those associated with the specific electrolyte imbalance. The presence of clinical manifestations and the severity depend on the degree of electrolyte imbalance and the acuity of onset. In addition, patients with underlying comorbidities are generally at higher risk of developing clinical manifestations associated with the electrolyte imbalances. For example, patients with heart failure tend to have a lower threshold for hypokalemia-induced dysrhythmias.[29] In addition, hypophosphatemia may have a significant impact on the success of mechanical ventilation weaning in patients with acute exacerbations of chronic obstructive pulmonary disease.[30]

In most cases, the diagnosis of a drug-induced electrolyte disorder is made based on laboratory findings in the presence of a medication(s) that may cause the observed electrolyte imbalance. However, when evaluating the laboratory results, it is important to rule out pseudo-electrolyte abnormalities in which the reported laboratory results do not reflect the actual patient electrolyte levels.[25] For example, pseudohyperkalemia may occur as a result of improper sample collection techniques resulting in cell lysis and release of intracellular potassium.[25] Pseudohypocalcemia has been described following the administration of certain types of gadolinium-based contrast agents used in MRI and angiography that interfere with the laboratory assays for calcium.[25] In patients receiving large doses of mannitol, pseudohypophosphatemia has been reported due to the binding of the drug with molybdate used in the assay, resulting in low detection of phosphate.[25]

Management

The management of drug-induced electrolyte disturbances depends on the severity, acuity of onset, and clinical manifestations. In mild and asymptomatic cases, the medication may be continued, if necessary, without the need for urgent treatment.[18,19] However, in moderate to severe electrolyte imbalances and/or the presence of symptoms or underlying comorbidities, management would typically involve stopping the medication and treating the electrolyte imbalance(s), along with managing the clinical manifestations.[18,19]

Although the common approach for managing electrolyte deficiencies is the administration of the deficient electrolyte, it is important to recognize that this may not be the ideal response for all cases. For example, hypomagnesemia may impair the release and activity of parathyroid hormone, thereby resulting in hypocalcemia. In such cases, management should start with correction of hypomagnesemia rather than the administration of calcium.[26] Furthermore, in the presence of hyperphosphatemia and hypocalcemia, administration of calcium is generally not recommended due to the concern of phosphate-calcium precipitation.[26]

Methemoglobinemia

Methemoglobinemia is a rare but serious and potentially fatal complication reported with the use of several medications. The most commonly reported cases involve dapsone, with both systemic and topical administration.[31,32] Other medications commonly used in the ICU that may cause methemoglobinemia include metoclopramide, nitroglycerin, nitroprusside, inhaled nitric oxide, and topical anesthetic agents, mainly benzocaine.[31,33] Procedures using topical anesthetic agents that are more frequently associated with methemoglobinemia are bronchoscopy and transesophageal echocardiography.[34]

Methemoglobinemia occurs when oxidizing medications, such as those mentioned previously, convert hemoglobin to methemoglobin by oxidizing the ferrous (Fe^{2+}) iron of the heme to the ferric (Fe^{3+}) state. This reduces the ability of hemoglobin to transport oxygen, leading to tissue hypoxemia.[35]

Clinical presentation and diagnosis

Clinical suspicion of methemoglobinemia is typically triggered by findings of cyanosis, dyspnea, and/or low oxygen saturation that does not improve with increased oxygen supplementation. Patients may exhibit additional signs and symptoms, depending on the level of methemoglobin and the underlying comorbidities, such as dysrhythmias, seizures, and coma.

In patients with methemoglobinemia, blood samples may appear chocolate brown in color and a saturation gap is usually observed between the calculated oxygen saturation obtained from the arterial blood gas and the results obtained from pulse oximetry. However, an elevated arterial or venous methemoglobin level measured by co-oximeter is necessary to confirm the diagnosis.[35]

Management

The management of methemoglobinemia requires discontinuation of the suspected medication and supportive care, as needed.[35] Initiating treatment may not be necessary for all patients and should be based on the severity of symptoms, methemoglobin level (if available), and the patient's underlying medical conditions.[35]

The mainstay of treatment for methemoglobinemia is methylene blue, which is recommended at a dose of 1 mg/kg intravenously. If the methemoglobin level remains above 30% or if clinical symptoms persist, a repeat dose may be given of up to 1 mg/kg, 1 hour after the first dose.[36] However, methylene blue should be avoided in individuals with deficiency in glucose-6-phosphate dehydrogenase and those taking serotonergic medications. In such situations, or in cases of refractory methemoglobinemia or where methylene blue may not be available, the administration of intravenous ascorbic acid, blood transfusions, or exchange transfusions has been suggested.[35,37] However, the use of these therapies is supported by weak evidence and may not be successful.[35,37]

Ototoxicity

Drug-induced ototoxicity, both reversible and irreversible, is an infrequent but serious and debilitating complication. Coexisting renal or liver failure, advanced age, and the administration of multiple drugs that are potentially ototoxic may put patients at increased risk. Medication-related factors that increase the risk of ototoxicity include the dose, duration of therapy, and infusion rate.[38]

Ototoxicity refers to the general concept of being toxic to the ear and ototoxic medications can be further subdivided into either cochleotoxic or vestibulotoxic, with the former resulting in hearing loss.[39,40] **Table 3** includes the most commonly encountered medications in critically ill patients that may cause ototoxicity along with the mechanism of toxicity.

Clinical presentation and diagnosis

Symptoms of ototoxicity may arise at any point during or after the end of therapy, which makes diagnosis and prevention problematic. Diagnosis may also be underestimated or delayed due to lack of appropriate evaluation and difficulty in assessment in sedated patients or those with delirium. Exposure to ototoxic medications may result

Table 3 Drug-induced ototoxicity	
Medication	**Mechanism of Toxicity**
Antibiotics[39–41]	
Aminoglycosides	Mechanism not well known, acute effects based on calcium antagonism and ion channel blockage; oxidative stress induces apoptosis and necrosis in the hair cells of inner ear; chronic due to formation of toxic metabolite
Macrolides	Mechanism largely unknown, dose dependent, reversible
Vancomycin	Mechanism not clearly understood, dose dependent, related to high peak serum concentrations (>30–45 mg/L)
Diuretics[42]	
Loop diuretics Ethacrynic acid	Edema of tissue in stria vascularis, dose related, usually reversible
Salicylates[43]	
Cyclooxygenase inhibitors	Decreased cochlear blood flow, inhibition of cochlear vasodilating prostaglandin synthesis; dose and concentration dependent

in high-frequency and/or low-frequency hearing loss and eventually higher degrees or complete hearing loss.

To establish a causal relationship, the time sequence between drug intake and symptom onset as well as duration of use should be evaluated. Typically, the high-frequency range is affected first with advancement to lower frequencies, particularly with aminoglycosides and platinum-based chemotherapies.[40] The 3 most common audiologic methods to assess cochlear ototoxicity include basic audiologic assessment, high-frequency audiometry, and otoacoustic emission tests.[44]

Management

A multimodal approach including mechanical, pharmacologic, and environmental strategies are necessary to decrease both the incidence and extent of hearing loss in the critically ill patient population. Patients with risk factors (eg, age, preexisting hearing loss, renal dysfunction) should be proactively identified to reduce the risk of hearing loss. Additional strategies to prevent hearing damage by ototoxic medications is to avoid concomitant dosing of ototoxic medications and using appropriate dosing strategies and monitoring in patients in whom these drugs are unavoidable. Dosing strategies also may be modified to reduce the risk of ototoxicity; for example, once-daily dosing of amikacin may reduce the rate of ototoxicity, while maintaining therapeutic efficacy.[45] Although ototoxicity of aminoglycosides generally results in irreversible damage, ototoxicity related to loop diuretics, macrolides, and quinine usually dissipates once the treatment is stopped.[43,46–48]

Propofol-Related Infusion Syndrome

Propofol-related infusion syndrome (PRIS) is a rare but potentially fatal complication in critically ill patients. It is generally associated with high propofol doses and/or prolonged propofol administration but can occur with lower doses and short exposures.[49]

The mechanism of PRIS appears to be multifactorial, which includes impairment of mitochondrial function, as well as increased production of catecholamines, glucocorticoids, creatinine kinase, and troponin-I, resulting in tissue necrotizing effects on the peripheral and cardiac muscles.[50,51]

Clinical presentation and diagnosis

Patients should be assessed for PRIS if they develop new or worsening metabolic acidosis or hypotension, changes on the echocardiogram, elevated lactic acid, or rhabdomyolysis, especially in the setting of high doses of propofol and/or prolonged infusions. Other manifestations include acute onset of bradycardia, renal failure, hypertriglyceridemia, and elevated liver enzymes.[49,50]

The diagnosis of PRIS in the critically ill patient is complicated by the overlap between the PRIS-related manifestations and the patient's underlying critical illnesses. It is typically a diagnosis by exclusion.[50]

Management

The management of PRIS requires discontinuation of propofol and providing supportive therapy to treat the specific PRIS-related complications, such as hemodynamic support, hemodialysis, and extracorporeal membrane oxygenation.[50]

Propylene Glycol Toxicity

Propylene glycol (PG) is used as a solvent in several parenteral medications commonly administered in the ICU, such as lorazepam, diazepam, phenobarbital, phenytoin, etomidate, and nitroglycerin.[52,53] Although PG is considered safe, the administration of large doses, especially if given over a short period, may result in toxicity.[53] Most of the reported drug-induced PG toxicities have involved lorazepam because intravenous (IV) lorazepam includes large amounts of PG and is typically given as a continuous infusion over several hours or days. However, clinically significant PG toxicities also have been reported with other medications containing PG.[53]

The precise mechanism by which PG causes toxicity is unclear, but appears to be related to the accumulation of lactic acid. Approximately half of PG is excreted unchanged by the kidneys, whereas the remainder is metabolized in the liver to lactate, which is then converted to acetate and pyruvate. PG toxicity has been reported mainly in patients who have underlying renal impairment and/or receive large PG doses. With normal kidney and liver functions, the half-life for PG is approximately 4 hours, but increases in the presence of any renal or hepatic impairment.[54]

Clinical presentation and diagnosis

Toxicity of PG is suspected in patients who have unexplained hyperosmolality, metabolic acidosis, or acute kidney injury and are receiving PG-containing medications.[53,55,56] Patients typically have anion gap metabolic acidosis due to the accumulation of lactic acid and may develop seizures and mental status changes, as well as sepsislike symptoms.

PG toxicity is usually a clinical diagnosis because a serum PG level may not be available or the result may be delayed. An elevated osmolar gap above 10 has been reported as a surrogate marker for elevated PG concentrations with lorazepam infusions.[55]

Management

The management of PG toxicity starts with discontinuation of the suspected drug. If the medication is necessary, one may switch to an alternative product that does not contain PG, such as the use of midazolam instead of lorazepam. In severe cases, intermittent hemodialysis may be considered, as it reduces the levels of PG and corrects the metabolic abnormalities.[53]

Renal Toxicity

Acute kidney injury (AKI) is common in critically ill patients, with up to 35% of the cases attributed to drug therapy.[57,58] The most common nephrotoxic medications used in the ICU are antibiotics, diuretics, and contrast media.[57] Nephrotoxic medications cause renal toxicity through 1 or more of the following major mechanisms: pre-renal, by altering the intraglomerular hemodynamics; intra-renal, mainly through acute tubular necrosis or acute interstitial nephritis (AIN); post-renal, through tubular obstruction.[59,60] **Table 4** provides a list of nephrotoxic medications commonly used in the ICU and their mechanism of renal toxicity.

Vancomycin is one of the commonly administered nephrotoxic antibiotics in the ICU, with a reported incidence of renal toxicity ranging from 5% to 43%.[62] The onset

Table 4
Drug-induced renal toxicity[59–61]

Medication	Mechanism of Toxicity
Acyclovir	Acyclovir crystals precipitate in the renal tubule resulting in tubular obstruction
Aminoglycosides	Binds to the acidic phospholipids brush border membrane of the proximal tubule, resulting in acute tubular necrosis. May also accumulate in the distal tubules and collecting ducts resulting in distal tubular dysfunction
Amphotericin B	Activates prostaglandins resulting in vasoconstriction of the afferent arterioles and decreased blood flow. Binds to the epithelial cells in the proximal and distal tubule-collecting ducts resulting in acute tubular necrosis and tubular dysfunction
Angiotensin-converting enzyme inhibitors Angiotensin receptor-blocking agents	Vasodilation of efferent arterioles, resulting in reduced transglomerular pressure and a decrease in glomerular filtration rate
Ascorbic acid	Tubular obstruction due to the precipitation of oxalate crystals
Calcineurin inhibitors	Vasoconstriction due to the increased production of vasoconstrictors, reduced renal vasodilatory prostaglandin release, and nitric oxide inhibition
Foscarnet	Acute tubular necrosis. Tubular obstruction due to the precipitation of crystals
Nonsteroidal anti-inflammatory drugs (both selective and nonselective drugs)	Alterations in intraglomerular hemodynamics due to prostaglandin inhibition. Allergic interstitial nephritis
Radio-contrast agents	Vasoconstriction due to the release of renal vasoconstrictors. Accumulates in the renal tubules and collecting ducts, causing direct cellular injury and acute tubular necrosis
Sulfa-based antibiotics	Acute interstitial nephritis
Vancomycin	Vancomycin-induced oxidative stress resulting in tubular damage. Acute interstitial nephritis

of nephrotoxicity usually occurs after 4 to 8 days of therapy, although early and late onset have been reported.[62,63] In most cases, nephrotoxicity is reversible.[62,63] Trough levels commonly targeted in critically ill patients ($\geq$15 mg/L) are associated with increased nephrotoxicity, compared with lower levels.[62] However, recent vancomycin dosing guidelines have been updated, recommending area under the curve–guided dosing, which appears to be associated with less AKI, compared with trough-guided dosing.[64]

Aminoglycosides are well known for their nephrotoxicity, with a prevalence that may exceed 50% in critically ill patients.[65] Nephrotoxicity associated with aminoglycosides typically manifests as nonoliguric AKI, after 5 to 7 days of treatment.[60,65] Other nephrotoxic medications include sulfa-based antimicrobials and polymyxins. Trimethoprim inhibits proximal tubular secretion of creatinine resulting in elevation of measured serum creatinine but this is unlikely a reflection of AKI.[60] Other antibiotics less commonly associated with renal toxicity include ciprofloxacin, penicillins, and cephalosporins.[60]

Among the antifungal agents, amphotericin B has the highest incidence of renal toxicity, reported in up to 80% of the patients on conventional amphotericin B. The incidence is lower with the use of lipid-based formulations.[66] Renal toxicity has also been reported with IV voriconazole, but this is primarily related to the nephrotoxic solubilizing agent, sulfobutylether-beta-cyclodextrin (SBECD), used in the IV formulation.[66]

Diuretics, mostly furosemide, are frequently used in critically ill patients for various indications, including the management of oliguric AKI. However, studies have suggested that diuretics are nephrotoxic. Most of the cases have been reported in the presence of underlying risk factors, such as other nephrotoxic medications, underlying comorbidities, and the critical illness.[67]

AKI associated with contrast has been reported in approximately 15% of critically ill patients, with onset within 48 hours of exposure and the peak effect seen at 72 hours.[60,68] In most cases, AKI is reversible and serum creatinine returns to baseline in 7 to 10 days, but some patients may not have complete recovery at discharge.[60,68]

Clinical presentation and diagnosis

The diagnosis of drug-induced nephrotoxicity is difficult and frequently complicated by the presence of other nephrotoxic medications and the underlying critical illness. Typically, assessing drug-induced AKI is triggered by an increase in the serum creatinine and/or decrease in urine output. An understanding of the characteristics and mechanism of nephrotoxicity associated with the suspected medication(s) is necessary to help in the assessment, but to confirm the diagnosis, renal biopsy is necessary.[69]

AIN is recognized in the presence of the classic triad of rash, fever, and eosinophilia occurring within a few days of the initiation of drug therapy. However, these findings and the timing of onset are not seen in most patients who develop drug-induced AIN and thus the diagnosis relies on clinical judgment.[70]

Kidney biomarkers have been proposed in the diagnosis of drug-induced AKI based on their higher sensitivity and specificity in detecting drug-induced nephrotoxicity compared with traditional methods, and their ability to provide a better prediction of the location of injury. However, the clinical utility of such biomarkers is not yet established.[69]

Management

Ideally, the management of drug-induced AKI is the discontinuation of the suspected drug. Although this may be possible in cases in which the medication is no longer needed or when there are less nephrotoxic alternative medications, in many cases, the continuation of the suspected medication is necessary.

In patients in whom the nephrotoxicity is related to AIN, discontinuation of the suspected drug is imperative. Corticosteroids may be considered in patients in whom there is no observed benefit after a few days of discontinuing the medication, although the evidence supporting their use is limited.[70]

Rhabdomyolysis

Rhabdomyolysis, a rare but potentially life-threatening condition of skeletal muscle destruction, has been reported with several medications commonly used in critically ill patients such as propofol, fluoroquinolones, daptomycin, linezolid, and trimethoprim/sulfamethoxazole.[71,72] The associated risk with these medications may increase with higher doses as with daptomycin, longer duration as with linezolid, or both as with propofol.[51,73,74] In addition, combining any of the previously mentioned medications will increase the rhabdomyolysis risk.[72]

Clinical presentation and diagnosis

The main symptoms of rhabdomyolysis are muscular pain and weakness, most prominent in the thighs, shoulders, calves, and lower back; however, it is often difficult to identify these symptoms in critically ill patients. Other symptoms may present in severely affected patients, including fever, tachycardia, and changes in mental status.[75] Elevation of serum creatine kinase level, typically greater than 5 times the upper normal limit, is the diagnostic hallmark for rhabdomyolysis. Metabolic complications of rhabdomyolysis can be life-threatening and include hyperkalemia, hyperphosphatemia, and hypocalcemia. Some patients may develop red to brown urine due to myoglobin being excreted in the urine.[76]

Management

The management of rhabdomyolysis starts with discontinuation of the suspected medication, as well as isotonic fluid administration and the correction of electrolyte abnormalities. The use of mannitol and fluids with sodium bicarbonate for AKI caused by rhabdomyolysis also has been reported despite limited clinical data.[77]

SUMMARY

This article discusses the mechanism, clinical presentation, diagnosis, and management of iatrogenic toxicities associated with medications that are commonly used in critically ill patients. The concurrent administration of several medications along with the underlying critical illnesses and comorbidities increases the risk of developing iatrogenic toxicities but also makes the diagnosis and management of such toxicities challenging.

CLINICS CARE POINTS

- Drugs commonly used in critically ill patients are associated with various types of iatrogenic toxicities.
- The underlying comorbidities and the patient's critical illness increase the risk of developing drug-induced toxicities, but also complicate the ability to diagnose and identify the contributing factor(s).

> • Management of drug-induced toxicities usually involves the discontinuation of the suspected medication(s), and if needed, supportive therapy to treat the underlying manifestations.

DISCLOSURE

No financial disclosures. No conflict of interest.

REFERENCES

1. Kane-Gill SL, Jacobi J, Rothschild JM. Adverse drug events in intensive care units: risk factors, impact, and the role of team care. Crit Care Med 2010;38(6 Suppl):S83–9.
2. Rothschild JM, Landrigan CP, Cronin JW, et al. The Critical Care Safety Study: the incidence and nature of adverse events and serious medical errors in intensive care. Crit Care Med 2005;33(8):1694–700.
3. Gauthier PM, Szerlip HM. Metabolic acidosis in the intensive care unit. Crit Care Clin 2002;18(2):289–308, vi.
4. Kitterer D, Schwab M, Alscher MD, et al. Drug-induced acid-base disorders. Pediatr Nephrol 2015;30(9):1407–23.
5. Liamis G, Milionis HJ, Elisaf M. Pharmacologically-induced metabolic acidosis: a review. Drug Saf 2010;33(5):371–91.
6. Wolf A, Weir P, Segar P, et al. Impaired fatty acid oxidation in propofol infusion syndrome. Lancet 2001;357(9256):606–7.
7. Kreisberg RA. Lactate homeostasis and lactic acidosis. Ann Intern Med 1980; 92(2 Pt 1):227–37.
8. Burgess JL, Birchall R. Nephrotoxicity of amphotericin B, with emphasis on changes in tubular function. Am J Med 1972;53(1):77–84.
9. Sawaya BP, Briggs JP, Schnermann J. Amphotericin B nephrotoxicity: the adverse consequences of altered membrane properties. J Am Soc Nephrol 1995;6(2):154–64.
10. Holt C, Hitchings A. Drug-induced metabolic acidosis. Adverse Drug React Bull 2017;304. 117V 1178.
11. Alappan R, Perazella MA, Buller GK. Hyperkalemia in hospitalized patients treated with trimethoprim-sulfamethoxazole. Ann Intern Med 1996;124(3):316–20.
12. Margassery S, Bastani B. Life threatening hyperkalemia and acidosis secondary to trimethoprim-sulfamethoxazole treatment. J Nephrol 2001;14(5):410–4.
13. Cannon PJ, Heinemann HO, Albert MS, et al. Contraction" alkalosis after diuresis of edematous patients with ethacrynic acid. Ann Intern Med 1965;62:979–90.
14. Gardner WN. The pathophysiology of hyperventilation disorders. Chest 1996; 109(2):516–34.
15. Berend K, de Vries AP, Gans RO. Physiological approach to assessment of acid-base disturbances. N Engl J Med 2014;371(15):1434–45.
16. Rhodes A, Evans LE, Alhazzani W, et al. Surviving sepsis campaign: international guidelines for management of sepsis and Septic Shock: 2016. Intensive Care Med 2017;43(3):304–77.
17. Galla JH. Metabolic alkalosis. J Am Soc Nephrol 2000;11(2):369–75.
18. Lee JW. Fluid and electrolyte disturbances in critically ill patients. Electrolyte Blood Press 2010;8(2):72–81.

19. Buckley MS, Leblanc JM, Cawley MJ. Electrolyte disturbances associated with commonly prescribed medications in the intensive care unit. Crit Care Med 2010;38(6 Suppl):S253–64.
20. Liamis G, Milionis H, Elisaf M. A review of drug-induced hyponatremia. Am J Kidney Dis 2008;52(1):144–53.
21. Wang N, Nguyen PK, Pham CU, et al. Sodium content of intravenous antibiotic preparations. Open Forum Infect Dis 2019;6(12):ofz508.
22. Liamis G, Milionis HJ, Elisaf M. A review of drug-induced hypernatraemia. NDT Plus 2009;2(5):339–46.
23. Ben Salem C, Badreddine A, Fathallah N, et al. Drug-induced hyperkalemia. Drug Saf 2014;37(9):677–92.
24. Grieff M, Bushinsky DA. Diuretics and disorders of calcium homeostasis. Semin Nephrol 2011;31(6):535–41.
25. Liamis G, Liberopoulos E, Barkas F, et al. Spurious electrolyte disorders: a diagnostic challenge for clinicians. Am J Nephrol 2013;38(1):50–7.
26. Liamis G, Milionis HJ, Elisaf M. A review of drug-induced hypocalcemia. J Bone Miner Metab 2009;27(6):635–42.
27. Megapanou E, Florentin M, Milionis H, et al. Drug-Induced hypophosphatemia: current insights. Drug Saf 2020;43(3):197–210.
28. Gröber U. Magnesium and drugs. Int J Mol Sci 2019;20(9):2094.
29. Skogestad J, Aronsen JM. Hypokalemia-induced arrhythmias and heart failure: new insights and implications for therapy. Front Physiol 2018;9:1500.
30. Zhao Y, Li Z, Shi Y, et al. Effect of hypophosphatemia on the withdrawal of mechanical ventilation in patients with acute exacerbations of chronic obstructive pulmonary disease. Biomed Rep 2016;4(4):413–6.
31. Ash-Bernal R, Wise R, Wright SM. Acquired methemoglobinemia: a retrospective series of 138 cases at 2 teaching hospitals. Medicine (Baltimore) 2004;83(5):265–73.
32. Swartzentruber GS, Yanta JH, Pizon AF. Methemoglobinemia as a complication of topical dapsone. N Engl J Med 2015;372(5):491–2.
33. Kane GC, Hoehn SM, Behrenbeck TR, et al. Benzocaine-induced methemoglobinemia based on the Mayo Clinic experience from 28 478 transesophageal echocardiograms: incidence, outcomes, and predisposing factors. Arch Intern Med 2007;167(18):1977–82.
34. Chowdhary S, Bukoye B, Bhansali AM, et al. Risk of topical anesthetic-induced methemoglobinemia: a 10-year retrospective case-control study. JAMA Intern Med 2013;173(9):771–6.
35. Cortazzo JA, Lichtman AD. Methemoglobinemia: a review and recommendations for management. J Cardiothorac Vasc Anesth 2014;28(4):1043–7.
36. Cenexi. Provayblue [methylene blue]. U.S. Food and Drug Administration Web site. 2016. Available at: https://www.accessdata.fda.gov/drugsatfda_docs/label/2016/204630s000lbl.pdf. Accessed December 14, 2020.
37. Sahu KK, Dhibar DP, Gautam A, et al. Role of ascorbic acid in the treatment of methemoglobinemia. Turk J Emerg Med 2016;16:119–20.
38. Halpern NA, Pastores SM, Price JB, et al. Hearing loss in critical care: an unappreciated phenomenon. Crit Care Med 1999;27(1):211–9.
39. Seligmann H, Podoshin L, Ben-David J, et al. Drug-induced tinnitus and other hearing disorders. Drug Saf 1996;14(3):198–212.
40. Campbell KCM, Le Prell CG. Drug-induced ototoxicity: diagnosis and monitoring. Drug Saf 2018;41(5):451–64.

41. Lanvers-Kaminsky C, Zehnhoff-Dinnesen AA, Parfitt R, et al. Drug-induced ototoxicity: mechanisms, pharmacogenetics, and protective strategies. Clin Pharmacol Ther 2017;101(4):491–500.

42. Rybak LP. Ototoxicity of loop diuretics. Otolaryngol Clin North Am 1993;26(5): 829–44.

43. Jung TT, Rhee CK, Lee CS, et al. Ototoxicity of salicylate, nonsteroidal antiinflammatory drugs, and quinine. Otolaryngol Clin North Am 1993;26(5):791–810.

44. American Academy of Audiology. Position statement and clinical practice guidelines: ototoxicity monitoring 2009. Available at: https://www.audiology.org/publications-resources/document-library/ototoxicity-monitoring. Accessed August 15, 2020.

45. Tulkens PM. Pharmacokinetic and toxicological evaluation of a once-daily regimen versus conventional schedules of netilmicin and amikacin. J Antimicrob Chemother 1991;27(Suppl C):49–61.

46. Brummett RE. Ototoxic liability of erythromycin and analogues. Otolaryngol Clin North Am 1993;26(5):811–9.

47. Ikeda K, Oshima T, Hidaka H, et al. Molecular and clinical implications of loop diuretic ototoxicity. Hear Res 1997;107(1–2):1–8.

48. Schacht J, Talaska AE, Rybak LP. Cisplatin and aminoglycoside antibiotics: hearing loss and its prevention. Anat Rec (Hoboken) 2012;295(11):1837–50.

49. Hemphill S, McMenamin L, Bellamy MC, et al. Propofol infusion syndrome: a structured literature review and analysis of published case reports. Br J Anaesth 2019;122(4):448–59.

50. Mirrakhimov AE, Voore P, Halytskyy O, et al. Propofol infusion syndrome in adults: a clinical update. Crit Care Res Pract 2015;2015:260385.

51. Vasile B, Rasulo F, Candiani A, et al. The pathophysiology of propofol infusion syndrome: a simple name for a complex syndrome. Intensive Care Med 2003; 29(9):1417–25.

52. Demey HE, Daelemans RA, Verpooten GA, et al. Propylene glycol-induced side effects during intravenous nitroglycerin therapy. Intensive Care Med 1988;14(3): 221–6.

53. Zar T, Graeber C, Perazella MA. Recognition, treatment, and prevention of propylene glycol toxicity. Semin Dial 2007;20(3):217–9.

54. Yu DK, Elmquist WF, Sawchuk RJ. Pharmacokinetics of propylene glycol in humans during multiple dosing regimens. J Pharm Sci 1985;74(8):876–9.

55. Barnes BJ, Gerst C, Smith JR, et al. Osmol gap as a surrogate marker for serum propylene glycol concentrations in patients receiving lorazepam for sedation. Pharmacotherapy 2006;26(1):23–33.

56. Wilson KC, Reardon C, Theodore AC, et al. Propylene glycol toxicity: a severe iatrogenic illness in ICU patients receiving IV benzodiazepines: a case series and prospective, observational pilot study. Chest 2005;128(3):1674–81.

57. Ehrmann S, Helms J, Joret A, et al. Nephrotoxic drug burden among 1001 critically ill patients: impact on acute kidney injury. Ann Intensive Care 2019;9(1):106.

58. Uchino S, Kellum JA, Bellomo R, et al. Acute renal failure in critically ill patients: a multinational, multicenter study. JAMA 2005;294(7):813–8.

59. Bentley ML, Corwin HL, Dasta J. Drug-induced acute kidney injury in the critically ill adult: recognition and prevention strategies. Crit Care Med 2010;38(6 Suppl): S169–74.

60. Pazhayattil GS, Shirali AC. Drug-induced impairment of renal function. Int J Nephrol Renovasc Dis 2014;7:457–68.

61. Sawada A, Kawanishi K, Morikawa S, et al. Biopsy-proven vancomycin-induced acute kidney injury: a case report and literature review. BMC Nephrol 2018; 19(1):72.
62. van Hal SJ, Paterson DL, Lodise TP. Systematic review and meta-analysis of vancomycin-induced nephrotoxicity associated with dosing schedules that maintain troughs between 15 and 20 milligrams per liter. Antimicrob Agents Chemother 2013;57(2):734–44.
63. Filippone EJ, Kraft WK, Farber JL. The nephrotoxicity of vancomycin. Clin Pharmacol Ther 2017;102(3):459–69.
64. Rybak MJ, Le J, Lodise TP, et al. Therapeutic monitoring of vancomycin for serious methicillin-resistant *Staphylococcus aureus* infections: a revised consensus guideline and review by the American Society of Health-System pharmacists, the Infectious Diseases Society of America, the Pediatric Infectious Diseases Society, and the Society of Infectious Diseases Pharmacists. Am J Health Syst Pharm 2020;77(11):835–64.
65. Oliveira JF, Silva CA, Barbieri CD, et al. Prevalence and risk factors for aminoglycoside nephrotoxicity in intensive care units. Antimicrob Agents Chemother 2009; 53(7):2887–91.
66. Mourad A, Perfect JR. Tolerability profile of the current antifungal armoury. J Antimicrob Chemother 2018;73(suppl_1):i26–32.
67. Wu X, Zhang W, Ren H, et al. Diuretics associated acute kidney injury: clinical and pathological analysis. Ren Fail 2014;36(7):1051–5.
68. Kim MH, Koh SO, Kim EJ, et al. Incidence and outcome of contrast-associated acute kidney injury assessed with Risk, Injury, Failure, Loss, and End-stage kidney disease (RIFLE) criteria in critically ill patients of medical and surgical intensive care units: a retrospective study. BMC Anesthesiol 2015;15:23.
69. Perazella MA. Diagnosing drug-induced AIN in the hospitalized patient: a challenge for the clinician. Clin Nephrol 2014;81(6):381–8.
70. Moledina DG, Perazella MA. Drug-induced acute interstitial nephritis. Clin J Am Soc Nephrol 2017;12(12):2046–9.
71. Oshima Y. Characteristics of drug-associated rhabdomyolysis: analysis of 8,610 cases reported to the U.S. Food and Drug Administration. Intern Med 2011;50(8): 845–53.
72. Teng C, Baus C, Wilson JP, et al. Rhabdomyolysis associations with antibiotics: a pharmacovigilance study of the FDA Adverse Event Reporting System (FAERS). Int J Med Sci 2019;16(11):1504–9.
73. Carroll MW, Choi H, Min S, et al. Rhabdomyolysis in a patient treated with linezolid for extensively drug-resistant tuberculosis. Clin Infect Dis 2012;54(11):1624–7.
74. Sbrana F, Di Paolo A, Pasanisi EM, et al. Administration interval and daptomycin toxicity: a case report of rhabdomyolysis. J Chemother 2010;22(6):434–5.
75. Giannoglou GD, Chatzizisis YS, Misirli G. The syndrome of rhabdomyolysis: pathophysiology and diagnosis. Eur J Intern Med 2007;18(2):90–100.
76. Huerta-Alardín AL, Varon J, Marik PE. Bench-to-bedside review: rhabdomyolysis—an overview for clinicians. Crit Care 2005;9(2):158–69.
77. Michelsen J, Cordtz J, Liboriussen L, et al. Prevention of rhabdomyolysis-induced acute kidney injury—a DASAIM/DSIT clinical practice guideline. Acta Anaesthesiol Scand 2019;63(5):576–86.

Toxic Alcohols

Jennifer A. Ross, MD, MPH, Heather A. Borek, MD,
Christopher P. Holstege, MD*

KEYWORDS

- Toxic alcohol • Methanol • Ethylene glycol • Diethylene glycol • Propylene glycol
- Isopropyl alcohol • Acetone

KEY POINTS

- Toxic alcohols are found in numerous products and significant exposure can lead to toxicity, which mimics other disease processes.
- Toxic alcohol poisoning requires specific and timely treatments to prevent long-term disability or death.
- The presence of toxic alcohol poisoning may be suggested by an anion gap metabolic acidosis and/or an increased osmole gap, depending on the specific toxic alcohol responsible and the timing of the laboratory analysis in relation to exposure.
- Clinicians must recognize the significance of an anion gap metabolic acidosis and the importance of timely trending of the chemistries to assure improvement with supportive care.
- An osmole gap can be useful in suggesting a toxic alcohol ingestion, but a normal osmole gap does not rule out the presence of a toxic alcohol.

INTRODUCTION

According to the Annual Report of the American Association of Poison Control Centers' National Poison Data System, there are thousands of toxic alcohol exposures in the United States each year with numerous deaths.[1] This article reviews the topic of toxic alcohols, specifically ethylene glycol, methanol, diethylene glycol, propylene glycol, and isopropyl alcohol. Patients poisoned with toxic alcohols often present without a history of exposure, and it is ancillary testing, specifically the anion and osmole gap, that enable clinicians to diagnose these toxins. This article also reviews the significance of an anion gap metabolic acidosis in the poisoned patient, which often is the common laboratory abnormality first noted in patients with specific toxic alcohols, and explore the utility as well as limitations of the osmole gap.

Ethylene Glycol

Ethylene glycol is present in numerous readily available products, including antifreeze, deicers, detergents, paints, and cosmetics. Ethylene glycol toxicity is associated with

Division of Medical Toxicology, Department of Emergency Medicine, University of Virginia School of Medicine, PO Box 800774, Charlottesville, VA 22908-0774, USA
* Corresponding author.
E-mail address: ch2xf@virginia.edu

Crit Care Clin 37 (2021) 643–656
https://doi.org/10.1016/j.ccc.2021.03.009
0749-0704/21/© 2021 Elsevier Inc. All rights reserved.

both accidental and intentional ingestions. It is a colorless, sweet-tasting liquid that can be disguised in other drinks, as has been reported with numerous criminal poisonings.[2] Sodium fluorescein dye is added to some preparations of antifreeze to facilitate identification of radiator leaks; however, this is product dependent, and fluorescence of the patient's oral pharynx or urine is not a reliable indicator of poisoning.[3]

Ethylene glycol is rapidly absorbed through the gastrointestinal (GI) tract, and the volume of distribution is 0.7 L/kg. Ethylene glycol undergoes first-order elimination when concentrations are less than 250 mg/dL, with a half-life of approximately 4 hours. When concentrations are greater than 250 mg/dL, elimination becomes zero-order, thereby prolonging the elimination half-life. When alcohol dehydrogenase (ADH) is competitively inhibited, such as with ethanol ingestion or the use of fomepizole, metabolism of ethylene glycol is delayed and becomes renally dependent, prolonging the elimination half-life to greater than 10 hours.

Metabolism of ethylene glycol occurs primarily in the liver through serial oxidation initially by ADH and aldehyde dehydrogenase (ALDH), with each step reducing NAD+ to NADH (**Fig. 1**). The rate-limiting step in metabolism occurs with the conversion of glycolic acid to glyoxylic acid, leading to the development of a marked anion gap metabolic acidosis due to the accumulation of glycolic acid. Glyoxylic acid undergoes conversion to oxalic acid, α-hydroxy-β-ketoadipic acid, or glycine. Thiamine is a cofactor in the production of α-hydroxy-β-ketoadipic acid, and pyridoxine and magnesium are cofactors in the production of glycine. These cofactors play a role in treating toxicity. Oxalic acid readily precipitates with calcium to form insoluble calcium oxalate crystals. Calcium oxalate crystals may be found in the patient's urine, and this finding, although nonspecific, may suggest ethylene glycol as a cause of toxicity. Organ injury, especially to the kidneys, is caused by the widespread deposition of oxalate crystals. The α-hydroxy-β-ketoadipic acid and glycine pathways are considered nontoxic.

Patients who ingest ethylene glycol may initially seem inebriated, mimicking ethanol intoxication. Immediately following the exposure, the patient will not be acidotic until

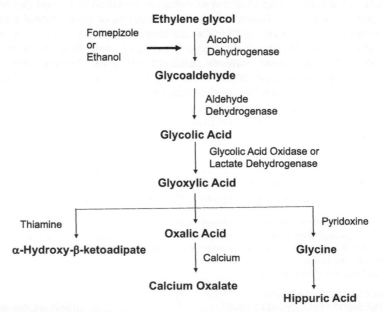

Fig. 1. Ethylene glycol metabolism.

enough time has passed to allow metabolism; however, an elevated osmole gap may be detected due to ethylene glycol. If ethanol is not coingested (which prevents metabolism of ethylene glycol), an anion gap metabolic acidosis will develop after a delay of hours, leading to potential compensatory hyperventilation. As the acidosis worsens and oxalic acid forms, hypocalcemia, creatinine elevation, seizures, and cardiac dysrhythmias may occur. If untreated, renal failure is common. Oxalic acid combining with calcium may lead to hypocalcemia with subsequent tetany, seizures, and QT interval prolongation. Cerebral edema has been reported with deposition of calcium oxalate crystals in the brain.

Patients with ethylene glycol poisoning can have elevations in serum lactate concentration. Elevations can be caused by true increases in the serum lactate, but some laboratory instruments may not be able to differentiate between lactate and glycolic acid due to its structural similarity to lactate.[4,5] This false lactate elevation is common when using blood gas analyzers and point-of-care testing.[6] A large difference in the reported lactate concentration using 2 different methods may help to determine an ethylene glycol poisoning.

The serum ethylene glycol concentration itself is not predictive of outcome but rather the serum concentration of glycolic acid, which correlates more closely with mortality. Because of the rapid elimination of ethylene glycol, its serum concentration may be low or undetectable at a time when glycolic acid remains elevated. If available, the determination of both ethylene glycol and glycolic acid concentrations provides useful clinical and confirmatory analytical information in ethylene glycol ingestion.[7] However, most hospital laboratories are unable to perform ethylene glycol or glycolic acid levels. According to Porter's study, an initial anion gap greater than 20 mmol/L and pH less than 7.30 are predictors for the development of acute renal failure in ethylene glycol toxicity (sensitivities of 95.6% and 100% and specificities of 94.4% and 88.5%, respectively).[7]

The mainstay of therapy for ethylene glycol toxicity includes administration of fomepizole (or ethanol if fomepizole is not available), thiamine, pyridoxine, and hemodialysis. Fomepizole has a higher affinity for ADH than ethylene glycol and will compete for metabolism, preventing the breakdown of ethylene glycol into toxic metabolites. Ethanol may also be used to inhibit ADH when fomepizole is unavailable. Fomepizole is the preferred treatment over ethanol, as it is more easily dosed, does not cause further inebriation or sedation, more strongly competitively inhibits ADH, and is associated with less administration errors.[8,9] Fomepizole has been used without dialysis in ethylene glycol poisoning if there is no significant acidosis or renal failure.[10,11] However, because of the significant prolongation of ethylene glycol's elimination half-life with fomepizole, fomepizole treatment without dialysis may prolong the time necessary for monitoring and intensive care unit care.[11] Fomepizole will not prevent the conversion of the acid metabolites to oxalate and the potential development of renal failure.

Fomepizole is administered intravenously with a loading dose of 15 mg/kg, followed by maintenance dosing of 10 mg/kg every 12 hours until the ethylene glycol concentration becomes less than 20 mg/dL.[12] If additional dosing is required beyond 4 maintenance doses, the dose should be increased to 15 mg/kg every 12 hours due to fomepizole's autoinduction of its own metabolism. During dialysis, fomepizole dosing should be increased to every 4 hours. If fomepizole is not available, ethanol can be used to competitively inhibit ADH and is administered via intravenous or oral routes with blood levels maintained at approximately 100 mg/dL. Ethanol therapy requires more frequent laboratory testing than with fomepizole to assure the ethanol level is maintained at appropriate levels and to ensure that hypoglycemia does not develop. The patient will require closer mental status and respiratory monitoring due to the additional inebriating effects of ethanol.

Pyridoxine and thiamine can theoretically aid in the metabolism of glyoxylic acid away from oxalic acid to nontoxic metabolites (glycine and α-hydroxy-β-ketoadipate). Sodium bicarbonate administration can be considered for patients with significant acidosis. Hemodialysis will remove both ethylene glycol and its acidic toxic metabolites. Ethylene glycol-toxic patients often present late with marked acidosis and developing renal failure associated with oxalate crystals in the urine. Such cases should not await confirmation of an ethylene glycol level, and instead hemodialysis should be pursued emergently. The indications for hemodialysis depend on the specific case and available local resources.[13] The clinician should discuss the case further with the local poison center (medical toxicologist) and nephrologist and include consideration of the total ethylene glycol level, the degree of metabolic acidosis (eg, anion gap >20 mmol/L or pH <7.30), and/or the presence of renal failure.[7]

Methanol

Methanol is found in numerous products, including as a solvent in several commercial products, as a constituent in windshield wiper fluid, copy machine fluids, fuel additives (octane boosters), paint remover or thinner, antifreeze, canned heating sources, deicing fluid, shellacs, and varnishes. Toxicity has been reported following consumption, both intentionally (eg, as an ethanol substitute or in suicide attempts) or accidently (eg, present as a contaminant in illegal whiskey).[14] Toxicity has also occurred via dermal and inhalational exposure.[15]

Methanol is slowly oxidized by ADH (at about one-tenth the rate of ethanol) to formaldehyde. Formaldehyde in turn is rapidly oxidized by ALDH to formic acid (**Fig. 2**).

Patients who ingest methanol may initially seem inebriated, similar to ethanol intoxication, although the degree of inebriation is often less due to methanol being a shorter chain alcohol than ethanol. The patient will not immediately develop acidosis due to methanol's slow metabolism; however, an elevated osmole gap may be present. If ethanol is not coingested (which prevents metabolism of

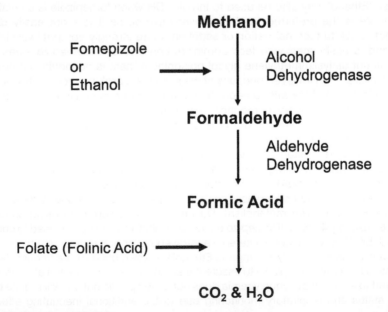

Fig. 2. Methanol metabolism.

methanol), the patient may develop a progressive anion gap metabolic acidosis after a delay of hours and subsequent optic neuropathy with reported visual disturbances potentially leading to blindness. Methanol toxicity can result in intracranial hemorrhages, as well as infarcts, especially of the basal ganglia, with an incidence of abnormal brain computed tomography findings in 67% of methanol-poisoned patients in one study.[16]

The mainstay of therapy for methanol toxicity includes administration of fomepizole (or ethanol if fomepizole is not available), folate or folinic acid, and hemodialysis.[17] As a competitive antagonist of ADH, fomepizole will prevent the metabolism of methanol into its toxic metabolite, formic acid.[18] Methanol levels greater than 20 mg/dL are considered toxic. Once ADH is blocked by fomepizole, the half-life of methanol increases to more than 50 hours.[17] Unlike ethylene glycol, there is no significant renal elimination of methanol, and it is thought to be eliminated through exhaled air. Because of its long elimination half-life as well as significant, often irreversible toxicity, treatment with fomepizole in combination with hemodialysis is often recommended. Folate or folinic acid can aid in the conversion of formic acid to nontoxic byproducts and can be considered an adjunct to treatment. Hemodialysis will rapidly remove both methanol and formic acid with indications and associated evidence found at *The Extracorporeal Treatments in Poisoning Working Group* (EXTRIP) Website (www.extrip-workgroup.org/methanol).

Diethylene Glycol

Diethylene glycol is an industrial solvent used in a variety of products, including antifreeze, brake fluid, wallpaper strippers, and fabric and dye manufacturing. Toxicity has been reported following oral ingestion. Diethylene glycol is metabolized by ADH and ALDH to 2-hydroxyethoxyacetic acid, after which it is oxidized to diglycolic acid (**Fig. 3**).[19] The development of an anion gap metabolic acidosis may be delayed for longer than 12 hours postingestion. Diglycolic acid causes both nephrotoxicity and neurotoxicity.[20,21]

Patients who ingest diethylene glycol may seem inebriated, similar to ethanol intoxication. Toxicity may further progress with metabolism to the development of gastritis, hepatitis, pancreatitis, metabolic acidosis, coma, and delayed neurologic sequelae. Nephrotoxicity is consistently reported in human cases.[19]

As with ethylene glycol and methanol, treatment with fomepizole (or ethanol if fomepizole is not available) prevents the breakdown to more toxic acidic metabolites.[22] If patients develop a significant anion gap metabolic acidosis or renal failure, hemodialysis is indicated.

Propylene Glycol

Propylene glycol is used as a diluent in many pharmaceutical medications, such as lorazepam, diazepam, phenobarbital, and phenytoin.[23] Propylene glycol toxicity is a potentially life-threatening iatrogenic complication that is preventable.[24,25] It is also used in other products, such as topical medications and cosmetics, and as a solvent. Propylene glycol is metabolized by ADH to lactaldehyde and then by ALDH to lactate and pyruvate (**Fig. 4**).

Propylene glycol ingestions can also cause inebriation similar to ethanol, and massive exposures have been reported to produce toxic adverse effects, including a marked lactic acidosis, hypoglycemia, seizures, and coma. Hypotension, dysrhythmias, and cardiovascular decompensation can also occur.[26]

Treatment is generally supportive care. If the patient develops acidosis, treatment with sodium bicarbonate may be indicated. In massive ingestions where the parent

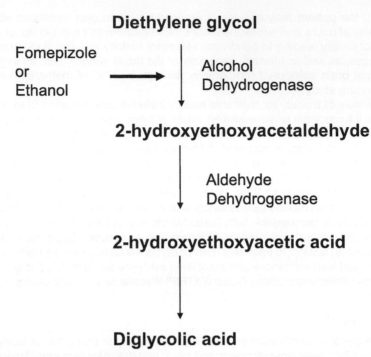

Fig. 3. Diethylene glycol metabolism.

compound is still considered to be present, fomepizole may be of benefit. Hemodialysis is effective but is rarely necessary, as these patients generally do well with supportive care.[23]

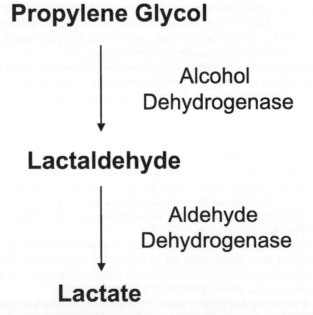

Fig. 4. Propylene glycol metabolism.

Isopropyl Alcohol (Isopropanol)

Isopropanol is readily available as an aqueous solution for use as rubbing alcohol but can also be found in other products such as cleaners, disinfectants, antifreezes, deicers, cosmetics, solvents, inks, and pharmaceuticals. It is used as an ethanol substitute by alcoholics because it is readily available and inexpensive.[27] With the emergence of COVID-19, hand cleansers containing greater than 60% isopropanol are more readily available to the public, and poison centers have documented increasing human exposure calls.[28]

Isopropanol has a short elimination half-life of 3 to 7 hours. It is rapidly metabolized by ADH to acetone, which is eliminated more slowly.[29] The kidneys excrete approximately 80% as acetone, and 20% of isopropyl alcohol is eliminated unchanged. Acetone has central nervous system (CNS) depressant activity similar to that of ethanol, and because of its longer elimination half-life, it may prolong the apparent CNS effects of isopropanol. Isopropanol is a secondary alcohol (the hydroxyl group is attached to a central, rather than a terminal carbon), and consequently it is metabolized by ADH to a dimethyl ketone (acetone) and not an acid. Ingestions of isopropyl alcohol will not cause significant metabolic acidosis unlike other toxic alcohols.

Patients who ingest isopropyl alcohol may present with inebriation similar to ethanol intoxication.[30] Isopropyl alcohol is a marked GI irritant and can cause hematemesis and hemorrhagic gastritis. Massive ingestions can lead to vasodilation and hypotension. Both isopropyl alcohol and acetone cause CNS depression.

The increased acetone can be detected in the patient's breath and results in a positive test for ketones in the serum and urine, potentially misleading the clinician into making a diagnosis of ethanol intoxication or diabetic ketoacidosis.[27] However, the presence of acetone in the breath (fruity odor) and urine in the absence of glycosuria or hyperglycemia provides a clue to the diagnosis of isopropyl alcohol intoxication.

Supportive care is the mainstay of treatment. Fomepizole or ethanol is not indicated. Hemodialysis is effective at removing both isopropyl alcohol and acetone but is rarely necessary, as these patients generally improve with supportive care.

LABORATORY TESTING

The history is notoriously unreliable in the poisoned patient. There are numerous reports of patients who presented with poisoning due to toxic alcohols that were only determined by clinicians who maintained such poisoning on their differential diagnosis. Case examples include the drinker of moonshine contaminated with methanol who was not forthcoming on a history of illicit whiskey due to fears of prosecution[14]; the substance user who was huffing toluene mixed with methanol who initially failed to give such history[31]; the suicidal patient who hid the fact that she drank a toxic alcohol along with medications taken in overdose; the patient presenting with altered mental status following the attempted murder by a spouse who surreptitiously placed ethylene glycol in a smoothie[2]; and the unrecognized medication error leading to a massive propylene glycol overdose.[23]

Two tests, the anion gap and osmole gap, are exceedingly important to consider as a critical care clinician.[32] These 2 tests help to increase toxic alcohols as a consideration in the differential diagnosis, result in the more rapid administration of appropriate treatment, and potentially save the patient from further harm or death.

ANION GAP METABOLIC ACIDOSIS

A basic metabolic panel should be obtained in all patients suspected of being poisoned. When a low serum bicarbonate is discovered, the clinician should determine if an elevated anion gap exists. The equation most commonly used for the serum anion gap calculation is as follows:[33]

$$\text{Anion gap} = Na^+ - (Cl^- + HCO_3^-)$$

The primary cation (sodium) and primary anions (chloride and bicarbonate) are represented in the equation.[34] Other serum cations are not commonly included in this calculation because either their concentrations are relatively low (eg, potassium), they may not have been assayed (eg, magnesium), or assigning a number to represent their respective contribution is difficult (eg, cationic serum proteins).[35] Similarly, there are a multitude of other serum anions (eg, sulfate, phosphate, organic anions) that are also difficult to measure or quantify in terms of charge-concentration units (mEq/L).[34,35] The anion gap represents these "unmeasured" ions. The normal range for the anion gap has conventionally been accepted to be 6 to 14 mEq/L.[34,35] Practically speaking, an increase in the anion gap beyond the normal range, accompanied by metabolic acidosis, represents an increase in unmeasured endogenous (eg, lactate) or exogenous (eg, glycolic acid) anions.[33] A list of the more common causes of this phenomenon is organized in the classic *MUDPILES* mnemonic (**Box 1**).

It is imperative that clinicians who care for poisoned patients presenting with an increased anion gap metabolic acidosis investigate the cause in a timely fashion. Many symptomatic poisoned patients may have an initial mild metabolic acidosis due to elevation of serum lactate. This finding can occur for a variety of reasons, including acidosis related to tissue hypoperfusion or a recent seizure. However, with adequate supportive care the anion gap acidosis should improve. If, despite adequate supportive care, an anion gap metabolic acidosis worsens, the clinician should consider either toxins that form acidic metabolites (eg, toxic alcohols) or toxins that cause worsening lactic acidosis by interfering with aerobic energy production (eg, cyanide, iron).[36] The failure to trend the anion gap in a timely fashion has led to numerous cases of adverse outcomes due to missed toxins, especially toxic alcohols, which would have been diagnosed earlier had the clinician performed serial testing (eg, every 2 hours) of the patient's chemistries.

OSMOLE GAP

The serum osmole gap is a laboratory test that may be useful when evaluating poisoned patients. This test is most often discussed in the context of evaluating the

---

Box 1
Potential toxic causes of increased anion gap metabolic acidosis

Methanol

Uremia

Diabetic, starvation, alcoholic ketoacidosis

Propylene glycol

Iron, inhalants (ie, carbon monoxide, cyanide, toluene), isoniazid, ibuprofen

Lactic acidosis

Ethylene glycol

Salicylates, sympathomimetics

patient suspected of toxic alcohol intoxication. Although this test may have utility in such situations, it has many pitfalls that limit its effectiveness.

Osmotic concentrations may be expressed in terms of either osmolality (milliosmoles per kilogram of solvent [mOsm/kg]) or osmolarity (milliosmoles per liter of solution [mOsm/L]).[37] Osmolality (Osm_M) is measured by an osmometer, a tool that most often uses the technique of freezing point depression.[38] Serum osmolarity (Osm_C) may be estimated clinically by several equations[39] involving the patient's serum glucose, sodium, and urea nitrogen, which normally account for almost all of the measured osmolality.[40] One of the most commonly used calculations is expressed as follows:

$$Osm_C = 2(sodium) + (urea\ nitrogen)/2.8 + (glucose)/18$$

The numerical factor in the sodium term (expressed in millimoles per liter) accounts for corresponding anions that contribute to osmolarity; the numerical factors in the other 2 terms convert their concentration units from milligrams per deciliter to millimoles per liter.[41] Finding the osmolar contribution of any other osmotically active substance that is reported in milligrams per deciliter (such as urea nitrogen or glucose) is accomplished by dividing by one-tenth of the substance's molecular weight in daltons.[41] For urea nitrogen this conversion factor is 2.8 and for glucose it is 18. Similarly, additional terms, along with corresponding conversion factors, may be added to this equation to account for ethanol and the various toxic alcohols (assuming they have been measured and their results are expressed in milligrams per deciliter):

$$Osm_C = 2(sodium) + (urea\ nitrogen)/2.8 + (glucose)/18 + (ethanol)/4.6 + (methanol)/3.2 + (ethylene\ glycol)/6.2 + (isopropanol)/6.0$$

The difference between the measured (Osm_M) and calculated (Osm_C) osmotic concentrations is the osmole gap:[41]

$$Osmole\ gap = Osm_M - Osm_C$$

One problem with this equation is that the units are different, as the measured form is in units of osmolality (mOsm/kg) and the calculated form is in units of osmolarity (mOsm/L). This unit difference is generally not considered significant for clinical purposes, and the gap may be expressed in either of the units.[39] Another important consideration is the timing of collection of samples. When comparing the measured and calculated osmoles, these samples should be collected at the same time from the same blood draw. Using older samples may not account for changes that have occurred to laboratory values over the course of treatment and could obscure interpretation of the osmole gap.

If a significant elevation of the osmole gap is discovered, the difference in the 2 values may represent presence of foreign substances in the blood.[39] Possible causes of an elevated osmole gap are listed in **Box 2**. Unfortunately, what constitutes a normal osmole gap is widely debated. Conventionally, a normal gap has been defined as less than or equal to 10 mOsm/kg. The original source of this value is an article from Smithline and Gardner, which declared this number as pure convention.[42] Further clinical study has not shown this assumption to be correct. A study of 56 healthy adults reported the normal osmole gap to range from −9 to +5 mOsm/kg.[43] A study examining a pediatric emergency department population (n = 192) found a range from −13.5 to 8.9.[44] Another study looked at the osmole gaps of 177 emergency department patients and reported the range to be from −10 to 20 mOsm/kg.[45] A vital point brought forth by the investigators of this study, however, is that the day-to-day coefficient of

> **Box 2**
> **Causes of an elevated osmole gap**
>
> Toxic alcohols
>   Ethanol
>   Isopropanol
>   Methanol
>   Ethylene glycol
>
> Drugs and excipients
>   Mannitol
>   Propylene glycol
>   Glycerol
>   Osmotic contrast dyes
>
> Other chemicals
>   Ethyl ether
>   Acetone
>   Trichloroethane
>
> Disease or illness
>   Chronic renal failure
>   Lactic acidosis
>   Diabetic ketoacidosis
>   Alcoholic ketoacidosis
>   Starvation ketoacidosis
>   Circulatory shock
>   Hyperlipidemia
>   Hyperproteinemia

variation for their laboratory in regard to sodium was 1%. They concluded that this level of imprecision translates to an analytical standard deviation of 9.1 mOsm/kg in regard to the osmole gap. This analytical imprecision alone may account for the variation found in osmole gaps of many patients. This concern that even small errors in sodium, urea nitrogen, glucose, and osmolality assays can result in large variations of the osmole gap has been voiced by other researchers.[46] Overall, the clinician should recognize that there is likely a wide range of variability in a patient's baseline osmole gap.

Several concerns exist in regard to using the osmole gap as a screening tool in the evaluation of the potentially toxic alcohol–poisoned patient. The lack of a well-established normal range is particularly problematic. For example, a patient may present with an osmole gap of 9 mOsm/kg, which is considered normal by the traditionally accepted upper normal limit of 10 mOsm/kg. If, however, this patient had an osmole gap of −5 mOsm/kg just before ingestion of a toxic alcohol, the patient's osmole gap must have increased by 14 mOsm/kg to reach the new gap of 9 mOsm/kg. If this increase was due to ethylene glycol, it would correspond to a toxic level of 86.8 mg/dL.[47] In addition, if a patient's ingestion of a toxic alcohol occurred at a time distant from the actual blood sampling, the osmotically active parent compound will have been metabolized to the acid metabolites. These metabolites do not influence the osmole gap because they are anions that displace bicarbonate and are accounted for by the doubled sodium term in the equation; hence no osmole gap elevation will be detected.[39,48] Therefore, it is possible that a patient may present at a point after ingestion with only a moderate increase in their osmole gap and anion gap. Steinhart reported a patient with ethylene glycol toxicity who presented with an osmole gap of 7.2 mOsm/L due to a delay in presentation.[49] Darchy and colleagues presented 2 other cases of significant ethylene glycol toxicity with osmole gaps of 4 and 7 mOsm/L.[46] The lack of an abnormal osmole gap in these cases was speculated to be due to either metabolism of the parent alcohol or a low baseline osmole gap that masked the toxin's presence.

The osmole gap should be used with caution as an adjunct to clinical decision-making and not as a primary determinant to rule out toxic alcohol ingestion. If the osmole gap obtained is particularly large, it suggests an agent from **Box 2** may be present. A "normal" osmole gap should be interpreted with caution, as it may not rule out the presence of such an ingestion. The test result must be interpreted within the context of the clinical presentation. If such a poisoning is suspected, appropriate therapy should be initiated presumptively (ie, fomepizole administration, hemodialysis, etc.) while confirmation from serum levels of the suspected toxin is pending.

SUMMARY

Toxic alcohol exposures can cause patients to become critically ill, and many products containing toxic alcohols are readily accessible. Ethylene glycol and methanol are found in numerous household products. Diethylene glycol, propylene glycol, and isopropyl alcohol, although less commonly ingested, can lead to unique clinical toxidromes that must be recognized and appropriately treated. It is important for critical care clinicians to know how to calculate, interpret, and identify the differential diagnosis for an anion gap metabolic acidosis. An osmole gap can be useful in identifying toxic alcohol ingestions; however, it has many limitations that must be recognized. It is important for critical care specialists to be familiar with these formulas as well as each toxic alcohol, so that an exposure can be identified promptly and treated appropriately.

CLINICS CARE POINTS

- Although classic teaching informs that toxic alcohol ingestions will present with an elevated osmole gap and anion gap, in reality this may not be the case and depends on the time of ingestion and which toxic alcohol is involved.

- Toxic alcohol levels are not readily available at many hospitals. If there is a high concern, dialysis and fomepizole (or ethanol) should be initiated for suspected poisoned patients with an unresolving anion gap metabolic acidosis who do not have an alternative cause for laboratory abnormalities.

- Laboratory interpretation and management recommendations for toxic alcohol poisonings are complex. Clinicians should consider discussing the case details with a regional poison center or clinical toxicologist.

DISCLOSURE

The authors do not have any commercial or financial conflicts of interest, and there are no funding sources for this article.

REFERENCES

1. Gummin DD, Mowry JB, Beuhler MC, et al. 2019 annual report of the American association of poison Control centers' National poison Data system (NPDS): 37th annual report. Clin Toxicol (Phila) 2020;58(12):1360–541.
2. Alsufyani A, Blackshaw A, Holstege C. Surreptitiously administered ethylene glycol resulting in murder. Clin Toxicol 2018;56(10):958–9.

3. Wallace KL, Suchard JR, Curry SC, et al. Diagnostic use of physicians' detection of urine fluorescence in a simulated ingestion of sodium fluorescein-containing antifreeze. Ann Emerg Med 2001;38(1):49–54.

4. Shirey T, Sivilotti M. Reaction of lactate electrodes to glycolate. Crit Care Med 1999;27(10):2305–7.

5. Eder AF, Dowdy YG, Gardiner JA, et al. Serum lactate and lactate dehydrogenase in high concentrations interfere in enzymatic assay of ethylene glycol. Clin Chem 1996;42(9):1489–91.

6. Brindley PG, Butler MS, Cembrowski G, et al. Falsely elevated point-of-care lactate measurement after ingestion of ethylene glycol. CMAJ 2007;176(8): 1097–9.

7. Porter WH, Rutter PW, Bush BA, et al. Ethylene glycol toxicity: the role of serum glycolic acid in hemodialysis. J Toxicol-clin Tox 2001;39(6):607–15.

8. Lepik KJ, Levy AR, Sobolev BG, et al. Adverse drug events associated with the antidotes for methanol and ethylene glycol poisoning: a comparison of ethanol and fomepizole. Ann Emerg Med 2009;53(4):439–50.

9. Lepik KJ, Sobolev BG, Levy AR, et al. Medication errors associated with the use of ethanol and fomepizole as antidotes for methanol and ethylene glycol poisoning. Clin Toxicol (Phila) 2011;49(5):391–401.

10. Buller GK, Moskowitz CB. When is it appropriate to treat ethylene glycol intoxication with fomepizole alone without hemodialysis? Semin Dial 2011;24(4):441–2.

11. Buchanan JA, Alhelail M, Cetaruk EW, et al. Massive ethylene glycol ingestion treated with fomepizole alone-a viable therapeutic option. J Med Toxicol 2010; 6(2):131–4.

12. Brent J, McMartin K, Phillips S, et al. Fomepizole for the treatment of ethylene glycol poisoning. Methylpyrazole for toxic alcohols study group. N Engl J Med 1999; 340(11):832–8.

13. Lavergne V, Nolin TD, Hoffman RS, et al. The EXTRIP (EXtracorporeal TReatments in Poisoning) workgroup: guideline methodology. Clin Toxicol (Phila) 2012;50(5): 403–13.

14. Holstege CP, Ferguson JD, Wolf CE, et al. Analysis of moonshine for contaminants. J Toxicol Clin Toxicol 2004;42(5):597–601.

15. Barceloux DG, Bond GR, Krenzelok EP, et al. American Academy of Clinical Toxicology practice guidelines on the treatment of methanol poisoning. J Toxicol-clin Tox 2002;40(4):415–46.

16. Taheri MS, Moghaddam HH, Moharamzad Y, et al. The value of brain CT findings in acute methanol toxicity. Eur J Radiol 2010;73(2):211–4.

17. Brent J, McMartin K, Phillips S, et al. Methylpyrazole for toxic alcohols study group. Fomepizole for the treatment of methanol poisoning. N Engl J Med 2001;344(6):424–9.

18. Hovda KE, Jacobsen D. Expert opinion: fomepizole may ameliorate the need for hemodialysis in methanol poisoning. Hum Exp Toxicol 2008;27(7):539–46.

19. Schep LJ, Slaughter RJ, Temple WA, et al. Diethylene glycol poisoning. Clin Toxicol (Phila) 2009;47(6):525–35.

20. Conrad T, Landry GM, Aw TY, et al. Diglycolic acid, the toxic metabolite of diethylene glycol, chelates calcium and produces renal mitochondrial dysfunction in vitro. Clin Toxicol (Phila) 2016;54(6):501–11.

21. Landry GM, Martin S, McMartin KE. Diglycolic acid is the nephrotoxic metabolite in diethylene glycol poisoning inducing necrosis in human proximal tubule cells in vitro. Toxicol Sci 2011;124(1):35–44.

22. Brent J. Fomepizole for the treatment of pediatric ethylene and diethylene glycol, butoxyethanol, and methanol poisonings. Clin Toxicol (Phila) 2010;48(5):401–6.
23. Zosel A, Egelhoff E, Heard K. Severe lactic acidosis after an iatrogenic propylene glycol overdose. Pharmacotherapy 2010;30(2):219.
24. Wilson KC, Farber HW. Propylene glycol accumulation during continuous-infusion lorazepam in critically ill patients. J Intensive Care Med 2008;23(6):413 [author reply: 414-5].
25. Wilson KC, Reardon C, Theodore AC, et al. Propylene glycol toxicity: a severe iatrogenic illness in ICU patients receiving IV benzodiazepines: a case series and prospective, observational pilot study. Chest 2005;128(3):1674–81.
26. Lim TY, Poole RL, Pageler NM. Propylene glycol toxicity in children. J Pediatr Pharmacol Ther 2014;19(4):277–82.
27. Zaman F, Pervez A, Abreo K. Isopropyl alcohol intoxication: a diagnostic challenge. Am J Kidney Dis 2002;40(3):E12.
28. Chang A, Schnall AH, Law R, et al. Cleaning and disinfectant chemical exposures and temporal associations with COVID-19 - National poison Data system, United States, January 1, 2020-March 31, 2020. MMWR Morb Mortal Wkly Rep 2020; 69(16):496–8.
29. Daniel DR, McAnalley BH, Garriott JC. Isopropyl alcohol metabolism after acute intoxication in humans. J Anal Toxicol 1981;5(3):110–2.
30. Rich J, Scheife RT, Katz N, et al. Isopropyl alcohol intoxication. Arch Neurol 1990; 47(3):322–4.
31. Frenia ML, Schauben JL. Methanol inhalation toxicity. Ann Emerg Med 1993; 22(12):1919–23.
32. Holstege CP, Borek HA. Toxidromes. Crit Care Clin 2012;28(4):479–98.
33. Chabali R. Diagnostic use of anion and osmolal gaps in pediatric emergency medicine. Pediatr Emerg Care 1997;13(3):204–10.
34. Ishihara K, Szerlip HM. Anion gap acidosis. Semin Nephrol 1998;18(1):83–97.
35. Gabow PA. Disorders associated with an altered anion gap. Kidney Int 1985; 27(2):472–83.
36. Judge BS. Metabolic acidosis: differentiating the causes in the poisoned patient. Med Clin North Am 2005;89(6):1107–24.
37. Kruse JA, Cadnapaphornchai P. The serum osmole gap. J Crit Care 1994;9(3): 185–97.
38. Erstad BL. Osmolality and osmolarity: narrowing the terminology gap. Pharmacotherapy 2003;23(9):1085–6.
39. Glaser DS. Utility of the serum osmol gap in the diagnosis of methanol or ethylene glycol ingestion. Ann Emerg Med 1996;27(3):343–6.
40. Worthley LI, Guerin M, Pain RW. For calculating osmolality, the simplest formula is the best. Anaesth Intensive Care 1987;15(2):199–202.
41. Suchard JR. Osmolal gap. In: Dart RC, editor. Medical toxicology. 3rd edition. Philadelphia: Lippincott Williams & Wilkins; 2004. p. 106–9.
42. Smithline N, Gardner KD Jr. Gaps–anionic and osmolal. JAMA 1976;236(14): 1594–7.
43. Glasser L, Sternglanz PD, Combie J, et al. Serum osmolality and its applicability to drug overdose. Am J Clin Pathol 1973;60(5):695–9.
44. McQuillen KK, Anderson AC. Osmol gaps in the pediatric population. Acad Emerg Med 1999;6(1):27–30.
45. Aabakken L, Johansen KS, Rydningen EB, et al. Osmolal and anion gaps in patients admitted to an emergency medical department. Hum Exp Toxicol 1994; 13(2):131–4.

46. Darchy B, Abruzzese L, Pitiot O, et al. Delayed admission for ethylene glycol poisoning: lack of elevated serum osmol gap. Intensive Care Med 1999;25(8): 859–61.
47. Hoffman RS, Smilkstein MJ, Howland MA, et al. Osmol gaps revisited: normal values and limitations. J Toxicol Clin Toxicol 1993;31(1):81–93.
48. Eder AF, McGrath CM, Dowdy YG, et al. Ethylene glycol poisoning: toxicokinetic and analytical factors affecting laboratory diagnosis. Clin Chem 1998;44(1): 168–77.
49. Steinhart B. Case report: severe ethylene glycol intoxication with normal osmolal gap–"a chilling thought". J Emerg Med 1990;8(5):583–5.

Carbon Monoxide Poisoning

James A. Chenoweth, MD, MAS[a,b,*], Timothy E. Albertson, MD, PhD[a,b,c],
Matthew R. Greer, MD[a]

KEYWORDS

- Carbon monoxide • Carboxyhemoglobin • CO poisoning • Hyperbaric oxygen
- Co-oximetry

KEY POINTS

- Carbon monoxide is a highly toxic gas produced through the incomplete combustion of organic material, with the most common sources of exposure being housefires, gas heaters, and combustion engines.
- Symptoms of carbon monoxide toxicity vary widely from mild headache to critical illness.
- The diagnosis of carbon monoxide poisoning is made via history and blood co-oximetry with a carboxyhemoglobin level of greater than 5% in nonsmokers and greater than 10% in smokers.
- The treatment of carbon monoxide toxicity consists of supportive care and either normobaric oxygen or hyperbaric oxygen.
- Hyperbaric oxygen therapy should be considered in patients with evidence of neurologic or cardiac toxicity, patients with underlying cardiac disease, and patients who are pregnant.

INTRODUCTION

Carbon monoxide (CO) is a colorless, odorless, and nonirritating gas that is highly toxic to humans. CO is primarily produced by incomplete combustion of organic material with motor vehicles being the largest anthropogenic source.[1] Natural sources exist, including forest fires and volcanos, although these are an uncommon source for human toxicity.[1–4] A rare form of CO toxicity can occur through hepatic metabolism of methylene chloride by cytochrome CYP2E1.[5–7] Additionally, volatile anesthetic agents can produce CO when used with carbon dioxide absorbents and can be a source of CO toxicity in the anesthesia suite.[8] Finally, a small amount of endogenous

The authors report no financial conflicts of interest.

[a] Department of Emergency Medicine, University of California – Davis, School of Medicine, 4150 V Street, PSSB Suite 2100, Sacramento, CA 95817, USA; [b] Department of Internal Medicine, Mather VA Medical Center, 10535 Hospital Way, Mather, CA 95655, USA; [c] Department of Internal Medicine, University of California – Davis, School of Medicine, 4150 V Street, PSSB Suite 3100, Sacramento, CA 95817, USA
* Corresponding author.
E-mail address: jachenoweth@ucdavis.edu

Crit Care Clin 37 (2021) 657–672
https://doi.org/10.1016/j.ccc.2021.03.010
0749-0704/21/Published by Elsevier Inc.

criticalcare.theclinics.com

> **Box 1**
> **Common sources of CO[1-8]**
>
> Endogenous production
>   Heme catabolism
>
> Combustion
>   Motor vehicle exhaust
>   Gas heaters
>   Wood- or coal-burning stoves
>   Indoor grills
>   Gas powered equipment (such as air compressors)
>   Boat engines
>   House fires
>   Cigarette or cigar smoking
>   Hookah and waterpipe smoking
>
> Industrial chemicals
>   Methylene chloride
>
> Medical sources
>   Volatile anesthetic agents
>
> Natural sources
>   Volcanic eruptions
>   Forest fires

CO is also produced through heme catabolism.[9] Common sources for CO toxicity are listed in **Box 1**.

Epidemiology

CO toxicity is estimated to be responsible for 30,000 to 50,000 emergency department visits each year.[10] In 2018, there were a total of 13,353 calls to poison control systems in the United States for CO exposure, which is similar to the average of 13,541 calls annually over the last 5 years.[11-15] The annual mortality from CO has been decreasing from 1874 deaths in 1999 to 1245 in 2014 (**Fig. 1**).[16] Most of this decline is due to a

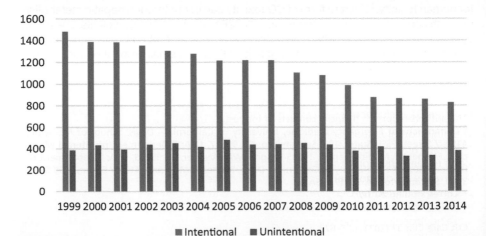

Fig. 1. Yearly intentional and unintentional CO deaths.[12]

decrease in mortality from intentional exposures.[16] Recently, there have been increasing reports of CO toxicity owing to waterpipe (hookah) smoking.[17–19] One recent study of patients undergoing treatment at a regional hyperbaric facility found waterpipe smoking to be the CO source in 22% of patients.[18] These patients tended to be younger than those exposed via other sources.[18]

BACKGROUND

CO typically enters the body through inhalation. The amount of CO absorbed depends on the concentration of CO in the inhaled air, minute ventilation, and duration of exposure.[20] Once absorbed, CO primarily binds to iron molecules in hemoglobin, myoglobin, and cytochrome C.[3] It is primarily excreted through exhalation with minimal in vitro conversion to carbon dioxide.[21] CO exerts its toxic effects through multiple mechanisms, some of which are incompletely understood.

Binding to Hemoglobin

The primary location of CO binding in the human body is to hemoglobin, which has an affinity for CO that is 200 to 250 times greater than that of oxygen.[22,23] Binding to hemoglobin forms carboxyhemoglobin (HgbCO) and results in conformational changes that shift the oxygen/hemoglobin dissociation curve to the left and decreases oxygen delivery to the tissues. This reaction has the effect of causing tissue hypoxia and increased anaerobic metabolism.

The HgbCO level does not completely explain the toxicity seen with CO. A study of CO poisoned canines found significant mortality owing to inhaled CO as compared with exchange transfusion with blood containing 90% HgbCO. This finding was despite the fact that both groups had similar blood HgbCO levels.[24] In a separate canine study, intraperitoneal injection of CO resulted in HgbCO levels as high as 80% with no resultant mortality.[24] The increased mortality with inhaled CO toxicity is postulated to be owing to the increased concentration of CO dissolved in serum, which can then act on tissue cytochromes and myoglobin.[25]

Binding to Other Heme Molecules

CO dissolved in serum (approximately 10%–15% of inhaled CO) can bind to tissue myoglobin, cytochromes, and nicotinamide adenine dinucleotide phosphate hydrogen reductase. Binding to mitochondrial cytochrome C oxidase in the electron transport chain inhibits oxidative phosphorylation resulting in anaerobic metabolism.[25,26] Binding to cytochrome C oxidase is greatest under hypoxic conditions owing to the fact that CO only has a 3 times greater affinity for this molecule than oxygen.[27] Organs with high energy requirements such as the heart and brain are particularly sensitive to this form of toxicity.

Reactive Oxygen Species

The inhibition of cytochrome C oxidase by CO results in oxidative stress through the continued action of other components of the electron transport chain.[25,28] This process leads to the activation of superoxide generation and oxidant damage to cells. Further superoxide production can occur through displacement of nitric oxide from circulating platelets activated by CO.[29] Activated platelets then stimulate neutrophils to release myeloperoxidase, which further exacerbates the inflammatory response by activating more neutrophils, leading to leukocyte adhesion.[25,30] Neutrophil actions on endothelial cells include oxidation of xanthine dehydrogenase to xanthine oxidase, further worsening oxidant stress.[30] Endothelial oxidant stress and xanthine oxidase are thought to contribute to the neurologic sequelae of CO poisoning.[30] Delayed neurologic sequelae may then occur through activation of lymphocytes and microglia by adducts of myeloperoxidase or reactive oxygen species with myelin basic protein.[31]

Effects on Clotting

CO toxicity leads to platelet activation and aggregation.[30] CO can also bind to heme molecules in fibrinogen, forming carboxyhemefibrinogen.[32] These effects, combined with the inflammatory effects described elsewhere in this article, can lead to a hypercoagulable state and intravascular thrombosis.[32,33]

CLINICAL EFFECTS

CO toxicity can cause a range of acute effects from mild symptoms to critical illness. The degree of illness and severity of symptoms seem to be correlated with the degree of CO exposure and the patient's underlying comorbidities.[34] Certain risk factors are associated with short term mortality, including a blood pH of less than 7.2 and need for endotracheal intubation.[35] In additional to the acute effects, delayed neurologic sequelae may also occur. The range of illnesses associated with CO toxicity is listed in **Table 1**.

Cardiovascular Effects

CO exposure leads to cardiac cellular hypoxia via decreased delivery of oxygen to the myocardial tissue and blockade of oxidative phosphorylation. This process can lead to chest pain, which may occur at low HgbCO levels in patients with underlying cardiovascular disease.[36] Tachycardia typically occurs owing to diffuse cellular hypoxia.[37] Myocardial necrosis may occur even in patients without underlying cardiovascular disease and has been reported in the absence of chest pain. In CO poisoned patients, an elevation in cardiac enzymes is associated with an increased 5-year mortality rate.[38] Prolongation of the QT interval has been reported along with cardiac dysrhythmias, including supraventricular tachycardias and premature ventricular contractions.[39,40]

Exposure to CO is also associated with abnormalities in cardiac function. Decreases in the ejection fraction are correlated with the degree of CO exposure. These changes can occur in the absence of myocardial infarction.[41] Changes in the ejection fraction typically resolve in 24 hours, but may persist in some patients.[41,42]

Neurologic Effects

The most common neurologic symptom of CO toxicity is headache, which is present in approximately 91% of patients.[3] More severely poisoned patients may have syncope,

Table 1	
Symptoms associated with CO toxicity[2–4,31]	
Severity	**Signs and Symptoms**
Mild (~5%–20% HgbCO)	Headache, nausea, vomiting, blurred vision, palpitations, dizziness
Moderate (~20%–50% HgbCO)	Syncope, chest pain, shortness of breath, altered coordination, altered mentation
Severe or life threatening (>50% HgbCO)	Cardiac dysrhythmias, cardiac ischemia, cerebral infarction, severe metabolic acidosis, seizures, pulmonary edema, coma, hemodynamic compromise

seizures, altered mentation (including coma), and cognitive difficulties.[3,26] In patients who survive the initial exposure, a significant number may suffer from delayed or persistent neurologic symptoms. These symptoms include depression, memory difficulties, ataxia, and motor deficits.[43,44]

Patient Presentation

One of the most challenging aspects of CO poisoning is the variety of clinical effects it can cause. This circumstance means that patients exposed to CO can present with a wide range of potential complaints, from mild headache and flulike illness to profound altered mental status with hemodynamic compromise. Clinicians must maintain a high level of suspicion for the disease in diverse patient presentations. It is commonly taught that neurologic findings such as headache are hallmark signs of CO poisoning. Unfortunately, these signs are not always present. Several studies have evaluated the prevalence of CO symptoms and found that headache (91% of patients), dizziness (77%), and weakness (53%) are the most commonly reported symptoms.[45–47] The classic findings of cherry red lips, cyanosis, and retinal hemorrhages are predominantly found in patients who are in extremis and tend to be rare in patients who present to the medical system.[48] Furthermore, many factors affect the severity of symptoms and disease sequalae in CO poisonings, namely, the frequency and duration of exposure, time between exposure and presentation, type of exposure, and the treatments that were rendered to the patient en route to the hospital (such as administration of supplemental oxygen) can all affect the patient's presentation.

Owing to the variability in patient presentation, a detailed and accurate history is crucial to determining the presence of CO poisoning. In some cases, a patient's history will obviously suggest CO poisoning. Patients pulled from burning buildings or from enclosed garages with a running motor vehicle (often the case in nonaccidental poisoning), for instance, immediately raise concern for CO poisoning. However, other common sources of CO poisoning will not lead to such transparent patient histories. Patients may be unaware of a leaky home furnace, a partially occluded vehicle exhaust pipe, or a potentially hazardous job site. In these cases, clinicians should look for clues in the patient history such as headaches that improve upon leaving the house or job site, recent similar ailments of family members or coworkers, or recent deaths or behavioral changes in pets. Additionally, patients suffering from chronic CO poisoning in cases like these may present with psychological symptoms, such as personality changes (which may have been detected by a friend or family) or memory loss.

Evaluation

The diagnosis of acute CO poisoning often depends on 3 factors[43,48]:

1. A history of potential exposure to a source of CO
2. Symptoms consistent with CO poisoning
3. HgbCO levels that are more than 5% in nonsmokers or more than 10% in smokers (although higher levels have been reported in cigar and waterpipe smokers)[49–51]

Although it may be necessary for the definitive diagnosis of CO toxicity, HgbCO levels are not reliably correlated with the severity of poisoning. Although it is true that extremely high levels are indicative of severe exposure (>50% HgbCO), it is not true that lower levels imply a less serious exposure. This circumstance is at least partially owing to spontaneous clearance of CO through respiration, which can be accelerated by the administration of supplemental oxygen, a common prehospital intervention.[52–54] There are case reports of patients with only mild symptoms but levels of 47% HgbCO, and at the same time there are reports of patients who are comatose with levels of 10%.[55] All this information suggests that, in diagnosing CO poisoning, the presence of HgbCO above the normal range is more important than the actual level.

Measuring HgbCO and oxygen saturation by pulse oximetry in a patient with CO poisoning has potential pitfalls. The standard pulse oximetry used in modern medical settings measures the absorption of light at a 660-nm wavelength. Both oxyhemoglobin and HgbCO have similar absorption properties at this wavelength of light and, as a result, the pulse oximeter will report a normal oxygen saturation.[56] Additionally, normal blood gas analyzers that measure the partial pressure of dissolved oxygen will also not detect the presence of CO owing to the minimal amounts dissolved in plasma. Like pulse oximetry, normal blood gas analyzers do not differentiate between oxyhemoglobin and HgbCO. Instead, they estimate the saturated O_2 based on the O_2 dissociation curve for the given pH, dissolved partial pressure of oxygen, and dissolved partial pressure of carbon dioxide. For this reason, when a clinician highly suspects CO poisoning, they should obtain a HgbCO level by ordering a co-oximetry study.[57] Co-oximetry uses several wavelengths of light, which allows it to differentiate between oxyhemoglobin, deoxyhemoglobin, HgbCO, methemoglobin, and in some cases sulfhemoglobin in a venous or arterial blood sample.[58] For the purposes of obtaining the HgbCO level, arterial and venous samples are equally reliable and may be used interchangeably. Additionally, a fingertip pulse co-oximeter has been available since 2005. Although some investigators have questioned the reliability of these devices, they may be a helpful early screening tool until definitive confirmatory laboratory testing can be performed.[43,59–61]

In addition to HgbCO measures, other laboratory tests also hold some value in diagnosis of CO poisoning and may assist in determining a patient's prognosis (**Box 2**). Because CO poisoning affects the electron transport chain, patients with the disease can be expected to shift to producing more lactate, leading to an elevated anion gap metabolic acidosis. Additionally, the effect that CO poisoning has on myoglobin and

---

Box 2
Common diagnostic tests in CO poisoning

Imaging
  Chest radiograph
  Cranial computed tomography scan
  Cranial MRI

Laboratory tests
  Complete blood count
  Basic chemistry
  Blood lactate
  Co-oximetry (critical for diagnosis)
  Urine or blood pregnancy test[a]

Neurologic testing
  Electroencephalogram
  Neuropsychiatric testing

Other
  Electrocardiogram

[a]In patients capable of getting pregnant.

subsequent muscle energy use can lead to increases in creatine kinase and troponin. Troponin elevation after CO exposure is associated with increased mortality.[38]

An electrocardiogram should be obtained to evaluate for signs of ischemia or cardiac dysrhythmias. Although there is no classic electrocardiogram pattern for CO toxicity, the presence of repolarization abnormalities such as ST depression, ST elevation, or supraventricular tachycardias can indicate more severe poisoning.[57] Imaging studies such as chest radiographs should be obtained, particularly if the patient has dyspnea or the source of exposure was a housefire. In patients with neurologic deficits, a cranial computed tomography scan may reveal alternative causes of their altered mentation, such as an intracranial hemorrhage. In more severe CO poisoning, a cranial computed tomography scan can reveal bilateral symmetric lesions in the globus pallidus, which may indicate a poor prognosis,[62–64] but is not specific to CO poisoning.[3] MRI is unlikely to be helpful in the initial presentation given the time it takes to administer the test, but there is some evidence that damage to a patient's globus pallidus and deep white matter may convey a risk of persistent neurologic symptoms from CO poisoning.[65]

TREATMENT

The initial steps for the resuscitation of any critically ill patient should follow a structured assessment and treatment for catastrophic failures in the areas of airway, breathing, and circulation. For any patient in whom CO poisoning is suspected, it is important to first remove the patient from the source of CO exposure and then administer the highest available concentration of oxygen, despite what the pulse oximeter reports (because, as noted elsewhere in this article, this measure will be unreliable in that it will report a falsely elevated number). Because CO binds to hemoglobin with a much greater affinity than oxygen, it likely limits the blood's capacity for oxygen transport to tissues.[22,23] The elimination of CO is related to minute ventilation, duration of exposure, atmospheric pressure, and fraction of inhaled oxygen.[3] On room air alone, the half-life of HgbCO is around 4 to 6 hours, but the quick administration of high-flow oxygen decrease this half-life considerably. By increasing the inhaled O_2 to 50% (as is achievable with a standard face mask), the half-life of HgbCO is decreased to around 2 hours, and using a well-fitting nonrebreather mask to administer 100% inhaled O_2 can decrease the half-life to 40 to 80 minutes.[66–68] A decrease in HgbCO alone does not guarantee avoidance of the sequela of the disease. Instead, the pathophysiology of the underlying cause of residual CO poisoning symptoms is complex and multifactorial, as noted elsewhere in this article. Removing CO from heme-containing enzymes will further decrease cellular changes in metabolism.

Hyperbaric Oxygen

A much-debated treatment for CO poisoning involves administration of oxygen under hyperbaric pressures. Hyperbaric oxygenation (HBO) first emerged as a possible treatment as early as 1895, when a report by Haldane[69] showed that HBO could prevent CO poisoning in mice. The treatment has since undergone decades of investigation, but its first use in humans was not reported until the 1960s.[70] There have also been several randomized trials comparing HBO to normobaric oxygen in patients with CO poisoning (**Table 2**).[71–77] After decades-long attempts to determine the exact set of circumstances in which HBO is indicated, it is now fairly well-accepted that HBO does decrease the half-life of HgbCO, typically, down to as low as 30 minutes. The ongoing controversy lies in that there is little evidence to show either (a) that HBO decreases morbidity or mortality in patients or (b) who will benefit most (a critical

Table 2
Randomized trials of hyperbaric oxygen (HBO) versus normobaric oxygen (NBO) in CO poisoning[68-74]

Trial (No. of Patients)	Groups and Intervention	Key Exclusion Criteria	Outcome	Results	Critiques
Raphael et al,[73] 1989 (n = 343)	Patients without history of loss of consciousness randomized to HBO at 2.0 ATA for 60 min followed by NBO for 4 h vs NBO for 6 h	Loss of consciousness, pregnancy, intoxication, hemodynamic instability	Self-assessment questionnaire and physical examination by neurologist at 1 month	Neurologic symptoms present in 50/158 patients (32%) treated with NBO vs 51/159 patients (32%) treated with HBO	Neither patient nor neurologist blinded to treatment allocation
Thom et al,[75] 1995 (n = 65)	Patients presenting within 6 h of removal from exposure randomized to HBO at 2.8 ATA for 30 min, then 2.0 ATA for 90 min vs NBO until all symptoms resolved	History of loss of consciousness, active ischemia	DNS self-reported as recurrent symptoms or new symptom consistent with DNS, plus deterioration in 1 or more subtest upon retesting	DNS present in 7/30 patients in NBO group vs 0/30 in HBO group	Neither patients nor investigators were blinded to treatment allocation, investigators did not report a prestudy primary outcome
Mathieu et al,[87] 1996 (n = 575)	Noncomatose patients without evidence of mixed poisoning and HgbCO level >10% randomized to HBO at 2.5 ATA for 90 min vs NBO for 12 h	Pregnant patients	Persistent neurologic manifestations determined by Neuropsychologic testing at 1, 3, 6, and 12 mo	Significant difference in persistent neurologic manifestations seen at 3 mo (HBO: 9.5% vs NBO: 15%; $P = .016$) but not at 1 mo (HBO: 23% vs NBO: 26%), 6 mo (HBO: 6.4% vs NBO: 9.5%), or 1 y (4.3% vs 5%)	Only data available are from an abstract of an interim analysis, trial was not registered, and full data are not available for independent review

Source	Description	Outcome definition	Results	Comments
Scheinkestel et al,[74] 1999 (n = 191)	Patients with CO poisoning randomized to 3 daily treatments with HBO at 2.8 ATA for 60 min vs NBO at 1 ATA for 100 min (sham treatment); all participants received NBO between treatments	Pregnant patients, burn victims	Poor outcome defined as PNS at hospital discharge or DNS defined as morbidity found at follow-up that was not obvious at hospital discharge, or deterioration of neuropsychological subtest scores by more than one standard deviation	No difference in PNS (HBO: 75% vs NBO 68%, P = .19) or DNS at 4 wk (HBO: 65% vs NBO: 59%, p = NS)	Large number of suicide attempts (69%), on 46% follow-up at 1 mo
Weaver et al,[76] 2002 (n = 152)	Patients with CO poisoning randomized to 3 sessions of HBO - 1 session 3 ATA for 1 h then 2 ATA for 1 h, followed by 2 sessions of 2 ATA for 2 h at 6–12 h intervals vs NBO 3 sessions at 1 ATA (sham treatment). NBO not routinely used between treatments	Pregnancy, >24 h since exposure	Structured questionnaire, serial neurologic testing, and other formalized assessments (for example, the Geriatric Depression Scale, Katz index of activities of daily living, Short Form-36) immediately after treatments 1 and 3, and then at 2- and 6-wk follow-up	Cognitive sequelae at 6 weeks were less frequent in the HBO group (HBO: 25.0% vs NBO: 46.1%; unadjusted odds ratio, 0.39 (95% CI, 0.20–0.78; P = .007)	Trial prematurely terminated owing to benefit; however, NBO group had a longer mean exposure (22 h vs 13 h) and a greater prevalence of cerebellar signs at baseline (15% vs 4%) Some concern the reported primary outcome was changed between initial reports and final study publication

(continued on next page)

Table 2
(*continued*)

Trial (No. of Patients)	Groups and Intervention	Key Exclusion Criteria	Outcome	Results	Critiques
Annane et al,[71] 2011 (n = 179)	Patients with transient loss of consciousness randomized to NBO for 4 h + HBO at 2.0 ATA for 2 h vs NBO for 6 h	Prolonged loss of consciousness, suicide attempt, pregnancy	Complete recover at 1 mo as determined by self-assessment questionnaire and physical examination (including neuropsychological testing)	No difference in the primary outcomes. Symptoms were present in 33/79 (42%) HBO patients 29/74 (39%) of control patients 1 month after poisoning/treatment	Patients and treatment team were not blinded, and no sham HBO was attempted Use of self-assessment questionnaire could be influenced by undergoing HBO
Cochrane Meta-analysis (Buckley et al,[77] 2011) (n = 1361)	Patients with CO poisoning randomized to HBO vs NBO	Studies comparing only different HBO treatments, studies involving other treatments, studies only using surrogate outcomes	Delayed or persistent neurologic symptoms at time of primary analysis	No difference in the presence of symptoms at time of primary analysis (HBO: 202/705 [28.7%] vs NBO: 219/65 [633.4%]; OR, 0.78; 95% CI, 0.54–1.12)	Significant heterogeneity between studies with some included studies having significant methodological flaws

Abbreviations: ATA, atmospheres; CI, confidence interval; DNS, delayed neurologic sequelae; HBO, hyperbaric oxygen; NBO, normobaric oxygen; OR, odds ratio; PNS, persistent neurologic sequelae.

question, given that few hospitals are equipped with hyperbaric chambers, meaning most patients will require transfer to receive HBO). Additionally, it is unclear what the appropriate HBO settings should be, including, but not limited to, (a) the time to initiation from exposure, (b) the duration of each session, (c) the number of sessions, (d) the pressure depth, and (e) the normal pressure O_2 concentration between sessions. Further complicating decisions is that the patient must be stable before undergoing a hyperbaric session because, once a "dive" is commenced, the risk of depressurizing too quickly inhibits the clinicians' ability to rapidly treat a decompensating patient. Additional complications specific to HBO include pneumothorax, barotrauma to ears, oxygen toxicity (including seizures), and gas embolization.

Considering this controversy, the American Academy of Clinical Toxicology and the American College of Medical Toxicology have not published guidelines on the use of HBO for CO poisoning. Emergency medicine and critical care texts do, however, list a few instances in which HBO is likely indicated (**Box 3**). These situations include syncope, persistent confusion or altered mental status, seizure, focal neurologic deficit, or evidence of acute myocardial ischemia.[57,78–80] Coma is also a highly accepted indication for HBO with limited resistance. Various sources also list a variety of HgbCO levels as potential thresholds for HBO indication, ranging from more than 25% to 40% for patients who are not pregnant and without prior cardiac disease.[81,82] This wide range is likely because the HgbCO level is not as important as the clinical presentation. Consultation with a specialist (such as a medical toxicologist or a hyperbaric physician) in the event of a HgbCO level or more than 10% coupled with neurologic sequalae is appropriate. There is even more uncertainty regarding special patient populations, such as children, pregnant patients, and those with prior cardiac disease. Fetal hemoglobin has an even greater affinity for CO than normal hemoglobin, and it has been shown that fetal morbidity occurs at relatively low levels of HgbCO.[83] For this reason, many groups recommend that HBO is indicated in pregnant patients with HgbCO levels of more than 15% to 20%.[84–86] Given the effects on myocardial tissue, some recommendations suggest a lower HgbCO threshold for HBO in patients with a prior history of ischemic heart disease.[3,75,82]

Special Considerations Regarding Hyperbaric Oxygen Treatment

In many parts of the United States and other countries, a shortage of multiperson HBO chambers exists. Patients who are most likely to benefit from HBO after CO poisoning are typically critically ill and require attendants in the HBO chamber during treatment.

Box 3
Indications for hyperbaric oxygen therapy in CO poisoning

Generally accepted indications
  Persistent altered mental status (including coma)
  Focal neurologic deficits
  Pregnancy with a HgbCO level of more than 15% to 20%
  Evidence of acute myocardial ischemia

Relative indications
  History of loss of consciousness
  Severe metabolic acidosis (pH <7.2) not owing to concomitant cyanide poisoning
  HgbCO level of more than 25% to 40%
  History of cardiac disease
  Hemodynamic instability
  Extremes of age
  Persistent symptoms despite normobaric oxygen

In such cases, transport would need to occur to a center with a multiperson HBO chamber. Air transport decreases atmospheric pressure and may add further risk early during the treatment of CO toxicity. Finally, for patients with cardiac dysrhythmias during HBO treatment, electrical cardioversion or defibrillation cannot be performed, meaning that treatment is limited to chest compressions and medication.

SUMMARY

CO toxicity is a common and potentially life-threatening case of acute and chronic illness. Patients may present with a wide variety of complaints and patient history is often key to making the proper diagnosis. The mainstay of treatment is normobaric oxygen via a nonrebreather mask along with supportive care. Some patients may benefit from HBO, but the indications for this treatment remain controversial. Consultation with a medical toxicologist or a physician specially trained in hyperbaric medicine may help when deciding if a patient should be transferred for treatment with hyperbaric oxygen.

CLINICS CARE POINTS

- Symptoms of CO toxicity vary widely from mild headache to critical illness.

- Resolution of symptoms upon leaving the source of exposure may delay diagnosis if this specific aspect of a patient history is not elucidated.

- A diagnosis of CO poisoning is made via blood co-oximetry with a HgbCO level of more than 5% in nonsmokers and of more than 10% in smokers.

- The treatment of CO toxicity consists of supportive care and supplemental oxygen.

- Hyperbaric oxygen therapy should be considered in patients with evidence of neurologic or cardiac toxicity, patients with underlying cardiac disease, and patients who are pregnant.

REFERENCES

1. Agency for Toxic Substances and Disease Registry. Toxicological profile of carbon monoxide. 2012. Available at: https://www.atsdr.cdc.gov/ToxProfiles/tp201.pdf. Accessed November 5, 2020.
2. Smollin C, Olson K. Carbon monoxide poisoning (acute). BMJ Clin Evid 2010; 2010:2103.
3. Ernst A, Zibrak JD. Carbon monoxide poisoning. N Engl J Med 1998;339(22): 1603–8.
4. Kao LW, Nanagas KA. Carbon monoxide poisoning. Med Clin North Am 2005; 89(6):1161–94.
5. Carlsson A, Hultengren M. Exposure to methylene chloride. III. Metabolism of 14C-labelled methylene chloride in rat. Scand J Work Environ Health 1975;1(2):104–8.
6. Kim SK, Kim YC. Effect of a single administration of benzene, toluene or m-xylene on carboxyhaemoglobin elevation and metabolism of dichloromethane in rats. J Appl Toxicol 1996;16(5):437–44.
7. Guengerich FP, Kim DH, Iwasaki M. Role of human cytochrome P-450 IIE1 in the oxidation of many low molecular weight cancer suspects. Chem Res Toxicol 1991;4(2):168–79.
8. Coppens MJ, Versichelen LF, Rolly G, et al. The mechanisms of carbon monoxide production by inhalational agents. Anaesthesia 2006;61(5):462–8.

9. Sjostrand T. Formation of carbon monoxide in connexion with haemoglobin catabolism. Nature 1951;168(4287):1118–9.

10. Hampson NB, Weaver LK. Carbon monoxide poisoning: a new incidence for an old disease. Undersea Hyperb Med 2007;34(3):163–8.

11. Gummin DD, Mowry JB, Spyker DA, et al. 2018 annual report of the American association of poison control centers' National poison Data system (NPDS): 36th annual report. Clin Toxicol (Phila) 2019;57(12):1220–413.

12. Gummin DD, Mowry JB, Spyker DA, et al. 2017 annual report of the American association of poison control centers' National poison Data system (NPDS): 35th annual report. Clin Toxicol (Phila) 2018;56(12):1213–415.

13. Gummin DD, Mowry JB, Spyker DA, et al. 2016 annual report of the American association of poison control centers' National poison Data system (NPDS): 34th annual report. Clin Toxicol (Phila) 2017;55(10):1072–252.

14. Mowry JB, Spyker DA, Brooks DE, et al. 2015 annual report of the American association of poison control centers' National poison Data system (NPDS): 33rd annual report. Clin Toxicol (Phila) 2016;54(10):924–1109.

15. Mowry JB, Spyker DA, Brooks DE, et al. 2014 annual report of the American association of poison control centers' National poison Data system (NPDS): 32nd annual report. Clin Toxicol (Phila) 2015;53(10):962–1147.

16. Hampson NBUS. Mortality due to carbon monoxide poisoning, 1999-2014. Accidental and intentional deaths. Ann Am Thorac Soc 2016;13(10):1768–74.

17. Ashurst JV, Urquhart M, Cook MD. Carbon monoxide poisoning secondary to hookah smoking. J Am Osteopath Assoc 2012;112(10):686–8.

18. Nguyen V, Salama M, Fernandez D, et al. Comparison between carbon monoxide poisoning from hookah smoking versus other sources. Clin Toxicol (Phila) 2020; 58(12):1320–5.

19. Retzky SS. Carbon monoxide poisoning from hookah smoking: an emerging public health problem. J Med Toxicol 2017;13(2):193–4.

20. Forbes WHSF, Roughton FJW. The rate of carbon monoxide uptake by normal men. Am J Physiol 1945;143:594–608.

21. Coburn RF. The carbon monoxide body stores. Ann N Y Acad Sci 1970;174(1): 11–22.

22. Sendroy JLS, Van Slyke DO. The gasometric estimation of the relative affinity constant for carbon monoxide and oxygen in whole blood at 38C. Am J Physiol 1929; 90:511–2.

23. Roughton FJW DR. The effect of carbon monoxide on the oxyhemoglobin dissociation curve. Am J Physiol 1944;141:17–31.

24. Goldbaum LR, Orellano T, Dergal E. Mechanism of the toxic action of carbon monoxide. Ann Clin Lab Sci 1976;6(4):372–6.

25. Rose JJ, Wang L, Xu Q, et al. Carbon monoxide poisoning: pathogenesis, management, and future directions of therapy. Am J Respir Crit Care Med 2017; 195(5):596–606.

26. Buboltz JB, Robins M. Hyperbaric treatment of carbon monoxide toxicity. Treasure Island (FL): StatPearls; 2020.

27. Wald G, Allen DW. The equilibrium between cytochrome oxidase and carbon monoxide. J Gen Physiol 1957;40(4):593–608.

28. Lo Iacono L, Boczkowski J, Zini R, et al. A carbon monoxide-releasing molecule (CORM-3) uncouples mitochondrial respiration and modulates the production of reactive oxygen species. Free Radic Biol Med 2011;50(11):1556–64.

29. Thom SR, Ohnishi ST, Ischiropoulos H. Nitric oxide released by platelets inhibits neutrophil B2 integrin function following acute carbon monoxide poisoning. Toxicol Appl Pharmacol 1994;128(1):105–10.

30. Thom SR, Bhopale VM, Han ST, et al. Intravascular neutrophil activation due to carbon monoxide poisoning. Am J Respir Crit Care Med 2006;174(11):1239–48.

31. Thom SR, Bhopale VM, Fisher D. Hyperbaric oxygen reduces delayed immune-mediated neuropathology in experimental carbon monoxide toxicity. Toxicol Appl Pharmacol 2006;213(2):152–9.

32. Nielsen VG, Arkebauer MR, Vosseller K. Redox-based thrombelastographic method to detect carboxyhemefibrinogen-mediated hypercoagulability. Blood Coagul Fibrinolysis 2011;22(8):657–61.

33. Nielsen VG, Pretorius E. Carbon monoxide: anticoagulant or procoagulant? Thromb Res 2014;133(3):315–21.

34. Aubard Y, Magne I. Carbon monoxide poisoning in pregnancy. BJOG 2000; 107(7):833–8.

35. Hampson NB, Hauff NM. Risk factors for short-term mortality from carbon monoxide poisoning treated with hyperbaric oxygen. Crit Care Med 2008;36(9):2523–7.

36. Balzan MV, Cacciottolo JM, Mifsud S. Unstable angina and exposure to carbon monoxide. Postgrad Med J 1994;70(828):699–702.

37. Thompson N, Henry JA. Carbon monoxide poisoning: poisons unit experience over five years. Hum Toxicol 1983;2(2):335–8.

38. Henry CR, Satran D, Lindgren B, et al. Myocardial injury and long-term mortality following moderate to severe carbon monoxide poisoning. JAMA 2006;295(4): 398–402.

39. Macmillan CS, Wildsmith JA, Hamilton WF. Reversible increase in QT dispersion during carbon monoxide poisoning. Acta Anaesthesiol Scand 2001;45(3):396–7.

40. Carnevali R, Omboni E, Rossati M, et al. [Electrocardiographic changes in acute carbon monoxide poisoning]. Minerva Med 1987;78(3):175–8.

41. Kalay N, Ozdogru I, Cetinkaya Y, et al. Cardiovascular effects of carbon monoxide poisoning. Am J Cardiol 2007;99(3):322–4.

42. Chamberland DL, Wilson BD, Weaver LK. Transient cardiac dysfunction in acute carbon monoxide poisoning. Am J Med 2004;117(8):623–5.

43. Hampson NB, Piantadosi CA, Thom SR, et al. Practice recommendations in the diagnosis, management, and prevention of carbon monoxide poisoning. Am J Respir Crit Care Med 2012;186(11):1095–101.

44. Weaver LKHR, Churchill SK, Deru K. Neurological outcomes 6 years after acute carbon monoxide poisoning [abstract]. Undersea Hyperb Med 2008;35:258–9.

45. Ely EW, Moorehead B, Haponik EF. Warehouse workers' headache: emergency evaluation and management of 30 patients with carbon monoxide poisoning. Am J Med 1995;98(2):145–55.

46. Myers RA, Snyder SK, Emhoff TA. Subacute sequelae of carbon monoxide poisoning. Ann Emerg Med 1985;14(12):1163–7.

47. Burney RE, Wu SC, Nemiroff MJ. Mass carbon monoxide poisoning: clinical effects and results of treatment in 184 victims. Ann Emerg Med 1982;11(8):394–9.

48. Hardy KR, Thom SR. Pathophysiology and treatment of carbon monoxide poisoning. J Toxicol Clin Toxicol 1994;32(6):613–29.

49. Radford EP, Drizd TA. Blood carbon monoxide levels in persons 3-74 years of age: United States, 1976-80. Adv Data 1982;(76):1–24.

50. Istvan JA, Cunningham TW. Smoking rate, carboxyhemoglobin, and body mass in the Second National health and Nutrition Examination Survey (NHANES II). J Behav Med 1992;15(6):559–72.

51. Dorey A, Scheerlinck P, Nguyen H, et al. Acute and chronic carbon monoxide toxicity from tobacco smoking. Mil Med 2020;185(1–2):e61–7.
52. Weaver LK, Valentine KJ, Hopkins RO. Carbon monoxide poisoning: risk factors for cognitive sequelae and the role of hyperbaric oxygen. Am J Respir Crit Care Med 2007;176(5):491–7.
53. Hampson NB, Hauff NM. Carboxyhemoglobin levels in carbon monoxide poisoning: do they correlate with the clinical picture? Am J Emerg Med 2008; 26(6):665–9.
54. Hampson NB, Dunn SL, Group UCCPS. Symptoms of carbon monoxide poisoning do not correlate with the initial carboxyhemoglobin level. Undersea Hyperb Med 2012;39(2):657–65.
55. Norkool DM, Kirkpatrick JN. Treatment of acute carbon monoxide poisoning with hyperbaric oxygen: a review of 115 cases. Ann Emerg Med 1985;14(12): 1168–71.
56. Hampson NB. Pulse oximetry in severe carbon monoxide poisoning. Chest 1998; 114(4):1036–41.
57. G M. Carbon monoxide. In: Tintinalli's emergency medicine manual. 7th edition. New York: McGraw-Hill Medical; 2012. p. 1410–3.
58. Mack E. Focus on diagnosis: co-oximetry. Pediatr Rev 2007;28(2):73–4.
59. Barker SJ, Curry J, Redford D, et al. Measurement of carboxyhemoglobin and methemoglobin by pulse oximetry: a human volunteer study. Anesthesiology 2006;105(5):892–7.
60. Touger M, Birnbaum A, Wang J, et al. Performance of the RAD-57 pulse CO-oximeter compared with standard laboratory carboxyhemoglobin measurement. Ann Emerg Med 2010;56(4):382–8.
61. Weaver LK, Churchill SK, Deru K, et al. False positive rate of carbon monoxide saturation by pulse oximetry of emergency department patients. Respir Care 2013;58(2):232–40.
62. Silver DA, Cross M, Fox B, et al. Computed tomography of the brain in acute carbon monoxide poisoning. Clin Radiol 1996;51(7):480–3.
63. Jones JS, Lagasse J, Zimmerman G. Computed tomographic findings after acute carbon monoxide poisoning. Am J Emerg Med 1994;12(4):448–51.
64. Miura T, Mitomo M, Kawai R, et al. CT of the brain in acute carbon monoxide intoxication: characteristic features and prognosis. AJNR Am J Neuroradiol 1985;6(5): 739–42.
65. Zagami AS, Lethlean AK, Mellick R. Delayed neurological deterioration following carbon monoxide poisoning: MRI findings. J Neurol 1993;240(2):113–6.
66. Pace N, Strajman E, Walker EL. Acceleration of carbon monoxide elimination in man by high pressure oxygen. Science 1950;111(2894):652–4.
67. Jay GD, McKindley DS. Alterations in pharmacokinetics of carboxyhemoglobin produced by oxygen under pressure. Undersea Hyperb Med 1997;24(3):165–73.
68. Araki R, Nashimoto I, Takano T. The effect of hyperbaric oxygen on cerebral hemoglobin oxygenation and dissociation rate of carboxyhemoglobin in anesthetized rats: spectroscopic approach. Adv Exp Med Biol 1988;222:375–81.
69. Haldane J. The relation of the action of carbonic oxide to oxygen tension. J Physiol 1895;18(3):201–17.
70. Smith G. The treatment of carbon monoxide poisoning with oxygen at two atmospheres absolute. Ann Occup Hyg 1962;5:259–63.
71. Annane D, Chadda K, Gajdos P, et al. Hyperbaric oxygen therapy for acute domestic carbon monoxide poisoning: two randomized controlled trials. Intensive Care Med 2011;37(3):486–92.

72. 1996 Undersea and hyperbaric medical Society annual scientific meeting. Anchorage, Alaska, 20 april-1-5 may 1996. Abstracts. Undersea Hyperb Med 1996;23(Suppl):7–97.

73. Raphael JC, Elkharrat D, Jars-Guincestre MC, et al. Trial of normobaric and hyperbaric oxygen for acute carbon monoxide intoxication. Lancet 1989;2(8660): 414–9.

74. Scheinkestel CD, Bailey M, Myles PS, et al. Hyperbaric or normobaric oxygen for acute carbon monoxide poisoning: a randomised controlled clinical trial. Med J Aust 1999;170(5):203–10.

75. Thom SR, Taber RL, Mendiguren II, et al. Delayed neuropsychologic sequelae after carbon monoxide poisoning: prevention by treatment with hyperbaric oxygen. Ann Emerg Med 1995;25(4):474–80.

76. Weaver LK, Hopkins RO, Chan KJ, et al. Hyperbaric oxygen for acute carbon monoxide poisoning. N Engl J Med 2002;347(14):1057–67.

77. Buckley NA, Juurlink DN, Isbister G, et al. Hyperbaric oxygen for carbon monoxide poisoning. Cochrane Database Syst Rev 2011;(4):CD002041.

78. Dinerman N, HJ. Inhalation injuries. In: Rosen P, editor. Emergency medicine: concepts and clinical practice. 2nd edition. St Louis (MO): Mosby; 1988. p. 585.

79. Jing JI, MA, Fontneau NM. Miscellaneous neurologic problems in the intensive care unit. In: Irwin RS, Rippe JM, editors. Irwin & Rippe's intensive care medicine. 7th edition. Philadelphia: Lippincott Williams and Wilkins; 2012. p. 1814–5.

80. American College of Emergency Physicians Clinical Policies Subcommittee on Carbon Monoxide P, Wolf SJ, Maloney GE, Shih RD, et al. Clinical Policy: critical issues in the evaluation and management of adult patients presenting to the emergency department with acute carbon monoxide poisoning. Ann Emerg Med 2017;69(1):98–107 e106.

81. Tibbles PM, Perrotta PL. Treatment of carbon monoxide poisoning: a critical review of human outcome studies comparing normobaric oxygen with hyperbaric oxygen. Ann Emerg Med 1994;24(2):269–76.

82. Myers RAM, TS. Carbon monoxide and cyanide poisoning. In: Hyperbaric medicine practice. Flagstaff (Ariz): Best Publishing; 1994. p. 357.

83. Di Cera E, Doyle ML, Morgan MS, et al. Carbon monoxide and oxygen binding to human hemoglobin F0. Biochemistry 1989;28(6):2631–8.

84. Silverman RK, Montano J. Hyperbaric oxygen treatment during pregnancy in acute carbon monoxide poisoning. A case report. J Reprod Med 1997;42(5): 309–11.

85. Elkharrat D, Raphael JC, Korach JM, et al. Acute carbon monoxide intoxication and hyperbaric oxygen in pregnancy. Intensive Care Med 1991;17(5):289–92.

86. Van Hoesen KB, Camporesi EM, Moon RE, et al. Should hyperbaric oxygen be used to treat the pregnant patient for acute carbon monoxide poisoning? A case report and literature review. JAMA 1989;261(7):1039–43.

87. Mathieu D, Wattel F, Mathieu-Nolf M, et al. Randomized prospective study comparing the effect of HBO vs. 12 hours NBO in non-comatose CO-poisoned patients: results of the preliminary analysis. Undersea & Hyperbaric Medicine 1996;23 Suppl:7 (abstract).

Management of Organophosphorus Poisoning: Standard Treatment and Beyond

Sakib Aman, MBBS, MCPS, FCPS[a], Shrebash Paul, MBBS, MCPS[b],
Fazle Rabbi Chowdhury, FCPS, MSc, PhD[b],*

KEYWORDS

- Organophosphorus • Poisoning • Atropine • Acetylcholine • Acetylcholinesterase

KEY POINTS

- Organophosphorus poisoning is the leading cause of self-poisoning and suicide across the globe.
- Atropine is still the only effective treatment.
- The clinical efficacy of pralidoxime is a debatable issue; however, it is widely administered as a part of standard treatment.
- Larger studies are needed to establish the efficacy of novel therapies for example, magnesium sulfate, calcium channel blockers, lipid emulsion, and others.

INTRODUCTION

Self-poisoning with organophosphorus (OP) pesticide contributes to around 110,000 deaths per year worldwide.[1] Globally, approximately 1 out of every 6 suicides is due to OP poisoning.[1] Countries in South East Asia, China, and Africa bear the brunt of most cases, reflecting the extensive use of OP compounds in agriculture-dependent economies.

The timely decision to ban the most hazardous OP insecticides (World Health Organization [WHO] class I toxicity compounds) has led to significant decreases in the global number of deaths owing to suicide with these compounds.[2–4] Marked economic growth and rapid urbanization, as well as improvement in medical care have also made significant contributions. However, the WHO class II insecticides such as

Conflict of Interest: None declared.
[a] Department of Medicine, Dhaka Medical College Hospital, Secretariat Road, Dhaka 1000, Bangladesh; [b] Department of Internal Medicine, Bangabandhu Sheikh Mujib Medical University, Shahbag, Dhaka 1000, Bangladesh
* Corresponding author.
E-mail address: masterfazlerabbi@gmail.com

dimethoate remain in extensive use in agriculture. As such, they are readily available as a means of suicide, especially involving the lower socioeconomic demographic group.

One would think that treatment of OP compound poisoning, which has claimed so many lives for so long, would see major advances in treatment especially in this modern era. However, apart from improvements in resuscitation and intensive care, very little has changed in terms of specific management of OP poisoning in the last 60 years. Antimuscarinics (mainly atropine) remain the mainstay of treatment, and the role of oximes is gradually diminishing.

This article reviews the evidence for treatments currently in standard use, as well as options that may complement traditional treatment in combating this global health problem.

ORGANOPHOSPHATE CHEMISTRY

A wide array of OP compounds are available for use as pesticides (**Table 1**). Central to the structure of an OP compound is a phosphorus atom bound to an oxygen atom (P=O) or a sulfur atom (P=S). OP compounds can be direct acting ("oxons") or indirect acting ("thions"). OP compounds can also be classified based on the attachment of methyl or ethyl groups to the phosphorus atom via an oxygen.

OP compounds exert their toxicity by inhibiting acetylcholinesterase.[5] Initially, the OP compounds cause phosphorylation of the enzyme, resulting in a compound that can still be reactivated by strong nucleophilic agents such as oximes.[5] However, the phosphorylated enzyme can undergo aging, a spontaneous time-dependent process where the enzyme is dealkylated, causing irreversible inhibition of acetylcholinesterase.[5] Acetylcholinesterase inhibited by dimethoxy compounds age much faster than inhibition by diethoxy compounds (3.7 hours vs 33 hours).[6] This difference in aging has important clinical implications as discussed elsewhere in this article in the section on oximes.

Table 1 Types of OP compounds	
Types	**Characteristics and Examples**
According to mode of activity	
Direct acting (oxons)	Have a P=O Bond Directly Inhibit Acetylcholinesterase Without Prior metabolism in the body Examples: Paraoxon, Malaoxon, Sarin, Tabun, tetraethyl pyrophosphate
Indirect acting (thions)	Have a P=S bond Undergo partial metabolism to active compounds that in turn inhibit acetylcholinesterase Examples: malathion, parathion
According to attachment of methyl or ethyl group	
Dimethoxy compounds	Methyl group is attached with phosphorus atom via oxygen Examples: parathion, paraoxon, quinalphos
Diethoxy compounds	Ethyl group is attached with phosphorus atom via oxygen Examples: monocrotophos, profenfos, prothiophos[6]

Note: Another group is S-alkyl OP compounds where an alkyl group is bound to the oxygen via a sulfur atom.

Other factors that may influence the severity of toxicity of these compounds include lipid solubility (hydrophilic vs lipophilic), rate of inhibition of acetylcholinesterase, the speed of conversion from thion to oxon, and prolonged storage in humid conditions. Highly lipophilic drugs often bind to fat stores and undergo a delayed and prolonged release into the systemic circulation resulting in mild early features and delayed cholinergic toxicity and respiratory failure.[7-9] Early acute features are usually seen in poisoning with hydrophilic compounds. Prolonged storage in warm conditions may result in conversion of the OP compound to even more toxic compounds as reported from Pakistan (2800 affected field workers in the malaria control program) and Egypt.[10-13]

CLINICAL COURSE

Acetylcholinesterase is responsible for the breakdown of acetylcholine in the cholinergic synapses that occurs throughout the central, peripheral, and autonomic nervous systems. The inhibition of acetylcholinesterase leads to accumulation of excessive acetylcholine in the cholinergic synapses, resulting in overstimulation of muscarinic and nicotinic cholinergic receptors. This overstimulation gives rise to clinical features collectively known as the acute cholinergic syndrome or acute cholinergic crisis (**Table 2**). These features usually appear within 24 hours of OP ingestion.

The commonest cause of death in the acute stage of OP poisoning is respiratory failure. Several factors contribute to respiratory failure (**Box 1**). The onset of respiratory failure from the time of poisoning depends on the chemical nature of the OP compound as well as the dose ingested. Deaths have occurred as soon as 5 minutes after ingestion of the compound mevinphos.[14,15] People poisoned by relatively less toxic WHO class II compounds generally do not require intubation until 2 to 4 hours after exposure. In cases of fenthion ingestion, recurrent cholinergic toxicity and respiratory failure may occur much later, owing to the high lipid solubility, its slow inhibition of acetylcholinesterase, and delayed conversion to the active compound.[7,8]

Two patterns of respiratory failure are observed in OP poisoning: respiratory failure occurring within the first 24 hours and occurring after 24 hours, commonly referred to as intermediate syndrome.[8] Respiratory failure occurring within the first 24 hours usually occurs in patients manifesting features of cholinergic crisis, usually owing to a loss of central respiratory drive and bronchorrhea, and is often associated with disturbances in consciousness. These patients usually require a shorter duration of ventilation. In contrast, failure occurring after 24 hours usually occurs in conscious patients, usually without any associated cholinergic features. Neuromuscular junction (NMJ) dysfunction is thought to play a key role in the pathogenesis, and these patients often require prolonged ventilation, leaving them at high risk of complications from immobility and mechanical ventilation.[8]

| Table 2 | | |
| Clinical manifestations of OP poisoning[16-18] | | |
Muscarinic Features	Nicotinic Features	Combined Features
Hypersalivation	Muscle weakness	Impaired consciousness
Vomiting	Fasciculation	Seizures
Diarrhea	Muscle paralysis	Central loss of respiratory drive
Bronchospasm	Tachycardia	
Miosis	Hypertension	
Bradycardia		
Hypotension		

> **Box 1**
> **Factors responsible for respiratory failure**
>
> Depression of central respiratory drive
>
> Bronchorrhea and bronchoconstriction leading to hypoxia
>
> Neuromuscular junction dysfunction leading to diaphragmatic paralysis
>
> Aspiration pneumonitis, as a consequence of unconsciousness and emesis
>
> Seizures (more common in cases of OP nerve agents)

In some cases, cardiovascular shock resistant to vasopressors and atropine is the cause of death. This clinical manifestation is sometimes seen in dimethoate ingestion, and the solvents combined with these compounds play some role in the pathogenesis.[16] Other causes of death include aspiration pneumonitis, acute respiratory distress syndrome, and irreversible hypoxic brain injury.

Initially described by Wadia and colleagues[17] and then Senanayake and Karalliedde,[18] the intermediate syndrome usually occurs 24 to 96 hours after OP exposure. The patient develops cranial nerve palsies, weakness of the neck flexors and proximal muscles, and ultimately diaphragmatic weakness leading to type II respiratory failure. Dimethyl OP compounds such as methyl parathion and fenthion are more commonly associated with intermediate syndrome than diethyl compounds.[19] Seizures are more common with OP nerve agents such as sarin and novichok.[20,21] Myocardial injury evidenced by modest increase in troponin may occur in some cases.[22,23] OP-induced delayed neuropathy usually occurs after several weeks giving rise to paralysis and involvement of the phrenic nerve, which may lead to respiratory failure.[24]

STANDARD ANTIDOTES
Atropine

As noted elsewhere in this article, an OP-poisoned patient presents with a myriad of clinical features, predominantly muscarinic in nature. It follows logically that antimuscarinics, especially atropine, have been used for a long time and with relative success in the management of pesticide poisoning. Atropine is a competitive nonspecific antagonist with good central nervous system penetration (**Fig. 1**), and has been the antidote of choice for OP poisoning since the 1950s.[25,26]

Atropine is given intravenously until the features of cholinergic excess have reversed and cardiorespiratory function is restored, a state known as atropinization. The standard clinical parameters of atropinization are (a) clear lungs on auscultation, (b) a systolic blood pressure of greater than 80 mm Hg, (c) a heart rate of greater than 80 beats/min, (d) dry axillae, and (e) pupils no longer pinpoint.[27] At least 4 end points, including all of the first 3, should be achieved before a patient is considered atropinized. Some caveats must be kept in mind: pneumonia secondary to aspiration will persist despite adequate atropinization and OP may be splashed in the eyes, causing prolonged constriction of pupils. As such, pupillary dilatation cannot be used as a guide to atropinization. Doses required for atropinization also do not prevent central apnea or NMJ dysfunction. Therefore, severely intoxicated patients still require mechanical ventilation in many cases.[28]

Surprisingly, the appropriate dose and duration of atropine have been determined only recently. As many as 33 different recommendations were found in a systematic review of existing literature.[27] Many of these regimens gave a fixed dose of atropine at timed intervals without any dose titration to effect, resulting in significant delay in

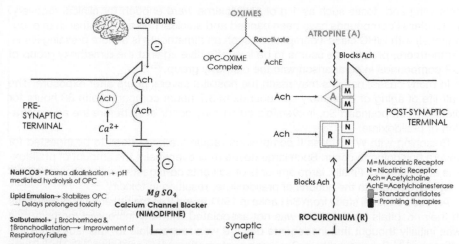

Fig. 1. Mechanism of action of standard and potential treatment options in acute OP and carbamate poisoning.

the time to reach atropinization (administering a dose of 23.4 mg took from 8 to 1380 minutes in various regimens).[27] Among these published regimens, incremental escalation of the dose of atropine[29] was prominent. In this type of regimen, atropine was started at 1 to 2 mg, and the dose was then doubled every 5 minutes. The dose necessary for atropinization was reached much more quickly (15–20 minutes to give a 23.4-mg dose), and atropine toxicity was also decreased. A randomized controlled trial (RCT) performed in Bangladesh compared this incremental dosage of atropine with conventional fixed dose atropine, with both regimens followed by a continuous infusion.[30] The results were quite significant. In comparison with patients on the conventional regimen, patients receiving the incremental dose regimen were atropinized much quicker (23.9 minutes vs 151.74 minutes), had decreased atropine toxicity (12.0% vs 28.4%), and required respiratory support less often (8.0% vs 24.7%). There was also significant decrease in mortality in the group receiving incremental dose regimens of atropine (8.0% vs 22.5%). Predictably, this incremental dose regimen is now recommended in most guidelines across the world.[31]

Once atropinized, patients receive an intravenous infusion at about 20% to 30% of the total dose needed for atropinization per hour. This dose is then titrated against effect and usually continued for 48 to 72 hours. The patient should be closely followed to assess for the development of atropine toxicity or reappearance of cholinergic toxicity (in which case repeat boluses of atropine may be needed), as well as the occurrence of intermediate syndrome needing ventilation.

Oximes

Along with atropine, pralidoxime is another drug that has been used in the management of OP poisoning. Pralidoxime (available as a chloride salt) is a drug that works by reactivating acetylcholinesterase in the cholinergic synapse, thereby enhancing breakdown of acetylcholine (see **Fig. 1**). In vitro studies in animals and humans show that pralidoxime does reactivate acetylcholinesterase.[32] Whether this reactivation translates into clinical efficacy, however, remains a matter of debate.

Oximes were first introduced against occupational poisoning with WHO class I diethoxy compounds.[33,34] In these cases, a small amount of ingestion led to severe poisoning and doses such as 1 g of pralidoxime were enough for clinical recovery. WHO class I compounds have been banned and suicidal poisoning (rather than occupational) with WHO class II compounds such as dimethoate is a more pressing issue. Furthermore, pralidoxime seems to be less effective against the dimethoxy group of OP compounds in comparison with the diethoxy group.[35,36]

In many cases, patients may reach the hospital several hours after exposure. The half-life of aging of dimethoxy compounds is 3.7 hours compared with 33 hours for diethoxy compounds.[6] So, irreversible aging may occur even before the administration of pralidoxime.

Poisoning with WHO class II compounds requires a large dose to be ingested for severe poisoning to occur. Such large doses may overwhelm the amount of pralidoxime administered. Finally, large amounts of solvents co-ingested with OP compounds may be resistant to the actions of pralidoxime, resulting in toxicity.

An observational study from Sri Lanka in 1991 found that the absence of pralidoxime in their hospitals for 6 months was not associated with any increased mortality.[37] It was initially thought that inadequate dosage was responsible for this lack of clinical efficacy.[38,39] Subsequently, a Cochrane systematic review analyzed 7 RCTs.[6] Three compared pralidoxime with placebo; the other 4 trials compared different doses. The single study that used the WHO recommended doses (30 mg/kg over 30 minutes followed by 8 mg/kg for 7 days) showed no clinical benefit of pralidoxime.[40] Most of the other studies that used pralidoxime in high doses (2 g followed by 0.5 g/h for 7 days) also failed to show any benefit. Thus, even when high doses were used, pralidoxime failed to show any benefit. Of note, an RCT of 200 patients performed in a private intensive care unit in India (pralidoxime 2 g loading dose followed by either 1 g/4 h for 2 days or 1 g/h for 2 days) showed decreased mortality.[41] In this RCT, patients presented early to the hospital, severely ill patients were excluded, and a majority were intubated at baseline. These factors need to be taken into account when interpreting the results.

It is possible that a certain subgroup of patients may benefit from pralidoxime, and larger studies are needed to identify this population. In the meantime, pralidoxime is widely given as a component of the standard treatment regimen along with atropine and other resuscitative measures.

Benzodiazepines

Benzodiazepines, such as diazepam and midazolam, are gamma amino butyric acid receptor agonists. They are used to treat seizures in the setting of OP poisoning. It is worth noting that seizures are relatively uncommon in OP pesticide self-ingestion (only 1%–3% cases).[7,17] They are more common in children[42,43] and in poisonings by OP nerve agents such as sarin. No animal or human clinical trial evidence exists that shows benzodiazepines to have any effect on mortality when used alone. Thus, they are not to be used routinely in the management of OP pesticide poisoning. Given intravenously, benzodiazepines are used to treat troublesome fasciculations occurring in OP poisoning and relief of agitation and anxiety, as well as the aforementioned management of seizures.[44]

PROMISING THERAPIES IN THE PIPELINE
Magnesium Sulfate and Calcium Channel Blockade

The role of presynaptic calcium channel blockade by calcium channel blockers (CCBs) and magnesium sulfate seems promising.[45,46] Calcium uptake via voltage-gated Ca^{++} channels in the presynaptic terminal causes release of acetylcholine in the synaptic cleft by exocytosis. Magnesium and CCBs decrease synaptic acetylcholine release by blocking these calcium channels (see **Fig. 1**). Rodent studies also suggest that CCBs reactivate OP inhibited Ca^{++} ATPase, reducing intracellular Ca^{++} concentrations and theoretically decreasing acetylcholine release.[47]

Preclinical studies of rodents suggested that, in addition to standard therapy, the administration of CCBs (nimodipine being used most commonly) and magnesium sulfate ($MgSO_4$) before or soon after OP exposure decrease mortality.[47] Small observational clinical studies and small case series have reported the use of these drugs in OP poisoning.[48–55] However, the effect of CCBs and $MgSO_4$ as an antidote to OP poisoning was not assessed, and neither were any data provided on mortality according to treatment. The drugs were used solely for the standard clinical uses of managing cardiac dysrhythmias and hypertonic uterine contractions ($MgSO_4$) occurring in OP poisoned patients.[48–55]

A total of 8 clinical studies or trials have now been performed with $MgSO_4$ (239 patients receiving $MgSO_4$ doses of up to 26 g/d and 202 control patients).[47] The dose most commonly used was 4 g, which is also the standard dose for treating cardiac dysrhythmias and needs no intensive monitoring of magnesium concentration. However, a small dose–response study suggested that doses of 4 g every 4 hours might offer greater benefit.[56] Importantly, a small phase II study performed in Bangladesh that tested 4 escalating (4, 8, 12, and 16 g) doses of $MgSO_4$ demonstrated good tolerance.[57] In only 1 study, 4 patients (11.1% of the sample) developed transient hypotension, which resolved after temporary discontinuation of the drug (Dawson and colleagues, unpublished, 2007).

Most studies showed decreases in mortality (pooled odds ratio, 0.55; 95% confidence interval [CI], 0.32–0.94) and/or need for intubation and ventilation (0.52; 95% CI, 0.34–0.79). However, all of these studies were small, had a marked risk of bias, and only $MgSO_4$ was used. Given the safety profile and encouraging findings, a large RCT might provide definitive evidence about its role in the management of OP poisoning.[47] To generate convincing evidence, a Medical Research Council –funded robust phase 3/4 RCT (NCT03925025) has been initiated in Bangladesh.

Plasma Alkalinization in Organophosphate Poisoning

The combination of hypoxia and hypotension often gives rise to acidosis, both metabolic and respiratory. Acidosis often resolves after standard therapy with fluid resuscitation, atropine, and oxygen supplementation. Nevertheless, many clinicians recommend the use of sodium bicarbonate for the alkalinization of plasma. Possible mechanisms by which plasma alkalinization may be beneficial are enhanced OP clearance through pH-mediated hydrolysis (see **Fig. 1**), a direct effect on the NMJ, or improved efficacy of oximes.[22,58]

To date, only 2 small RCT's have been conducted, one using high dose (5 mEq/kg over 1 hour, followed by 5–6 mEq/kg until recovery or death) and the other using low dose $NaHCO_3$.[58] Although the trial using low-dose $NaHCO_3$ showed no clinical benefit, the high-dose study showed promise in terms of decreasing the atropine requirement and the duration of hospital stay.[59] However, it was a small study involving only 26 patients. No large RCT has been performed. A systematic Cochrane review found insufficient evidence to support its routine clinical use.[58]

In Sri Lanka, district hospitals faced difficulties while attempting to study the use of $NaHCO_3$, which shows that this treatment is best considered in modern intensive care units, something that is not always available or affordable for the subset of population who ingest OP pesticides.[60]

Salbutamol (Albuterol)

There are β-2 adrenergic receptors present throughout the lungs, including the alveolar epithelium. These receptors, via cyclic adenosine monophosphate–dependent pathways, upregulate Na^+ transport across alveolar epithelium. This process helps in clearing excess fluid from the alveoli (see **Fig. 1**).[61] Key clinical features of OP poisoning are bronchorrhea and bronchoconstriction, often leading to respiratory failure and ultimately death. Although atropine is effective in decreasing bronchial secretion, it cannot clear the fluid that already accumulated in the alveolar cavity.[62] Keeping these processes in mind, it was hoped that salbutamol, a safe and effective β-2 agonist, would complement atropine by increasing the removal of fluid from the alveolar airspace and expedite the return of effective oxygen exchange.[62]

A single-blind phase II study explored whether the addition of nebulized salbutamol had any influence on oxygen saturation.[63] Salbutamol was compared against placebo in doses of 2.5 and 5.0 mg. Although it was a small pilot study and conducted in a resource-poor hospital, they found no evidence to support adding salbutamol to the standard treatment in OP poisoning. Larger phase III RCTs are needed to determine whether β-2 agonists have a role in OP pesticide poisoning management in the future.

Nicotinic Receptor Antagonism

Intermediate syndrome is a well-recognized complication of OP poisoning. It is thought that excess acetylcholine causes overstimulation of presynaptic and postsynaptic nicotinic receptors. This stimulation results in downregulation of nicotinic receptors and subsequent failure of neurotransmission (see **Fig. 1**).[18,64] Because atropine is an antimuscarinic drug, it plays no role in the treatment of intermediate syndrome. Mechanical ventilation remains the mainstay of therapy.

Rocuronium causes reversible, nondepolarizing blockade of nicotinic receptors in presynaptic and postsynaptic membranes of NMJs. As a result, there was hope that given early, rocuronium might prevent the development of intermediate syndrome. A pilot phase II trial was conducted in Sri Lanka comparing 3 groups of patients. Two groups received rocuronium bolus titrated to achieve greater than 95% (rocuronium >95) and 50% (rocuronium 50) inhibition of the NMJ, whereas the third group did not receive rocuronium. Unfortunately, the addition of rocuronium to standard therapy did not shorten the duration of intubation; instead, patients receiving rocuronium had significantly longer durations of intubation compared with controls (median duration for rocuronium >95 was 259 hours, for rocuronium 50 was 226.8 hours, and for controls was 88.5 hours).[65] Further studies are needed to determine whether nicotinic receptor antagonists have a role in the management of OP poisoning.

Clonidine

Clonidine is a centrally acting α-2 agonist that acts on the presynaptic membrane to reduce acetylcholine synthesis (see **Fig. 1**) and release in the synaptic membrane.[66] Owing to its excellent central nervous system penetration, this presynaptic effect is more prominent in the central nervous system compared with the peripheral system.[67] An open-label, multicenter phase II trial was conducted to evaluate the safety of clonidine in OP poisoning.[68] Three loading doses of clonidine (0.15, 0.30, and 0.45 mg) were given at sequential levels. All of the loading doses were followed by an infusion of 0.5 mg over 24 hours. At loading doses of 0.45 mg, 42% of patients (5/12) developed hypotension that was reversed with intravenous fluids. Another study from Egypt also reported that 43% of patients developed hypotension without adding any benefit over standard treatment.[69]

Lipid Emulsion

Lipid emulsion was first used to treat life-threatening toxicity with local anesthetics. Over time, it has also been used to manage poisoning by lipid-soluble agents, such as antidepressants and antipsychotics.[70] The exact mechanism of action is unclear. The most widely accepted hypothesis is the lipid sink phenomenon. Lipid emulsion creates an expanded intravascular lipid phase that causes lipophilic agents to be extracted from the target tissue and bind to the lipid, thereby reversing toxicity.[71] Because many OP compounds are highly lipid soluble and formulated in lipid solvents, lipid emulsion has been suggested as a treatment modality for OP poisoning.

A rodent study suggested a benefit of lipid emulsion in OP poisoning,[72] but no high-quality evidence exists showing benefit in humans. Rather, a study conducted by Wellen and colleagues suggested that high dose lipid emulsion may actually stabilize the OP compound from degradation.[73]

An open label pilot study of 40 patients reported no adverse effects of lipid emulsion when compared with controls. Although no difference in mortality was noted, there was a decreased duration of mechanical ventilation, hospital stay, and early resolution of hypernatremia.[74] Large RCTs are need to assess whether lipid emulsion will be clinically beneficial in management of OP poisoned patients.

SUMMARY

The fact that atropine is still the only effective treatment for OP poisoning after so many years indicates a failure of the medical community to properly deal with this prevalent problem. Larger trials are needed to evaluate whether treatments such as $MgSO_4$, nimodipine, sodium bicarbonate, and other novel therapies can complement atropine in the standard management. A total understanding of the pathophysiology of OP toxicity is still lacking. It is time that OP pesticide poisoning is given more attention, and funds are allocated to conduct high-quality trials.

CLINICS CARE POINTS

- Stomach wash is now prohibited and discouraged in acute pesticide poisoning. Gastric lavage can be given if the patient arrives within 1 hour of ingestion.

- Incremental dosage of atropine is more effective and safer than the conventional fixed dose regimen.

- There are 5 signs of atropinization: (1) clear lungs on auscultation, (2) systolic blood pressure of more than 80 mm Hg, (3) a heart rate of greater than 80 beats/min, (4) dry axillae, and (5) pupils no longer pinpoint.

- Dilated pupils are not a sign of atropinization; rather, they are a sign of atropine toxicity.

- There is no role of atropine in the treatment of intermediate syndrome and in organophosphate-induced delayed neuropathy. Mechanical ventilation remains the mainstay of treatment for intermediate syndrome.

- Oximes are less effective against the dimethoxy group of OP compound (parathion, paraoxon, quinalphos, etc), especially when patients comes late (after 4 hours) to the hospital.

- Critical fluid balance is important in overall management. Benzodiazepines (midazolam, diazepam) are effective in relief of agitation, anxiety, muscle fasciculation, and seizures in OP poisoning compared with haloperidol.
- Adjuvant therapies such as $MgSO_4$, lipid emulsion, and CCBs could help; however, their efficacy is yet to be established by larger trials.

REFERENCES

1. Mew EJ, Padmanathan P, Konradsen F, et al. The global burden of fatal self-poisoning with pesticides 2006;15: systematic review. J Affect Disord 2017; 219:93–104.
2. Knipe DW, Gunnell D, Eddleston M. Preventing deaths from pesticide self-poisoning-learning from Sri Lanka's success. Lancet Glob Heal 2017;5(7): e651–2.
3. Chowdhury FR, Dewan G, Verma VR, et al. Bans of WHO Class I pesticides in Bangladesh-suicide prevention without hampering agricultural output. Int J Epidemiol 2018;47(1):175–84.
4. Organization WH. The WHO Recommended Classification of Pesticides by Hazard and Guidelines to Classification: 2009. Vol 66.; 2010.
5. Li H, Schopfer LM, Nachon F, et al. Aging pathways for organophosphate-inhibited human butyrylcholinesterase, including novel pathways for isomalathion, resolved by mass spectrometry. Toxicol Sci 2007;100(1):136–45.
6. Eddleston M, Szinicz L, Eyer P, et al. Oximes in acute organophosphorus pesticide poisoning: a systematic review of clinical trials. QJM 2002;95(5): 275–83.
7. Eddleston M, Eyer P, Worek F, et al. Differences between organophosphorus insecticides in human self-poisoning: a prospective cohort study. Lancet 2005; 366(9495):1452–9.
8. Eddleston M, Mohamed F, Davies JOJ, et al. Respiratory failure in acute organophosphorus pesticide self-poisoning. QJM 2006;99(8):513–22.
9. Davies JE, Barquet A, Freed VH, et al. Human pesticide poisonings by a fat-soluble organophosphate insecticide. Arch Environ Health 1975;30(12): 608–13.
10. Casida JE, Sanderson DM. Toxic hazard from formulating the insecticide dimethoate in methyl "Cellosolve". Nature 1961;189:507–8.
11. Baker ELJ, Warren M, Zack M, et al. Epidemic malathion poisoning in Pakistan malaria workers. Lancet 1978;1(8054):31–4.
12. Soliman SA, Sovocool GW, Curley A, et al. Two acute human poisoning cases resulting from exposure to diazinon transformation products in Egypt. Arch Environ Health 1982;37(4):207–12.
13. Meleney WP, Peterson HO. The relationship of shelf age to toxicity of dimethoate to sheep. J Am Vet Med Assoc 1964;144:756–8.
14. Lokan R, James R. Rapid death by mevinphos poisoning while under observation. Forensic Sci Int 1983;22(2):179–82.
15. Erratum. Respiratory complications of organophosphorus nerve agent and insecticide poisoning. Implications for respiratory and Critical care. Am J Respir Crit Care Med 2019;200(7):946–8.
16. Davies J, Roberts D, Eyer P, et al. Hypotension in severe dimethoate self-poisoning. Clin Toxicol (Phila) 2008;46(9):880–4.

17. Wadia RS, Sadagopan C, Amin RB, et al. Neurological manifestations of organo-phosphorous insecticide poisoning. J Neurol Neurosurg Psychiatry 1974;37(7): 841–7.
18. Senanayake N, Karalliedde L. Neurotoxic effects of organophosphorus insecti-cides. An intermediate syndrome. N Engl J Med 1987;316(13):761–3.
19. De Bleecker J, Van den Neucker K, Colardyn F. Intermediate syndrome in organ-ophosphorus poisoning: a prospective study. Crit Care Med 1993;21(11): 1706–11.
20. Sidell FR, Takafuji ET, Franz DR. Medical aspects of chemical and biological war-fare. Falls Church (VA): Office of the Surgeon General (Army); 1997.
21. Eddleston M, Chowdhury FR. Organophosphorus poisoning: the wet opioid tox-idrome. Lancet 2021;397(10270):175–7.
22. Eddleston M, Chowdhury FR. Pharmacological treatment of organophosphorus insecticide poisoning: the old and the (possible) new. Br J Clin Pharmacol 2016;81(3):462–70.
23. Cha YS, Kim H, Go J, et al. Features of myocardial injury in severe organophos-phate poisoning. Clin Toxicol (Phila) 2014;52(8):873–9.
24. Rivett K, Potgieter PD. Diaphragmatic paralysis after organophosphate poisoning. A case report. S Afr Med J 1987;72(12):881–2.
25. Freeman G, Epstein MA. Therapeutic factors in survival after lethal cholines-terase inhibition by phosphorus insecticides. N Engl J Med 1955;253(7): 266–71.
26. DurhamWF, Hayes WJJ. Organic phosphorus poisoning and its therapy. With special reference to modes of action and compounds that reactivate inhibited cholinesterase. Arch Environ Health 1962;5:21–47.
27. Eddleston M, Buckley NA, Checketts H, et al. Speed of initial atropinisation in sig-nificant organophosphorus pesticide poisoning–a systematic comparison of rec-ommended regimens. J Toxicol Clin Toxicol 2004;42(6):865–75.
28. Eddleston M. Novel clinical toxicology and pharmacology of organophos-phorus insecticide self-poisoning. Annu Rev Pharmacol Toxicol 2019;59(1): 341–60.
29. Roberts DM, Aaron CK. Management of acute organophosphorus pesticide poisoning. BMJ 2007;334(7594):629–34.
30. Abedin MJ, Sayeed AA, Basher A, et al. Open-label randomized clinical trial of atropine bolus injection versus incremental boluses plus infusion for organophos-phate poisoning in Bangladesh. J Med Toxicol 2012;8(2):108–17.
31. Connors NJ, Harnett ZH, Hoffman RS. Comparison of current recommended reg-imens of atropinization in organophosphate poisoning. J Med Toxicol 2014;10(2): 143–7.
32. Eyer P. The role of oximes in the management of organophosphorus pesticide poisoning. Toxicol Rev 2003;22(3):165–90.
33. Namba T, Hiraki K. PAM (pyridine-2-aldoxime methiodide) therapy for alkyl-phosphate poisoning. J Am Med Assoc 1958;166(15):1834–9.
34. Namba T, Taniguchi Y, Okazaki S, et al. Treatment of severe organophosphorus poisoning by large doses of PAM. Naika No Ryoiki (Domain Intern Med 1959;7: 709–13.
35. Thiermann H, Szinicz L, Eyer F, et al. Modern strategies in therapy of organophos-phate poisoning. Toxicol Lett 1999;107(1–3):233–9.
36. Worek F, Bäcker M, Thiermann H, et al. Reappraisal of indications and limitations of oxime therapy in organophosphate poisoning. Hum Exp Toxicol 1997;16(8): 466–72.

37. de Silva HJ, Wijewickrema R, Senanayake N. Does pralidoxime affect outcome of management in acute organophosphorus poisoning? Lancet 1992;339(8802): 1136–8.

38. Johnson MK, Jacobsen D, Meredith TJ, et al. Evaluation of antidotes for poisoning by organophosphorus pesticides. Emerg Med 2000;12(1):22–37.

39. Johnson MK, Vale JA, Marrs TC, et al. Pralidoxime for organophosphorus poisoning. Lancet 1992;340(8810):64.

40. Syed S, Gurcoo S, Farooqui A, et al. Is the World Health Organization-recommended dose of pralidoxime effective in the treatment of organophosphorus poisoning? A randomized, double-blinded and placebo-controlled trial. Saudi J Anaesth 2015;9(1):49–54.

41. Pawar KS, Bhoite RR, Pillay CP, et al. Continuous pralidoxime infusion versus repeated bolus injection to treat organophosphorus pesticide poisoning: a randomised controlled trial. Lancet 2006;368(9553):2136–41.

42. Levy-Khademi F, Tenenbaum AN, Wexler ID, et al. Unintentional organophosphate intoxication in children. Pediatr Emerg Care 2007;23(10):716–8.

43. Panda M, Hutin YJ, Ramachandran V, et al. A fatal waterborne outbreak of pesticide poisoning caused by damaged pipelines, Sindhikela, Bolangir, Orissa, India, 2008. J Toxicol 2009;2009:692496.

44. Ford MD. Clinical toxicology. Philadelphia: WB Saunders Company; 2001.

45. Dretchen KL, Bowles AM, Raines A. Protection by phenytoin and calcium channel blocking agents against the toxicity of diisopropylfluorophosphate. Toxicol Appl Pharmacol 1986;83(3):584–9.

46. Petroianu G, Toomes LM, Petroianu A, et al. Control of blood pressure, heart rate and haematocrit during high-dose intravenous paraoxon exposure in mini pigs. J Appl Toxicol 1998;18(4):293–8.

47. Brvar M, Chan MY, Dawson AH, et al. Magnesium sulfate and calcium channel blocking drugs as antidotes for acute organophosphorus insecticide poisoning - a systematic review and meta-analysis. Clin Toxicol (Phila) 2018;56(8):725–36.

48. Fang JL, Shao QPQX. Application of calcium channel blocker in rescue of severe organophosphate pesticide poisoning. Chin Med Fact Mine 1997;3:201–2.

49. Tao XSZJ. The experience of using diltiazem hydrochloride for sinus tachycardia in nine cases of severe organophosphate pesticide poisoning. Fujian Med J 2010;32:138–9.

50. Zhu YCMX. Resuscitation experience of sudden cardiac arrest during recovery phase of acute organophosphate poisoning - a report of 7 cases. Chin J Indust Med 1990;4:28–9.

51. Zhang JY, Zhao JYZC. Clinical observation of diazepam and verapamil in preventing heart damage caused by acute organophosphate poisoning. Occup Heal Damage 2001;16:13–4.

52. Ru X. Study on the protective effect of verapamil on myocardial injury induced by organophosphate pesticide poisoning. Cent Plains Med J 2003;30:21–2.

53. Singh G, Avasthi G, Khurana D, et al. Neurophysiological monitoring of pharmacological manipulation in acute organophosphate (OP) poisoning. The effects of pralidoxime, magnesium sulphate and pancuronium. Electroencephalogr Clin Neurophysiol 1998;107(2):140–8.

54. Nel L, Hatherill M, Davies J, et al. Organophosphate poisoning complicated by a tachyarrhythmia and acute respiratory distress syndrome in a child. J Paediatr Child Health 2002;38(5):530–2.

55. Wang MH, Tseng CD, Bair SY. Q-T interval prolongation and pleomorphic ventricular tachyarrhythmia ('Torsade de pointes') in organophosphate poisoning: report of a case. Hum Exp Toxicol 1998;17(10):587–90.

56. Pajoumand A, Shadnia S, Rezaie A, et al. Benefits of magnesium sulfate in the management of acute human poisoning by organophosphorus insecticides. Hum Exp Toxicol 2004;23(12):565–9.

57. Basher A, Rahman SH, Ghose A, et al. Phase II study of magnesium sulfate in acute organophosphate pesticide poisoning. Clin Toxicol (Phila) 2013;51(1):35–40.

58. Roberts D, Buckley NA. Alkalinisation for organophosphorus pesticide poisoning. Cochrane Database Syst Rev 2005;1:CD004897.

59. Balali-Mood M, Ayati M-H, Ali-Akbarian H. Effect of high doses of sodium bicarbonate in acute organophosphorous pesticide poisoning. Clin Toxicol (Phila) 2005;43(6):571–4.

60. Roberts DM, Dawson AH, Hittarage A, et al. Letter to the editor: "Plasma alkalinization for acute organophosphorus poisoning - is it a reality in the developing world?" [1]. Clin Toxicol 2007;45(1):90–1 [author reply: 92–3].

61. Mutlu GM, Factor P. Alveolar epithelial beta2-adrenergic receptors. Am J Respir Cell Mol Biol 2008;38(2):127–34.

62. Moriña P, Herrera M, Venegas J, et al. Effects of nebulized salbutamol on respiratory mechanics in adult respiratory distress syndrome. Intensive Care Med 1997;23(1):58–64.

63. Chowdhury FR, Rahman MM, Ullah P, et al. Salbutamol in acute organophosphorus insecticide poisoning - a pilot dose-response phase II study. Clin Toxicol (Phila) 2018;56(9):820–7.

64. De Bleecker JL. The intermediate syndrome in organophosphate poisoning: an overview of experimental and clinical observations. J Toxicol Clin Toxicol 1995;33(6):683–6.

65. Dhanarisi J, Shihana F, Harju K, et al. A pilot clinical study of the neuromuscular blocker rocuronium to reduce the duration of ventilation after organophosphorus insecticide poisoning. Clin Toxicol (Phila) 2020;58(4):254–61.

66. Wu-Fu L. A symptomatological assessment of organophosphate-induced lethality in mice: comparison of atropine and clonidine protection. Toxicol Lett 1991;56(1):19–32.

67. Buccafusco JJ, Graham JH, Vanlingen J, et al. Protection afforded by clonidine from the acute and chronic behavioral toxicity produced by the cholinesterase inhibitor soman. Neurotoxicol Teratol 1989;11(1):39–44.

68. Perera PMS, Jayamanna SF, Hettiarachchi R, et al. A phase II clinical trial to assess the safety of clonidine in acute organophosphorus pesticide poisoning. Trials 2009;10(1):73.

69. El-Ebiary AA, Gad SA, Wahdan AA, et al. Clonidine as an adjuvant in the management of acute poisoning by anticholinesterase pesticides. Hum Exp Toxicol 2016;35(4):371–6.

70. Jamaty C, Bailey B, Larocque A, et al. Lipid emulsions in the treatment of acute poisoning: a systematic review of human and animal studies. Clin Toxicol (Phila) 2010;48(1):1–27.

71. Zhou Y, Zhan C, Li Y, et al. Intravenous lipid emulsions combine extracorporeal blood purification: a novel therapeutic strategy for severe organophosphate poisoning. Med Hypotheses 2010;74(2):309–11.

72. Dunn C, Bird SB, Gaspari R. Intralipid fat emulsion decreases respiratory failure in a rat model of parathion exposure. Acad Emerg Med 2012;19(5):504–9.

73. Bhalla A, Chhabria B, Shafiq N, Kumar S SN. Role of lipid emulsion in management of organophosphate compound poisoning. In: 14th Annual Meeting of the American College of Medical Toxicology (ACMT). San Juan, Puerto Rico, March 31-April 2, 2017.

74. Von Der Wellen J, Worek F, Thiermann H, et al. Investigations of kinetic interactions between lipid emulsions, hydroxyethyl starch or dextran and organophosphorus compounds. Clin Toxicol (Phila) 2013;51(10):918–22.

Inhalants

Evan S. Schwarz, MD

KEYWORDS

- Irritants • Asphyxiants • Toxicants • Inhalation • Vaping
- Electronic cigarette or vaping use-associated lung injury

KEY POINTS

- Irritants are classified according to their water solubility. High water solubility agents tend to cause upper respiratory tract injuries, while low water solubility agents cause lower tract injuries.
- Simple asphyxiants displace oxygen, while chemical asphyxiants interfere with cellular respiration. Cyanide and hydrogen sulfide are classic chemical asphyxiants. Hydroxocobalamin is the preferred treatment for cyanide intoxication.
- Electronic cigarette or vaping use-associated lung injury is associated with vaping cannabis products. Patients present with predominately respiratory symptoms. Steroids may be beneficial.

INTRODUCTION

Inhalants include a broad range of xenobiotics that differ in structure, clinical effects, and treatments. Exposures can be accidental or intentional and occur at work, at home, during terroristic events, or when using a substance in a harmful or hazardous way. Although this article will focus on pulmonary irritants, pulmonary asphyxiants, and inhaled intoxicants, there are many other toxic inhalants.

Work is a common source of exposure to inhalational toxicants. Metal fume fever develops in workers exposed to metals such as zinc oxide and cadmium. Workers develop fever, shortness of breath, myalgias, and headaches. Cadmium fumes are particularly worrisome, as workers also develop noncardiogenic pulmonary edema. Exterminators are exposed to multiple inhalants. Organophosphates cause a cholinergic, specifically a muscarinic, toxidrome, which includes bronchorrhea, bradycardia, bronchospasm, emesis and diarrhea, and seizures (see Sakib Aman and colleagues' article, "Management of Organophosphorus Poisoning: Standard Treatment and Beyond," in this issue). Pyrethrins, although generally safe, do cause allergic reactions and central nervous system (CNS) depression in high doses. Inorganic hydrides such

Washington University School of Medicine, 660 South Euclid, Campus Box 8072, St Louis, MO 63110, USA
E-mail address: schwarze@wustl.edu
Twitter: @TheSchwarziee (E.S.S.)

Crit Care Clin 37 (2021) 687–702
https://doi.org/10.1016/j.ccc.2021.03.014
0749-0704/21/© 2021 Elsevier Inc. All rights reserved.

criticalcare.theclinics.com

as arsine and phosphine used in industry have unique toxicities including hemolysis and inhibition of oxidative phosphorylation, respectively.

PULMONARY IRRITANTS

Irritants are a common class of toxic inhalants (**Table 1**). Water solubility is the primary characteristic that predicts their pattern of injury. Highly water-soluble or hydrophilic agents dissolve in the mucosal secretions of the eyes, nose, and upper airways. Noxious symptoms develop nearly instantaneously leading victims to rapidly escape, thus minimizing injuries. Victims who cannot escape develop more severe toxicity, including lower respiratory tract injury. Poorly water-soluble irritants tend not to significantly injure the upper airway, so people do not experience immediate symptoms, remain in contaminated areas longer, and sustain more severe injuries. Prolonged or large exposures may damage the entire respiratory tract. Additional injury occurs from the inflammatory response generated by cytokines and other inflammatory mediators. Irritants can also act like asphyxiants in very large exposures by displacing oxygen.

Signs and symptoms of exposure to highly water-soluble agents include coughing, sore throat, rhinorrhea, lacrimation, ocular irritation, and wheezing. Hypoxia, rales, tracheobronchitis, bronchospasm, pneumonitis, and acute respiratory distress syndrome (ARDS) develop after exposure to poorly water-soluble irritants or very large or prolonged exposures to highly water-soluble irritants. Patients rarely develop burns involving the skin or eyes.

General Care

Care should initially focus on airway support and breathing as most victims will only develop inhalational injuries. Airway hyperreactivity is treated with bronchodilators. If intubation is necessary following exposure to highly water-soluble agents, a larger endotracheal tube is recommended to avoid obstruction from mucosal sloughing and facilitate bronchoscopy if needed.[1]

Ocular irritation is treated with copious irrigation and continued until the pH of the corneal surface is neutral (7.4).[2] Relying solely on symptomatology is problematic, as irrigation causes additional irritation. Cycloplegics decrease pain and prevent morbidity from synechia.[3] Formal ophthalmology consultation is warranted for severe injuries.[1] Prolonged or severe dermal exposures may result in significant burns. Patients should undergo decontamination, which includes removal of clothing and copious irrigation with water.

Table 1 Irritants		
High Water Solubility	**Medium Water Solubility**	**Low Water Solubility**
Ammonia	Chlorine	Phosgene
Chloramine	Hydrogen sulfide	Nitrogen oxides
Formaldehyde		Ozone
Hydrogen chloride		
Hydrogen fluoride		
Riot control agents		
Sulfur dioxide		

Corticosteroids

The use of corticosteroids is controversial. Trials investigating the utility of corticosteroids in ARDS rarely included patients exposed to pulmonary irritants. Thus, recommendations generally rely on expert opinion.

A meta-analysis that included 9 randomized trials demonstrated a reduction in time to extubation and duration of hospitalization in patients with ARDS who received glucocorticoids.[4] Patients with ARDS from all causes were included. The DEXA-ARDS trial concluded that early dexamethasone reduced the duration of mechanical ventilation and overall mortality in patients with ARDS.[5] However, the etiology of ARDS was nontoxicologic in 98% of patients.

Two sisters were treated in the emergency department following an exposure to chlorine.[6] One was admitted and received corticosteroids for 4 days, while the other did not receive corticosteroids. One year later, the sister who received steroids had a normal forced expiratory volume in 1 second (FEV_1), while the other sister's FEV_1 was only 80% to 85% of predicted value. Other authors discussed the utility of corticosteroids in toxic inhalant-induced ARDS,[1,7–11] with 1 review discouraging their use due to concerns of unspecified adverse events.[1]

High Water Solubility Agents

Ammonia

Anhydrous ammonia (ammonia [NH_3]) is the third most abundantly produced chemical in the world. It is a colorless gas with an extremely pungent odor that is detected when the concentration is at least 5 ppm.[12] Ammonia has many uses including in the production of paper, plastics, and dyes; in the petroleum industry; and as an intermediate in the illicit production of methamphetamine.[1,9,13]

Following an exposure, irritant symptoms begin almost immediately. The odor threshold of approximately 5 to 50 ppm is well below the irritant threshold of 400 ppm, allowing victims to escape before developing significant toxicity.[14] When ammonia contacts mucous membranes, it combines with water to form ammonium hydroxide (NH_4OH), a strong base. Ammonium hydroxide further dissociates into hydroxyl ions, causing tissue damage and liquefactive necrosis. Collectively, this causes edema, hemorrhage, smooth muscle contraction, and formation of cellular debris that results in airway obstruction. Injuries occur initially to the eyes, oropharynx, and upper respiratory tract. Patients may develop conjunctivitis, ulceration, iritis, cataracts, blepharospasm, and glaucoma as a direct effect from ammonia or its sequelae.

Hydrogen fluoride

Hydrogen fluoride dissolves in the mucosa to form the weak acid, hydrofluoric acid (HF). Victims experience typical signs and symptoms of respiratory irritants.[15] Patients also develop life-threatening hypocalcemia and hyperkalemia similar to exposures to HF from other routes (eg, dermal or oral).[16] Nebulized and intravenous calcium should be administered.[16,17] Extracorporeal membrane oxygenation (ECMO) was successfully used in 2 patients.[16,18]

Intermediate Water Solubility Agents

Chlorine

Chlorine is a pungent, green-yellow gas. When bleach containing hypochlorite is mixed with an acid, chlorine gas is formed. Outside of the home, chlorine is used in water purification, textile and paper bleaching, and manufacturing.[11]

Chlorine damages the respiratory tract at all levels. When it combines with water on mucous membranes, hypochlorous and hydrochloric acids are formed. Animal models demonstrate increased pulmonary microvascular permeability.[19] This permeability results in edema and hemorrhage of the respiratory tract, bronchiolar mucosal destruction, and alveoli filled with exudates. Clinically, patients develop cough, chest pain, dyspnea, sore throat, bronchospasm, ocular irritation, rales, tachypnea, and hypoxia.

Treatment is supportive. Nebulized sodium bicarbonate (NSB) may be administered to neutralize the hydrochloric acid. Although controversial, NSB is unlikely be harmful.[20] Case reports describe rapid improvement following a single treatment.[7,8] In a retrospective review from poison centers, no adverse events were reported in 86 patients.[21] Only 17 patients required admission, with a mean hospital length of stay of 1.4 days. Although the number of NSB treatments and other adjunctive treatments varied, the authors concluded that NSB was beneficial. A double-blind pseudorandomized study of emergency department patients exposed to chlorine gas concluded that NSB was beneficial, as administration was associated with higher FEV_1 values.[22]

Low water solubility agents

Irritants that are poorly water soluble cause injuries to the lower respiratory tract. Because these agents are less reactive with water, victims may not experience the sudden and unpleasant symptoms to the same degree as with highly soluble agents. Gas penetrates deeper in the bronchopulmonary system and results in lower respiratory tract injury and potentially delayed toxicity. Lower respiratory tract injuries include tracheobronchitis, bronchiolitis, and ARDS.

Phosgene

Phosgene ($COCl_2$ or carbonyl chloride) is a colorless gas with an odor described as being similar to freshly mown hay and has a low odor threshold, 0.4 to 1.5 ppm.[23] Phosgene's minor, acute irritant effects, combined with these other factors lead to prolonged exposures. It is used in the synthesis of plastics and industrial materials and forms when chlorofluorocarbons are accidently heated.

Phosgene forms hydrochloric acid (HCl) upon reacting with mucous membranes.[24] Phosgene denatures proteins and irreversibly disrupts cellular membranes while depleting glutathione and other endogenous antioxidants.[23,25] The resultant effect is pulmonary edema, hypoxia, and ARDS.[26]

Initially, patients experience minor upper respiratory tract irritation. Although victims may improve clinically, in actuality, they enter a latent phase with ongoing injury.[23] The duration of the latent phase can last hours and is inversely proportional to the inhaled dose.[23] In time, patients may develop pulmonary edema and ARDS, so prolonged observation is warranted. In general, patients without signs or symptoms of respiratory illness and a clear chest radiograph may be discharged after 8 hours of observation.[23] Lung-protective ventilation strategies are recommended for patients requiring intubation.[26]

Other suggested treatment strategies aim to reduce the inflammation produced by phosgene.[26] N-acetylcysteine (NAC), leukotriene receptor inhibitors, aminophylline, isoproterenol, ibuprofen, colchicine, cyclophosphamide, and corticosteroids were tested in animal studies.[27–33] Case reports anecdotally demonstrate improvement following treatment with nebulized NAC in people.[34] One recommendation is to nebulize 1 to 10 mL of 20% NAC with administration every 2 to 6 hours. Intravenous methylprednisolone did not improve mortality in a porcine model.[31] Although dietary supplements have been studied in animals, data do not support their use in people.[35]

Nitrogen oxides

Nitrogen oxides (NO_x) are a series of oxidized compounds, including NO_2 and NO.[36] NO_2 is generated during welding and by propane-driven ice resurfacing vehicles.[37] Silo filler disease is the result of NO_2 formed during decomposition in improperly vented silos. Cases of delayed toxicity are reported hours to weeks after even brief exposures.[38,39]

NO_x directly injure respiratory mucosa, form free radicals,[16] and generate nitric acid (HNO_3).[37] Patients may have minimal upper respiratory tract irritation before developing lower respiratory symptoms up to 12 hours later.[16] The initial phase of the injury and recovery is potentially followed by a more severe injury, including bronchiolitis obliterans, weeks later.[40] Patients may also develop methemoglobinemia.[36] Treatment is supportive, with the use of corticosteroids remaining controversial.[37] Nebulized or intravenous NAC may inhibit damage from free radicals.[16,41]

ASPHYXIANTS

Asphyxiants are divided into simple and chemical asphyxiants (**Table 2**). Simple asphyxiants displace oxygen causing hypoxia and do not have other physiologic effects. Common simple asphyxiants include methane, propane, hydrogen, and helium. Carbon dioxide and nitrogen are generally categorized as simple asphyxiants even though they cause vasoconstriction and encephalopathy, respectively.

Chemical asphyxiants displace oxygen but also disrupt the body's ability to use oxygen and undergo aerobic metabolism. Chemical asphyxiants include carbon monoxide (CO), cyanide (CN), and hydrogen sulfide (H_2S). CO is further discussed in James Chenoweth and colleagues' article, "Carbon Monoxide Poisoning," elsewhere in this issue.

Cyanide

Cyanide is an incredibly rapid and lethal poison that gained infamy from use in mass murders by the Nazis and Jim Jones in the 1970s.[42] Although there are multiple other sources of exposure (**Table 3**), smoke inhalation is the most common source in the United States and Western countries.[43] Hydrogen cyanide forms following the combustion of carbon- and nitrogen-based materials including plastics, synthetic fibers, and polymers.[44] Cyanide should also be suspected in laboratory or industrial workers who suddenly collapse, have an unexplained coma, or present with severe metabolic acidosis.[42,45] Up to 50% of the population cannot appreciate its bitter almond odor.[43]

Mechanism of Action

Cyanide binds the ferric iron portion of cytochrome oxidase, inhibiting cytochrome a_3 and poisoning the electron transport chain.[42] Organ systems such as the heart and CNS are most susceptible given their high demands for oxygen. Cyanide also effects

Table 2 Asphyxiants	
Simple	**Chemical**
Carbon dioxide	Carbon monoxide
Hydrocarbons	Cyanide
Nitrogen gas	Hydrogen sulfide
Noble gases	

Table 3 Sources of cyanide	
Sources of Cyanide	Professions Where Exposures May Occur
Acetonitrile	Electroplating
Acrylonitrile	Fumigation
Amygdalin	Jeweler
Cassava (Manihut esculenta)	Laboratory worker
Fruits (Prunus species)	Manufacturing (textiles, plastics)
Laetrile	Metallurgy
Nitroprusside	Photography
Smoke inhalation	

the GABAergic and glutamatergic pathways.[46] Onset of symptoms following a gaseous exposure occurs in seconds, but is delayed following exposure to liquids or solids, up to hours if requiring metabolism or degradation to form cyanide such as with nitriles and nitroprusside.

Signs and Symptoms

Initially, patients experience transient bradycardia and hypertension followed by tachycardia and hypotension before cardiac arrest.[42] Early on, patients are tachypneic and hyperpneic; later symptoms are respiratory depression and apnea without cyanosis. Neurologic symptoms include syncope, headaches, altered mental status, encephalopathy, and seizures.[42] Cherry-red complexion and bright red retinal veins are late findings.

Diagnosis

Severe metabolic acidosis with an elevated lactate concentration is the hallmark of cyanide poisoning.[43] Concentrations greater than 10 mmol/L suggest cyanide poisoning in fire victims independent of co-occurring CO toxicity.[47] The oxygen content of venous blood is abnormally high because of inhibition of aerobic metabolism, leading to the arterialization of venous blood.[43] The arteriovenous oxygen saturation difference reflected by arterial and venous blood gasses obtained simultaneously may be less than 10 mm Hg. Cyanide concentrations are not useful in the acute management.[42]

Treatment

Hydroxocobalamin is the preferred treatment, and it binds cyanide to form cyanocobalamin, which is renally excreted.[48] It temporarily causes an erythroderma-like appearance that interferes with the co-oximeter and colorimetric laboratory tests.[49,50] It also causes hypertension, which is likely beneficial.[49] The dose is 70 mg/kg intravenously up to 5 g. Sodium thiosulfate and hydroxocobalamin may be administered together.[49]

An older cyanide antidote kit contains amyl nitrite, sodium nitrite, and sodium thiosulfate. The nitrites induce methemoglobinemia, with cyanide preferentially binding to methemoglobin, forming cyanomethemoglobin.[48–51] Amyl nitrite ampules are inhaled if intravenous access is not available. Sodium nitrite 300 mg is administered intravenously to induce a methemoglobin concentration of 20% to 30%. Dose adjustment is required in children and patients with anemia. Nitrites cause additional hypotension in patients who are already hemodynamically unstable.[49] Additionally, fire victims may have a significant carboxyhemoglobinemia, further complicating the induction of methemoglobin. Sodium thiosulfate acts as a substrate to convert cyanide to thiocyanate but has a delayed onset of action.[48] Adult dosing is 12.5 g administered intravenously over 30 minutes. Thiocyanate can accumulate in patients with renal failure, causing neurotoxicity.[52]

Hydrogen Sulfide

Hydrogen sulfide (H_2S) acts as a chemical asphyxiant by inhibiting the electron transport chain, and itis also an irritant.[53] It is a colorless gas with a rotten egg odor. It is a byproduct produced by the decay of organic material.[53,54] Around 2007, H_2S was produced in a series of detergent suicides.[55]

H_2S has an odor threshold of 3 to 30 ppm, with olfactory paralysis (inability to smell) occurring at 100 to 150 ppm.[56–58] Patients present with headache, cough, dyspnea, bronchitis, pulmonary edema, syncope, nausea and vomiting, cardiac dysrhythmias, myocardial infarction, and seizures.[59] Keratoconjunctivitis, or gas eye, also occurs.[57] Similar to cyanide, it is considered a knock down gas, and patients may present with sudden collapse and death.[53] No specific diagnostic laboratory tests are available.

Treatment with nitrites (3% sodium nitrite) is proposed, as methemoglobin has a high affinity for hydrogen sulfide, allowing resumption of aerobic metabolism.[54,59,60] There may be benefit if used early following the exposure.[60,61] Case reports discuss the use of hyperbaric oxygen,[59,62] but further research is necessary.[60]

INTOXICANTS

Many xenobiotics used as inhalants to become high are hydrocarbons. They can be straight or branched chains, aliphatic, or aromatic.[63] The exact mechanism behind their effects on the CNS remains unknown.[63] Substituted hydrocarbons containing halogen groups can produce sudden cardiac death. Some hydrocarbons are nephrotoxic or hepatotoxic.[64,65] All inhalants can cause anoxic injuries by displacing oxygen, while some have unique toxicities (**Table 4**).

Acute cardiotoxicity from inhalants is referred to as sudden sniffing death, cardiac sensitization syndrome, and sudden cardiac death syndrome. Halogenated or aromatic hydrocarbons are most likely to produce dysrhythmias by sensitizing the myocardium to catecholamines.[63] The syndrome may also be caused by blocking the potassium current (I_{KR}), thereby prolonging repolarization; other ion channels are also implicated.[63,66]

Pulseless ventricular tachycardia and ventricular fibrillation are treated with basic advanced cardiac life support (ACLS) principles including defibrillation. However, instead of epinephrine, patients should receive ß-adrenergic antagonists including propranolol or esmolol.[67,68] Perfusing tachyarrhythmias should also be treated with ß-adrenergic antagonists.

Volatile Hydrocarbons

Volatile hydrocarbons are organic compounds comprised of carbon and hydrogen atoms.[63] Gasoline, methane, propane, and butane are all examples. Many hydrocarbon-containing products are mixtures of multiple hydrocarbons. Their lipophilicity is generally proportional to their intoxicating effects, with the acute presentation varying depending on the specific inhalant.[63] Dusting refers to inhaling halogenated hydrocarbons from compressed air cleaners (**Table 5**). Patients can rapidly develop ventricular dysrhythmias. This diagnosis should be considered in a young person who suddenly collapses in an electronics store.

Table 4
Inhalants

Inhalant	Chemical	Specific Considerations
Carburetor cleaner	Methanol	May not cause the same toxicity as ingested methanol
Dry cleaning agents	Tetrachlorethylene, trichloroethylene	Hepatotoxicity, nephrotoxicity, neuropathy
Dusters	Difluorethane, tetrafluorethane, chlorinated hydrocarbons	Cardiac sensitization syndrome
Gasoline, air fresheners	Aliphatic and aromatic hydrocarbons (eg, butane, ethane)	Lung injury if aspirated, gastritis
Glue, Adhesives, Spray paint	Toluene	Severe hypokalemia, leukoencephalopathy
Paint thinner	Methylene chloride	Delayed carbon monoxide toxicity
Poppers	Amyl nitrite	Methemoglobinemia
Salvia diviner leaves	Salvadoran A	Hallucinations
Degreaser/solvent	Trichloroethylene	Neuropathy, degreasers flush, disulfiram reaction
Whipped cream dispensers (whippets)	Nitrous oxide	Myeloneuropathy of the dorsal columns of the spinal cord similar to vitamin B12 deficiency
Solvent	Xylene	Ototoxicity

Patients develop a defatting syndrome in areas where the hydrocarbon contacts the skin.[69] The rash appears as an erythematous dermatitis. Hydrocarbons are sensitizers and may cause eczema or glue sniffer's rash.[70] If they are aspirated, hydrocarbons cause a direct pulmonary injury leading to ARDS. Cardiomyopathy is also reported.[71]

Freon is a brand name referring to specific fluorinated hydrocarbons, although it commonly refers to any fluorocarbon refrigerant.[72] Toxicity consists of CNS depression, headache, syncope, and respiratory depression along with cardiotoxicity.[72,73]

Xylene (dimethyl benzene) is an aromatic hydrocarbon with a sweet odor.[74] Methyl hippuric acid is a metabolite found in the urine.[75] Patients develop respiratory tract irritation, CNS depression, vomiting, and hematuria.[76] Confusion and slurred speech occur at concentrations greater than 800 ppm with syncope and death at concentrations greater than 10,000 ppm.[74] It is also ototoxic.[77]

Toluene

Toluene is an aromatic hydrocarbon found in paints, glues, cleaning products, and other solvents. It is metabolized into benzoic acid and hippuric acid, with the latter being useful to diagnose an exposure.[78] Chronic exposure results in a permanent

Table 5
Types of hydrocarbon inhalation

Bagging	Placed into a bag for rebreathing
Dusting	Inhaling compressed air cleaners
Huffing	Poured onto material and placed over the mouth or nose
Sniffing	Sniffed directly from the container

leukoencephalopathy. MRI demonstrates atrophy of the cerebrum, cerebellum, and brainstem, and white matter changes.[79,80]

Acute intoxication results in altered mental status, nausea, and vomiting.[65] Patients develop weakness and dysrhythmias caused by profound hypokalemia from a distal renal tubular acidosis-like syndrome.[63,64,81] Patients develop a nonanion gap hyperchloremic metabolic acidosis and an anion gap metabolic acidosis. In 22 patients presenting to an emergency department with toluene intoxication, mean serum bicarbonate was 10 mmol/L with a blood pH of 7.15 and a mean potassium of 1.87 mmol/L.[81] All patients received parenteral potassium doses between 400 and 800 mEq/d. Toluene is also a known hepatotoxin.[65]

Nitrous Oxide

Nitrous oxide (N_2O) is commonly used as an anesthetic. Whippits is a common slang term for N_2O, as whipped cream canisters contain nitrous oxide as a propellant, which can be inhaled.[82]

N_2O causes nausea, vomiting, intoxication, irritant effects, and death from asphyxiation.[83] Bone marrow function can be impaired.[84] Chronic use causes irreversible oxidation of the cobalt ion of cyanocobalamin (vitamin B_{12}).[85] This prevents formation of methylcobalamin and formation of succinyl coenzyme A, resulting in the development of a myeloneuropathy resembling the subacute combined degeneration seen with B_{12} deficiency. Patients develop numbness; tingling; diminished pinprick, light touch, and vibratory sensation; proprioception and gait disturbances; and weakness and paralysis.[82,85] Vitamin B_{12} concentrations are normal or low, and methylmalonic acid and homocysteine concentrations may be elevated.[82,85] Supplementation with Vitamin B_{12} may be beneficial.[85,86]

ELECTRONIC CIGARETTE OR VAPING USE-ASSOCIATED LUNG INJURY

Electronic cigarettes are battery operated devices that allow the user to inhale a superheated complex of semiliquid particulates.[87] While initially marketed as a safer alternative to traditional cigarettes, this claim is dubious with little actual support.[88] Newer-generation devices allow the user to customize them, for instance adding nonstandard e-liquids, and increasing the amount of nicotine delivered.[87]

In addition to nicotine, e-liquids contain a variety of chemicals including humectants and flavoring agents. Propylene glycol and glycerin or vegetable glycerin are common humectants in e-liquids.[87] Although regarded as "generally recognized as safe," this designation does not apply when they are inhaled, which is associated with toxicity.[89,90] Additionally, other known harmful chemicals such as diacetyl, the compound responsible for popcorn worker's lung, are found in e-liquids.[91] Vitamin E acetate (VEA) was detected in all 29 samples of bronchoalveolar lavage (BAL) in 1 convenience sample of patients with electronic cigarette or vaping use-associated lung injury (EVALI), so this may be the cause of EVALI.[92] VEA was also found in multiple cannabis-containing products.[93–95] In vape cartridges, VEA serves to dilute the tetrahydrocannabinol (THC) without affecting the fluid's viscosity so that the bubble test (ability of trapped air bubbles to move in less viscous fluid) is comparable to unadulterated fluid.[87]

Although cases of lung injury date back to 2006 in North America, the association was not well recognized until July 2019.[91,96] Case definitions were generated to improve surveillance (**Box 1**). Patients presented with a combination of respiratory, gastrointestinal (GI), and constitutional symptoms with a median duration of symptoms until presentation of 6 days (range 0–155 days). Ninety-seven percent presented

> **Box 1**
> **Case definition for E-cigarette, or vaping, product use-associated lung injury**
>
> Use of an e-cigarette or dabbing in 90 d prior to symptoms
>
> Pulmonary infiltrate including opacity on plain film and ground glass opacity on chest computed tomography
>
> Absence of pulmonary infection on work-up
>
> Probable case: either there is an infection or one has not been completely ruled out, but the clinical team does not believe that the infection is solely responsible for the respiratory illness

with respiratory symptoms, with nearly two-thirds reporting nausea and vomiting and all but five requiring hospitalization. Of those with complete data, 88% used e-cigarettes daily, while 73% reported vaping nicotine products and 89% THC-containing products. As of February 18, 2020, 2807 patients were hospitalized with EVALI, with approximately 80% of patients reporting vaping THC-containing liquids.[97,98] In 1 survey of people who vaped THC e-liquid, 501 respondents reported using 732 different THC-containing products.[99] Nicotine-containing vape fluid is not reported to contain VEA, so it is not clear why patients who deny vaping THC developed EVALI, although under-reporting and recall errors are possible.

Patients present with a combination of respiratory, GI, and constitutional symptoms.[87,96,100] Data from the Centers for Disease Control and Prevention suggest that patients with fatal cases were more likely to be older and have pre-existing respiratory and cardiac disease compared with nonfatal cases.[101] No specific diagnostic test is recommended, with the diagnosis being one of exclusion. Nearly all patients will have infiltrates or opacities on chest imaging. Current recommendations include respiratory panels to exclude viral and fungal or other opportunistic or atypical infections.[102] If BAL is obtained, the fluid may have a neutrophilic or macrophage predominance.[103] Lipid-laden macrophages detected with oil-red-O staining are reported.[103] Care is supportive. Some evidence suggests corticosteroids are beneficial, although the optimal dosing is unknown.[87,96,100] Use of veno-venous extracorporeal membrane oxygenation has been reported, and a 17 year old received a double lung transplant.[87,96]

CLINICS CARE POINTS

- Highly water soluble agents generally injure the upper respiratory tract and respond to general supportive care.

- Nebulized sodium bicarbonate is a therapeutic option in patients with pulmonary injury from chlorine gas.

- Patients with injuries from inhaled hydrofluoric acid are at the same risk of electrolyte abnormality and sudden death as patients exposed via other routes. Aggressive care with calcium is recommended.

- Inhalation of hydrocarbons in an attempt to get high can result in sudden cardiac death. The use of beta adrenergic antagonists, and not epinephrine, is recommended in addition to standard ACLS.

- Cyanide toxicity should be considered in victims of fires with lactate concentrations greater than 10 mmol/L.

- Toluene can cause neurologic symptoms similar to those of B-12 deficiency; however, it is not clear that supplementation with vitamin B-12 is beneficial.

- In the treatment of cyanide intoxication, hydroxocobalamin is the preferred treatment, as nitrites cause other complications including hypotension and methemoglobinemia, and sodium thiosulfate acts in a delayed fashion.
- EVALI is associated with the use of vape or e-liquid fluid that contains VEA. Steroids may be beneficial once infectious etiologies have been excluded.

DISCLOSURE

The author has nothing to disclose.

REFERENCES

1. White CE, Park MS, Renz EM, et al. Burn center treatment of patients with severe anhydrous ammonia injury: case reports and literature review. J Burn Care Res 2007;28(6):922–8.
2. Welch A. Exposing the dangers of anhydrous ammonia. Nurse Pract 2006; 31(11):40–5.
3. Amshel CE, Fealk MH, Phillips BJ, et al. Anhydrous ammonia burns case report and review of the literature. Burns J Int Soc Burn Inj 2000;26(5):493–7.
4. Meduri GU, Siemieniuk RAC, Ness RA, et al. Prolonged low-dose methylpred-nisolone treatment is highly effective in reducing duration of mechanical ventilation and mortality in patients with ARDS. J Intensive Care 2018;6:53.
5. Villar J, Ferrando C, Martínez D, et al. Dexamethasone treatment for the acute respiratory distress syndrome: a multicentre, randomised controlled trial. Lancet Respir Med 2020;8(3):267–76.
6. Chester EH, Kaimal J, Payne CB, et al. Pulmonary injury following exposure to chlorine gas. Possible beneficial effects of steroid treatment. Chest 1977; 72(2):247–50.
7. Douidar SM. Nebulized sodium bicarbonate in acute chlorine inhalation. Pediatr Emerg Care 1997;13(6):406–7.
8. Vinsel PJ. Treatment of acute chlorine gas inhalation with nebulized sodium bicarbonate. J Emerg Med 1990;8(3):327–9.
9. O'Kane GJ. Inhalation of ammonia vapour. A report on the management of eight patients during the acute stages. Anaesthesia 1983;38(12):1208–13.
10. Winder C. The toxicology of chlorine. Environ Res 2001;85(2):105–14.
11. Babu RV, Cardenas V, Sharma G. Acute respiratory distress syndrome from chlorine inhalation during a swimming pool accident: a case report and review of the literature. J Intensive Care Med 2008;23(4):275–80.
12. Makarovsky I, Markel G, Dushnitsky T, et al. Ammonia–when something smells wrong. Isr Med Assoc J 2008;10(7):537–43.
13. Bloom GR, Suhail F, Hopkins-Price P, et al. Acute anhydrous ammonia injury from accidents during illicit methamphetamine production. Burns 2008;34(5): 713–8.
14. Pirjavec A, Kovic I, Lulic I, et al. Massive anhydrous ammonia injury leading to lung transplantation. J Trauma 2009;67(4):E93–7.
15. Lee T-K, Yoo H-W, Bae S-H, et al. Reactive airways dysfunction syndrome after hydrofluoric acid inhalation. Allergol Int 2016;65(3):343–4.
16. Shin JS, Lee S-W, Kim N-H, et al. Successful extracorporeal life support after potentially fatal pulmonary oedema caused by inhalation of nitric and hydrofluoric acid fumes. Resuscitation 2007;75(1):184–8.

17. Steverlynck L, Baert N, Buylaert W, et al. Combined acute inhalation of hydrofluoric acid and nitric acid: a case report and literature review. Acta Clin Belg 2017; 72(4):278–88.

18. Pu Q, Qian J, Tao W, et al. Extracorporeal membrane oxygenation combined with continuous renal replacement therapy in cutaneous burn and inhalation injury caused by hydrofluoric acid and nitric acid. Medicine (Baltimore) 2017; 96(48):e8972.

19. Traub SJ, Hoffman RS, Nelson LS. Case report and literature review of chlorine gas toxicity. Vet Hum Toxicol 2002;44(4):235–9.

20. Sexton JD, Pronchik DJ. Chlorine inhalation: the big picture. J Toxicol Clin Toxicol 1998;36(1–2):87–93.

21. Bosse GM. Nebulized sodium bicarbonate in the treatment of chlorine gas inhalation. J Toxicol Clin Toxicol 1994;32(3):233–41.

22. Aslan S, Kandiş H, Akgun M, et al. The effect of nebulized NaHCO3 treatment on "RADS" due to chlorine gas inhalation. Inhal Toxicol 2006;18(11):895–900.

23. Borak J, Diller WF. Phosgene exposure: mechanisms of injury and treatment strategies. J Occup Environ Med 2001;43(2):110–9.

24. Lim SC, Yang JY, Jang AS, et al. Acute lung injury after phosgene inhalation. Korean J Intern Med 1996;11(1):87–92.

25. Sciuto AM, Clapp DL, Hess ZA, et al. The temporal profile of cytokines in the bronchoalveolar lavage fluid in mice exposed to the industrial gas phosgene. Inhal Toxicol 2003;15(7):687–700.

26. Parkhouse DA, Brown RF, Jugg BJ, et al. Protective ventilation strategies in the management of phosgene-induced acute lung injury. Mil Med 2007;172(3): 295–300.

27. Guo YL, Kennedy TP, Michael JR, et al. Mechanism of phosgene-induced lung toxicity: role of arachidonate mediators. J Appl Physiol (1985) 1990;69(5): 1615–22.

28. Sciuto AM, Hurt HH. Therapeutic treatments of phosgene-induced lung injury. Inhal Toxicol 2004;16(8):565–80.

29. Sciuto AM, Strickland PT, Kennedy TP, et al. Protective effects of N-acetylcysteine treatment after phosgene exposure in rabbits. Am J Respir Crit Care Med 1995;151(3 Pt 1):768–72.

30. Konukoğlu D, Cetinkale O, Bulan R. Effects of N-acetylcysteine on lung glutathione levels in rats after burn injury. Burns J Int Soc Burn Inj 1997;23(7–8): 541–4.

31. Smith A, Brown R, Jugg B, et al. The effect of steroid treatment with inhaled budesonide or intravenous methylprednisolone on phosgene-induced acute lung injury in a porcine model. Mil Med 2009;174(12):1287–94.

32. Sciuto AM, Stotts RR, Hurt HH. Efficacy of ibuprofen and pentoxifylline in the treatment of phosgene-induced acute lung injury. J Appl Toxicol 1996;16(5): 381–4.

33. Ghio AJ, Kennedy TP, Hatch GE, et al. Reduction of neutrophil influx diminishes lung injury and mortality following phosgene inhalation. J Appl Physiol (1985) 1991;71(2):657–65.

34. Gutch M, Jain N, Agrawal A, et al. Acute accidental phosgene poisoning. BMJ Case Rep 2012;2012.

35. Hardison LS, Wright E, Pizon AF. Phosgene exposure: a case of accidental industrial exposure. J Med Toxicol 2014;10(1):51–6.

36. Malatinský J, Kadlic T, Kovácik V. Acute poisoning by higher nitrogen oxides. Anesth Analg 1973;52(1):94–9.

37. Karlson-Stiber C, Höjer J, Sjöholm A, et al. Nitrogen dioxide pneumonitis in ice hockey players. J Intern Med 1996;239(5):451–6.
38. Ramirez J, Dowell AR. Silo-filler's disease: nitrogen dioxide-induced lung injury. Long-term follow-up and review of the literature. Ann Intern Med 1971;74(4): 569–76.
39. Sriskandan K, Pettingale KW. "Numismatist's pneumonitis." A case of acute nitrogen dioxide poisoning. Postgrad Med J 1985;61(719):819–21.
40. Ramírez RJ. The first death from nitrogen dioxide fumes. The story of a man and his dog. JAMA 1974;229(9):1181–2.
41. Lachmanová V, Hnilicková O, Povýsilová V, et al. N-acetylcysteine inhibits hypoxic pulmonary hypertension most effectively in the initial phase of chronic hypoxia. Life Sci 2005;77(2):175–82.
42. Baud FJ. Cyanide: critical issues in diagnosis and treatment. Hum Exp Toxicol 2007;26(3):191–201.
43. Borron SW. Recognition and treatment of acute cyanide poisoning. J Emerg Nurs 2006;32(4 Suppl):S12–8.
44. Shepherd G, Velez LI. Role of hydroxocobalamin in acute cyanide poisoning. Ann Pharmacother 2008;42(5):661–9.
45. Kales SN, Christiani DC. Acute chemical emergencies. N Engl J Med 2004; 350(8):800–8.
46. Persson SA, Cassel G, Sellström A. Acute cyanide intoxication and central transmitter systems. Fundam Appl Toxicol 1985;5(6 Pt 2):S150–9.
47. Baud FJ, Barriot P, Toffis V, et al. Elevated blood cyanide concentrations in victims of smoke inhalation. N Engl J Med 1991;325(25):1761–6.
48. Mégarbane B, Delahaye A, Goldgran-Tolédano D, et al. Antidotal treatment of cyanide poisoning. J Chin Med Assoc 2003;66(4):193–203.
49. Hall AH, Saiers J, Baud F. Which cyanide antidote? Crit Rev Toxicol 2009;39(7): 541–52.
50. Fortin JL, Ruttiman M, Domanski L, et al. Hydroxocobalamin: treatment for smoke inhalation-associated cyanide poisoning. Meeting the needs of fire victims. JEMS 2004;29(8):suppl 18–21.
51. Barillo DJ. Diagnosis and treatment of cyanide toxicity. J Burn Care Res 2009; 30(1):148–52.
52. Morris AA, Page RL, Baumgartner LJ, et al. Thiocyanate accumulation in critically ill patients receiving nitroprusside infusions. J Intensive Care Med 2017; 32(9):547–53.
53. Ago M, Ago K, Ogata M. Two fatalities by hydrogen sulfide poisoning: variation of pathological and toxicological findings. Leg Med (Tokyo) 2008;10(3):148–52.
54. Hall AH, Rumack BH. Hydrogen sulfide poisoning: an antidotal role for sodium nitrite? Vet Hum Toxicol 1997;39(3):152–4.
55. Morii D, Miyagatani Y, Nakamae N, et al. Japanese experience of hydrogen sulfide: the suicide craze in 2008. J Occup Med Toxicol 2010;5:28.
56. Gabbay DS, De Roos F, Perrone J. Twenty-foot fall averts fatality from massive hydrogen sulfide exposure. J Emerg Med 2001;20(2):141–4.
57. Reiffenstein RJ, Hulbert WC, Roth SH. Toxicology of hydrogen sulfide. Annu Rev Pharmacol Toxicol 1992;32:109–34.
58. Beauchamp RO, Bus JS, Popp JA, et al. A critical review of the literature on hydrogen sulfide toxicity. Crit Rev Toxicol 1984;13(1):25–97.
59. Yalamanchili C, Smith MD. Acute hydrogen sulfide toxicity due to sewer gas exposure. Am J Emerg Med 2008;26(4):518, e5-7.

60. Gerasimon G, Bennett S, Musser J, et al. Acute hydrogen sulfide poisoning in a dairy farmer. Clin Toxicol (Phila) 2007;45(4):420–3.
61. Guidotti TL. Hydrogen sulphide. Occup Med Oxf Engl 1996;46(5):367–71.
62. Lindenmann J, Matzi V, Neuboeck N, et al. Severe hydrogen sulphide poisoning treated with 4-dimethylaminophenol and hyperbaric oxygen. Diving Hyperb Med 2010;40(4):213–7.
63. Tormoehlen LM, Tekulve KJ, Nañagas KA. Hydrocarbon toxicity: a review. Clin Toxicol (Phila) 2014;52(5):479–89.
64. Carlisle EJ, Donnelly SM, Vasuvattakul S, et al. Glue-sniffing and distal renal tubular acidosis: sticking to the facts. J Am Soc Nephrol 1991;1(8):1019–27.
65. Camara-Lemarroy CR, Rodríguez-Gutiérrez R, Monreal-Robles R, et al. Acute toluene intoxication–clinical presentation, management and prognosis: a prospective observational study. BMC Emerg Med 2015;15:19.
66. Jiao Z, De Jesús VR, Iravanian S, et al. A possible mechanism of halocarbon-induced cardiac sensitization arrhythmias. J Mol Cell Cardiol 2006;41(4): 698–705.
67. Gindre G, Le Gall S, Condat P, et al. [Late ventricular fibrillation after trichloro-ethylene poisoning]. Ann Fr Anesth Reanim 1997;16(2):202–3.
68. Mortiz F, de La Chapelle A, Bauer F, et al. Esmolol in the treatment of severe arrhythmia after acute trichloroethylene poisoning. Intensive Care Med 2000; 26(2):256.
69. Rauber-Lüthy C, Kupferschmidt H. Household chemicals: management of intoxication and antidotes. EXS 2010;100:339–63.
70. Flanagan RJ, Ruprah M, Meredith TJ, et al. An introduction to the clinical toxicology of volatile substances. Drug Saf 1990;5(5):359–83.
71. Wiseman MN, Banim S. "Glue sniffer's" heart? Br Med J Clin Res Ed 1987; 294(6574):739.
72. Harris WS. Toxic effects of aerosol propellants on the heart. Arch Intern Med 1973;131(1):162–6.
73. Lamba PS, Karanwal R, Sahni TK, et al. Gas poisoning with Freon-12 (A report of three cases). Med J Armed Forces India 1994;50(1):69–70.
74. Kandyala R, Raghavendra SPC, Rajasekharan ST. Xylene: an overview of its health hazards and preventive measures. J Oral Maxillofac Pathol 2010; 14(1):1–5.
75. Lavon O. Acute inhaled xylene poisoning confirmed by methylhippuric acid urine test. J Clin Toxicol 2015;05(06).
76. Morley R, Eccleston DW, Douglas CP, et al. Xylene poisoning: a report on one fatal case and two cases of recovery after prolonged unconsciousness. Br Med J 1970;3(5720):442–3.
77. Fuente A, McPherson B, Cardemil F. Xylene-induced auditory dysfunction in humans. Ear Hear 2013;34(5):651–60.
78. Benignus VA. Health effects of toluene: a review. Neurotoxicology 1981;2(3): 567–88.
79. Filley CM, Halliday W, Kleinschmidt-DeMasters BK. The effects of toluene on the central nervous system. J Neuropathol Exp Neurol 2004;63(1):1–12.
80. Wang Y-J, Yang H, Zeng F, et al. Toluene-induced leukoencephalopathy with characteristic magnetic resonance imaging findings. Neuroimmunol Neuroin-flammation 2014;1(2):92.
81. Cámara-Lemarroy CR, Gónzalez-Moreno EI, Rodriguez-Gutierrez R, et al. Clinical presentation and management in acute toluene intoxication: a case series. Inhal Toxicol 2012;24(7):434–8.

82. Thompson AG, Leite MI, Lunn MP, et al. Whippits, nitrous oxide and the dangers of legal highs. Pract Neurol 2015;15(3):207–9.
83. Wagner SA, Clark MA, Wesche DL, et al. Asphyxial deaths from the recreational use of nitrous oxide. J Forensic Sci 1992;37(4):1008–15.
84. Weimann J. Toxicity of nitrous oxide. Best Pract Res Clin Anaesthesiol 2003; 17(1):47–61.
85. Williamson J, Huda S, Damodaran D. Nitrous oxide myelopathy with functional vitamin B 12 deficiency. BMJ Case Rep 2019;12(2):e227439.
86. Hughes G, Moran E, Dedicoat MJ. Encephalitis secondary to nitrous oxide and vitamin B12 deficiency. BMJ Case Rep 2019;12(12):e229380.
87. Cao DJ, Aldy K, Hsu S, et al. Review of health consequences of electronic cigarettes and the outbreak of electronic cigarette, or vaping, product use–associated lung injury. J Med Toxicol 2020;16(3):295–310.
88. Bozier J, Chivers EK, Chapman DG, et al. The evolving landscape of e-cigarettes: a systematic review of recent evidence. Chest 2020;157(5):1362–90.
89. Wieslander G, Norbäck D, Lindgren T. Experimental exposure to propylene glycol mist in aviation emergency training: acute ocular and respiratory effects. Occup Environ Med 2001;58(10):649–55.
90. Pankow JF, Kim K, McWhirter KJ, et al. Benzene formation in electronic cigarettes. PLoS One 2017;12(3):e0173055.
91. Landman ST, Dhaliwal I, Mackenzie CA, et al. Life-threatening bronchiolitis related to electronic cigarette use in a Canadian youth. Can Med Assoc J 2019;191(48):E1321–31.
92. Blount BC, Karwowski MP, Morel-Espinosa M, et al. Evaluation of bronchoalveolar lavage fluid from patients in an outbreak of E-cigarette, or vaping, product use–associated lung injury — 10 states, August–October 2019. MMWR Morb Mortal Wkly Rep 2019;68(45):1040–1.
93. Taylor J, Wiens T, Peterson J, et al. Characteristics of E-cigarette, or vaping, products used by patients with associated lung injury and products seized by law enforcement — Minnesota, 2018 and 2019. MMWR Morb Mortal Wkly Rep 2019;68(47):1096–100.
94. Lewis N, McCaffrey K, Sage K, et al. E-cigarette use, or vaping, practices and characteristics among persons with associated lung injury — Utah, April–October 2019. MMWR Morb Mortal Wkly Rep 2019;68(42):953–6.
95. New York State Department of Health announces update on investigation into vaping-associated pulmonary illness. Available at: https://health.ny.gov/press/releases/2019/2019-09-05_vaping.htm.
96. Layden JE, Ghinai I, Pray I, et al. Pulmonary illness related to E-cigarette use in Illinois and Wisconsin — final report. N Engl J Med 2020;382(10):903–16.
97. Ghinai I, Pray IW, Navon L, et al. E-cigarette product use, or vaping, among persons with associated lung injury — Illinois and Wisconsin, April–September 2019. MMWR Morb Mortal Wkly Rep 2019;68(39):865–9.
98. Centers for Disease Control and Prevention. Outbreak of lung injury associated with the use of E-cigarette, or vaping, products. Available at: https://www.cdc.gov/tobacco/basic_information/e-cigarettes/severe-lung-disease.html#overview.
99. Navon L, Ghinai I, Layden J. Notes from the field: characteristics of tetrahydrocannabinol–containing E-cigarette, or vaping, products used by adults — Illinois, September–October 2019. MMWR Morb Mortal Wkly Rep 2020;69(29):973–5.
100. Billa R, Tigges C, Vijayakumar N, et al. E-cigarette, or vaping, product use associated lung injury (EVALI) with acute respiratory failure in three adolescent

patients: a clinical timeline, treatment, and product analysis. J Med Toxicol 2020;16(3):248–54.
101. Werner AK, Koumans EH, Chatham Stephens K, et al. Hospitalizations and deaths associated with EVALI. N Engl J Med 2020;382(17):1589–98.
102. Siegel DA, Jatlaoui TC, Koumans EH, et al. Update: interim guidance for health care providers evaluating and caring for patients with suspected E-cigarette, or vaping, product use associated lung injury — United States, October 2019. MMWR Morb Mortal Wkly Rep 2019;68(41):919–27.
103. Maddock SD, Cirulis MM, Callahan SJ, et al. Pulmonary lipid-laden macrophages and vaping. N Engl J Med 2019;381(15):1488–9.

Moving?

Make sure your subscription moves with you!

To notify us of your new address, find your **Clinics Account Number** (located on your mailing label above your name), and contact customer service at:

Email: journalscustomerservice-usa@elsevier.com

800-654-2452 (subscribers in the U.S. & Canada)
314-447-8871 (subscribers outside of the U.S. & Canada)

Fax number: 314-447-8029

**Elsevier Health Sciences Division
Subscription Customer Service
3251 Riverport Lane
Maryland Heights, MO 63043**

*To ensure uninterrupted delivery of your subscription, please notify us at least 4 weeks in advance of move.

Printed and bound by CPI Group (UK) Ltd, Croydon, CR0 4YY

03/10/2024

01040405-0006